# ESSENTIALS OF
# ENDOCRINOLOGY

# ESSENTIALS OF ENDOCRINOLOGY

EDITED BY

*J. L. H. O'Riordan* DM FRCP

*P. G. Malan* PhD

*R. P. Gould* MSc

*University College and*
*Middlesex School of Medicine*
*London*

SECOND EDITION

OXFORD

**Blackwell Scientific Publications**

LONDON EDINBURGH BOSTON

PARIS BERLIN VIENNA MELBOURNE

First published 1982
Reprinted 1984, 1985
Second edition 1988
Reprinted 1988, 1992

Set by Setrite Typesetters
Hong Kong
Printed and bound in Great Britain
by Redwood Press Limited
Melksham, Wiltshire

DISTRIBUTORS

Marston Book Services Ltd
PO Box 87
Oxford OX2 0DT
(*Orders:* Tel: 0865 791155
        Fax: 0865 791927
        Telex: 837515)

USA
Blackwell Scientific
  Publications, Inc.
238 Main Street
Cambridge, MA 02142
(*Orders:* Tel: 800 759–6102
              617 225–0401)

Canada
Times Mirror Professional
  Publishing, Ltd.
5240 Finch Avenue East
Scarborough, Ontario M1S 5A2
(*Orders:* Tel: 800 268–4178
              416 298–1588)

Australia
Blackwell Scientific
  Publications (Australia) Pty Ltd
54 University Street
Carlton, Victoria 3053
(*Orders:* Tel: 03 347–0300)

British Library
Cataloguing in Publication Data

Essentials of endocrinology.—2nd ed.
  1. Clinical endocrinology
  I. O'Riordan, J.L.H.  II. Malan, P.G.
  III. Gould, R.P.
  616.4    RC648

ISBN 0–632–02112–8

# Contents

# Contributors to first edition

*J. Bell* PhD
Research Associate, Department of Physics Applied to Medicine
*Chapter 3*

*S. R. Bloom* MD FRCP
Reader in Medicine, Royal Postgraduate Medical School,
Hammersmith Hospital
*Chapter 7*

*C. G. D. Brook* MA MD FRCP DCH
Consultant, Department of Child Health
*Chapter 4*

*B. L. Brown* PhD
Senior Lecturer, Department of Human Metabolism and Chemical
Pathology, University of Sheffield
*Chapter 2*

*W. F. Coulson* PhD FRSC
Senior Lecturer, Department of Biochemistry
*Chapter 4*

*M. L. Forsling* PhD
Senior Lecturer, Department of Physiology
*Chapters 2 & 3*

*R. P. Gould* MSc
Reader in Histology, Department of Anatomy
*Chapters 1—7*

*P. Heffron* MB BS PhD
Senior Lecturer, Department of Pharmacology
*Chapter 3*

*S. J. Holt* PhD DSc FRSC FIBiol
Professor of Biochemistry
*Chapter 7*

*P. Hyatt* PhD
Research Associate, Department of Physics Applied to Medicine
*Chapter 3*

*A. B. Kurtz* PhD FRCP
Senior Lecturer, Department of Medicine and Consultant Physician
*Chapter 5*

*P. McLean* PhD DSc
Professor of Biochemistry
*Chapter 7*

*P. G. Malan* PhD
Senior Lecturer, Department of Nuclear Medicine
*Chapters 1−7*

*J. D. N. Nabarro* MD FRCP
Consultant Physician
*Chapters 2 & 7*

*J. L. H. O'Riordan* DM (Oxon) FRCP
Professor, Department of Medicine and Consultant Physician
*Chapters 1−7*

*J. D. H. Slater* MA MD FRCP
Consultant Physician
*Chapter 3*

*A. D. Smith* PhD
Senior Lecturer, Department of Biochemistry
*Chapter 7*

*S. J. Steele* MA FRCS FRCOG
Reader, Department of Obstetrics and Gynaecology
*Chapter 4*

*E. K. Symes* PhD
Research Associate, Department of Biochemistry
*Chapter 4*

*All contributors were members of the staff of the Middlesex Hospital Medical School, Mortimer Street, London W1N 8AA, unless stated otherwise.*

# Contributors to second edition

*C. G. D. Brook* MA MD FRCP DCH
Reader in Paediatric Endocrinology
*Chapters 2 and 3*

*B. L. Brown* PhD
Reader, Department of Human Metabolism and Chemical
Pathology, University of Sheffield
*Chapters 1 and 2*

*W. F. Coulson* PhD FRSC
Senior Lecturer, Department of Biochemistry
*Chapters 1 and 4*

*M. L. Forsling* PhD
Senior Lecturer, Department of Physiology
*Chapter 2*

*R. P. Gould* MSc
Emeritus Reader in Histology
*Chapter 1—7*

*T. A. Howlett* MA MB BS BChir MRCP
Lecturer in Endocrinology, Medical College of St Bartholomew's
Hospital London
*Chapter 2*

*A. B. Kurtz* PhD FRCP
Senior Lecturer, Department of Medicine and Consultant
Physician
*Chapter 5*

*P. G. Malan* PhD
Amersham Laboratories, White Lion Road, Amersham, Bucks
*Chapters 1—7*

*N. J. Marshall* MSc PhD
Principal Biochemist, University College Hospital, London
*Chapter 5*

*P. McLean* PhD DSc
Professor of Biochemistry
*Chapter 7*

*J. L. H. O'Riordan* DM FRCP
Professor of Metabolic Medicine and Consultant Physician
*Chapters 1—7*

*L. H. Rees* MSc MD FRCP MRCPath
Professor of Chemical Endocrinology, Medical College of St
Bartholomew's Hospital, London
*Chapter 2*

*P. A. Sanford* PhD
Associate Professor of Physiology, King Saud University, Riyadh
*Chapter 7*

*J. D. H. Slater* MA MD FRCP
Consultant Physician
*Chapter 3*

*E. K. Symes* PhD
Research Associate in Biochemistry
*Chapter 4*

*G. P. Vinson* PhD DSc
Professor of Biochemistry, Medical College of St Bartholomew's
Hospital, London
*Chapter 3*

*All contributors are members of the staff of The University College
and Middlesex School of Medicine unless stated otherwise.*

# Preface to second edition

In the five years since the book was first published there have been major advances in endocrinology and it is important for the student to be aware of many of these. Preparation of a new edition has allowed us to take account of the impact of molecular biology on endocrinology and to incorporate new information on the mode of action of hormones. Thus the major changes in the text are in Chapter 1 but the impact of these and other advances has required changes throughout the text. The advances in reproductive endocrinology have required changes in Chapter 4 to allow description of the principles of *in vitro* fertilization for example. The bulk of the original text, of course, remains intact and in modifying it we have attempted to avoid increasing its length greatly.

We have taken the opportunity of incorporating nineteen new illustrations and, in addition, the style of all the original pictures has been altered by close collaboration with the artist to increase their impact. We hope, therefore, that this book will continue to be of use to students of endocrinology in many disciplines.

We are grateful to all the contributors to the second edition: in addition we would like to thank Professor H. S. Jacobs Professor R. Craig and Dr. D. J. Chiswell who made useful suggestions. Any virtues of the book must be credited to the original contributors and to those who helped subsequently, while any defects must be attributed to the editors.

*July 1987*                                    *J. L. H. O'Riordan*
*Middlesex Hospital*                                *P. G. Malan*
*London W1*                                       *R. P. Gould*

# Preface to first edition

This book is intended for those beginning to study endocrinology. The authors approach the subject from their different viewpoints, morphological, physiological, biochemical, pharmacological and clinical, and the text brings together these diverse views. It is based on the teaching given during the second year of the Basic Medical Sciences Course at The Middlesex Hospital Medical School, and we hope that it will appeal to medical students and those taking a science degree.

The opening chapter describes the underlying principles of modern endocrinology, at cellular, biochemical and physiological levels. The ensuing chapters are based on single glands or functional groups of glands. No attempt has been made to impose a rigid format on these chapters as each system lends itself to a slightly different emphasis. In general, however, in each chapter the introduction is an outline of the history of the subject, to provide an inkling of the basic, long established principles. Then the morphological and embryological basis for function is presented, and this leads onto the biochemical and physiological aspects. Clinical disorders are then considered from the viewpoint of the insight they give to the understanding of endocrine physiology. The link between basic endocrinology and clinical endocrinology is so close, that it seems very reasonable to do that, while attempting at the same time, to show that a knowledge of the scientific basis of endocrinology helps to explain the consequences of endocrine disease and the rationale of its treatment.

We would like to thank all those who contributed to this book. The authors have been very patient with us as we have brought together and edited the work of so many people and have striven to help the reader avoid the pitfalls of a multi-author book. The authors can justly claim credit for the virtues of this book, while the editors must accept responsibility for any faults that may be detected. Apart from authors, there are many to whom we are indebted. Dr Howard Jacobs very kindly advised in the writing on the chapter on reproductive endocrinology and many useful comments and suggestions were received from Professors J. F. Tait FRS, F. Hobbiger and E. Neil and Drs N. J. Marshall and P. Sanford on the chapters in their specialist fields. The many secretaries who contributed to the typing of manuscripts for this book are also gratefully acknowledged.

We hope that this book will stimulate its readers in endocrinology and that they will see how the various endocrine glands form a closely regulated, integrated system that is essential for homeostasis.

*February 1982*                                      *J. L. H. O'Riordan*
*Middlesex Hospital*                                      *P. G. Malan*
*London W1*                                      *R. P. Gould*

# 1  The endocrine system and the molecular basis for hormone action

The endocrine system is one of the two great control systems of the body, the other being the nervous system. These two regulatory systems are responsible for monitoring changes in an animal's internal and external environments and directing the body to make any necessary adjustments to its activities so that it adapts itself to these environmental changes. The nervous system mediates its activity through nerves directly supplying the organs and structures concerned, while the endocrine system operates through chemical messengers, or hormones, which circulate in the blood to their respective target organs and modify their activity. The term 'hormone' was introduced in 1905 by Starling and is derived from the Greek, meaning 'to arouse' or 'to excite', though it should be stressed that not all hormonal effects are stimulatory; some are inhibitory. The endocrine glands secrete hormones into the circulation and therefore differ from exocrine glands which secrete their products into ducts, rather than the circulation.

Unicellular organisms and simple multicellular organisms are exposed to their environment and react to it, but they cannot control it or insulate themselves from it. In contrast, in higher organisms such as man (in whom there are about $10^{14}$ cells and 200 or more cell types), only relatively few cells are exposed to the outside world. Nevertheless, all the cells are affected directly or indirectly by external changes and can only survive if the constancy of their internal environment is controlled. For this, the endocrine system is important. It responds to recurrent environmental changes, such as meals, and helps the organism to adapt to changing habits. The endocrine system is also important for controlling development and growth, puberty and sexual maturation. Thus the secretion of hormones, apart from maintaining the body's internal environment, can also induce important long-term changes in an organism's behaviour.

In their original experiments in 1902, Bayliss and Starling studied the control of the exocrine secretion of the pancreas. They collected pancreatic secretions and showed that introduction of acid into a denervated segment of jejunum increased the production of alkaline pancreatic juice. Since this occurred after denervation, it could not be the result of a nerve reflex and they postulated that there must in fact be a chemical reflex. They

1

then prepared extracts of intestinal mucosa, and injected them intravenously into test animals and showed that these extracts could also stimulate pancreatic secretion. They gave the name 'secretin' to the active principle in these extracts.

With this experiment they introduced an important approach into the investigation of endocrine function, which was to study the effects of the injection of tissue extracts into the bloodstream. Another approach is to investigate the effects of removal of a putative endocrine organ. Berthold used this in studies on the effect of castration, and showed that the testes were necessary for the maintenance of male characteristics in the cock and eventually the hormone testosterone was isolated from the testes. It also follows that the disturbance produced by removal of an endocrine organ should be correctable by injection of extracts from the organ; for example, insulin extracted from the pancreas can control the diabetes mellitus that follows pancreatectomy. Transplantation or re-implantation of the endocrine gland should also correct the effects of deficiency.

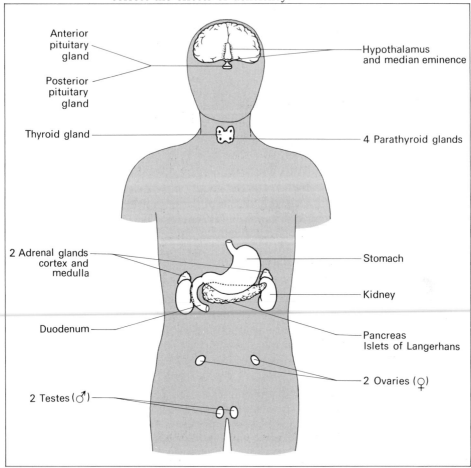

**Fig. 1.1**   The sites of the principal endocrine glands.

Clinical studies can also be valuable in understanding the function of an endocrine gland since disease can cause over-production or underproduction of hormones. Thus in 1500 BC

**Table 1.1** The principal endocrine glands of the body and the hormones they produce.

| Gland | Hormone | Molecular characteristics |
|---|---|---|
| Hypothalamus/median eminence | *Releasing and inhibiting hormones:* Thyrotrophin releasing hormone Somatostatin Gonadotrophin releasing hormone Corticotrophin releasing hormone Growth hormone releasing hormone | Peptides |
| | Prolactin inhibiting factor (dopamine) | Biogenic amine |
| Anterior pituitary | Thyrotrophin or thyroid stimulating hormone Luteinizing hormone Follicle stimulating hormone | Glycoproteins |
| | Growth hormone Prolactin Adrenocorticotrophin | Proteins |
| Posterior pituitary | Vasopressin (antidiuretic hormone) Oxytocin | Peptides |
| Thyroid | Thyroxine and triiodothyronine | Tyrosine derivatives |
| | Calcitonin | Peptide |
| Parathyroid | Parathyroid hormone | Peptide |
| Adrenal cortex | Aldosterone and cortisol | Steroids |
| Adrenal medulla | Adrenaline and noradrenaline (also called epinephrine and norepinephrine) | Catecholamines |
| Stomach | Gastrin | Peptide |
| Pancreas (Islets of Langerhans) | Insulin Glucagon Somatostatin | Proteins |
| Duodenum and jejunum | Secretin Cholecystokinin | Proteins |
| Ovary | Oestrogens and progesterone | Steroids |
| Testis | Testosterone | Steroid |

the clinical features of diabetes mellitus were described and this was long before the isolation of insulin by Banting and Best in 1921. Similarly, the features of thyrotoxicosis were described and associated with disease of the thyroid gland in the 19th century before it was realized that there was overproduction of the thyroid hormones, thyroxine and triiodothyronine, which were only isolated many years later. Another example of the value of clinical observation was Addison's description of the effects of deficient secretion of the adrenal cortex; he associated the condition with disease of the adrenal glands long before the isolation of the adrenal hormones cortisol and aldosterone which are steroids secreted by the adrenal cortex. Another example of the usefulness of clinical studies in characterizing the role of a hormone concerns prolactin. Its importance in fertility was only recognized after it became possible to measure circulating prolactin, when it was then found that some cases of infertility were due to overproduction of prolactin. In other cases, of course, it has been understanding the physiology of a hormone which has led to the recognition of the effects of disordered secretion. Thus, in the case of aldosterone, the effects of overproduction were only recognized once the hormone had been isolated and then it was found that some cases of muscle weakness with potassium deficiency were a consequence of overproduction of aldosterone.

## THE ROLE OF HORMONES

Hormones belong to a class of regulatory molecules that are synthesized in special cells. The cells either may be collected into distinct endocrine glands or are found as single cells within some other organ, e.g. the gastrointestinal tract. Hormones are released from the cells that make them into the adjacent extracellular space (Fig. 1.2a and c) from where they enter a local blood vessel. They then circulate in the blood to their target cells. Some cells secrete hormones that act locally on nearby cells without entering the bloodstream: they are called paracrine hormones (Fig. 1.2b). Molecules secreted by neurones that excite or inhibit other neurones or muscle by means of synapses are called neurotransmitters (Fig. 1.2d). Often, however, both neurotransmitters and hormones are secreted by neurones; they form the neuroendocrine system (Fig. 1.2c).

Hormones act by binding to specific receptors either on the target cell surface or within the cell. The result is a cascade of intracellular reactions within the target cell that frequently amplifies the original stimulus and leads ultimately to a response by the target cell. Some hormones have a general importance in the body as a whole rather than acting on a specific target tissue.

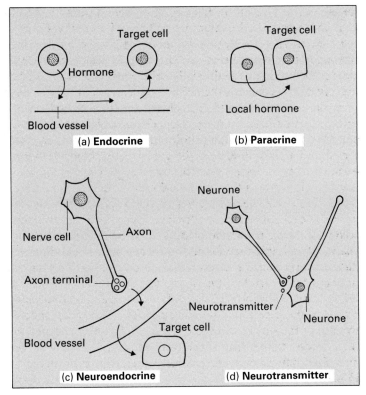

**Fig. 1.2** Illustration of cells that secrete regulatory substances to reach their target organs.

(**a**) Endocrine cells secrete hormone into the blood vessel where it is carried to the target cell which may be a considerable distance from the secreting cell, such as the anterior pituitary hormones which act, for example, on the thyroid.

(**b**) Paracrine cells secrete local hormones which act on a nearby cell, e.g. glucagon and somatostatin act on the adjacent pancreatic cells that secrete insulin.

(**c**) Neuroendocrine cells secrete molecules from the neural axon terminals in response to some neural signal, and the hormone (e.g. adrenaline) is released into the bloodstream to travel to its target organ such as the liver or adipose tissue.

(**d**) Neurotransmitter cells secrete molecules from the axon terminals to activate adjacent neurones.

These include growth hormone, underproduction of which in children leads to dwarfism while overproduction causes gigantism. In adults overproduction of growth hormone causes acromegaly, with enlargement, for example, of the hands and feet and coarsening of the facial appearance. Thyroxine, too, acts on most tissues of the body, and if present in excess the basal metabolic rate increases, while if there is a deficiency of the hormone the metabolic rate declines. Insulin also acts on most if not all tissues, including the liver, muscle and adipose tissue; this implies that receptors for the hormone are widespread. The importance of insulin is illustrated by the fact that it is an important component for the maintenance of cells in tissue culture.

In contrast, many other hormones only act on one tissue, for example, thyrotrophin, adrenocorticotrophin and the gonadotrophins are secreted by the anterior pituitary and have specific target tissues, namely, the thyroid gland, the adrenal cortex and the gonads, respectively. A further example of a hormone with specific target tissues is parathyroid hormone; this is secreted from the parathyroid glands which are located in the neck close to the thyroid gland and it controls the concentration of calcium in the circulation, acting particularly on bone and the kidney.

## Types of hormones

From the chemical standpoint, there are three groups of hormones. Firstly, there are derivatives of the amino acid tyrosine; secondly, peptide and protein hormones and thirdly, steroid hormones.

### HORMONES DERIVED FROM TYROSINE

These include adrenaline (Fig. 1.3), which is secreted by the adrenal medulla, and noradrenaline, which can be produced in the adrenal medulla but is also produced at sympathetic nerve endings where it acts as a neurotransmitter. Dopamine is another derivative of tyrosine which is a neurotransmitter that can also act as a hormone. It is released from the median eminence and suppresses the secretion of prolactin from the anterior pituitary. The thyroid hormones, thyroxine and triiodothyronine, each have two molecules of tyrosine fused together; thyroxine itself has four iodine atoms attached to the amino acid rings while triiodothyronine has three iodine atoms (see Chapter 5).

### PROTEIN AND PEPTIDE HORMONES

These vary considerably in size and may be quite small and consist of only a single chain of amino acids. For example, thyrotrophin releasing hormone, secreted from the hypothalamus, has only three amino acid residues. Many of the hormones from the gastrointestinal tract, such as secretin from the duodenum and gastrin from the stomach, are larger with up to 34 amino acids, while parathyroid hormone is larger still with 84. Ring structures linked by disulphide bridges are present in some hormones, including the two hormones from the pituitary gland, oxytocin and vasopressin (Fig. 1.4): oxytocin is important for the contraction of the uterus in labour and vasopressin regulates water excretion. Thus, they have very different physiological roles, even though structurally they are remarkably similar with only small differences in their amino acid sequence. An intrachain

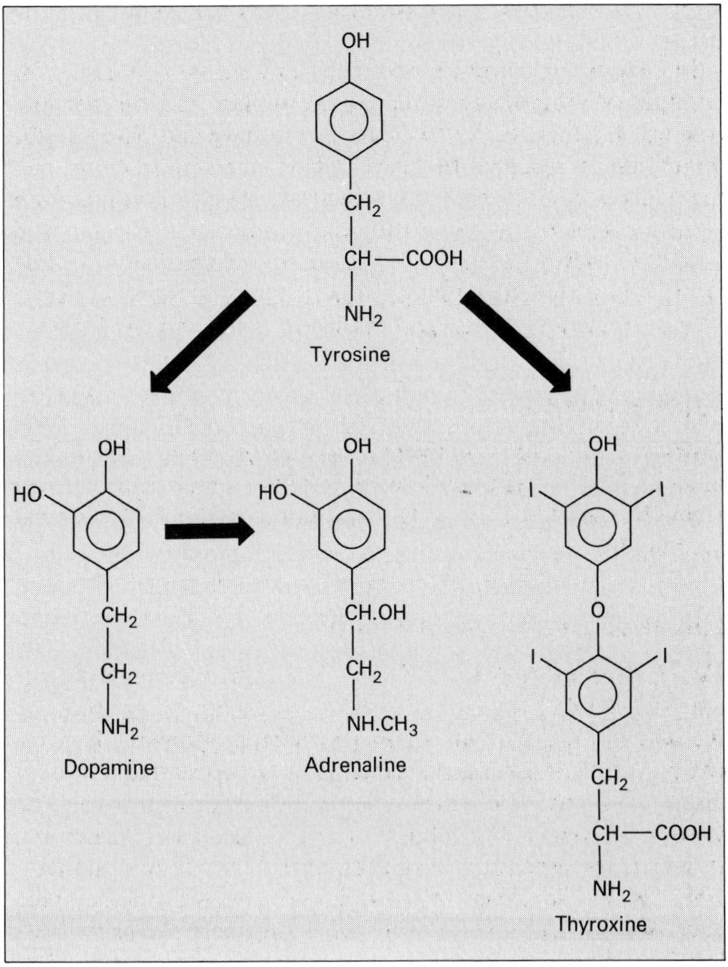

**Fig. 1.3** Some of the hormones derived from tyrosine. Dopamine exists as a hormone in its own right, but it also occurs as an intermediate in the synthesis from tyrosine of adrenaline and noradrenaline. Noradrenaline lacks the methyl group in the amino position of adrenaline. Triiodothyronine has only one of the two iodine atoms (I) present on the upper ring of thyroxine.

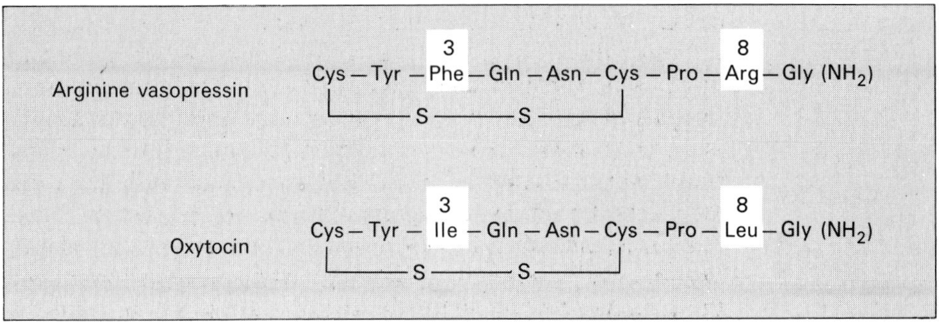

**Fig. 1.4** The structures of arginine vasopressin and of oxytocin. The small differences in their chemical structure are highlighted. They profoundly influence the physiological effects of the two hormones.

disulphide bond to form a ring of seven amino acids at the amino terminus is also found in calcitonin, a hormone which can lower serum calcium.

Insulin may be regarded as a small protein or a large peptide and it has two chains, the A- and the B-chains which are linked by interchain disulphide bonds. Initially, insulin is made as a single chain peptide and subsequently a section of the chain is removed; this is referred to as the C-peptide or connecting peptide which is removed by enzymatic hydrolysis after the disulphide bonds have been formed, and once the C-peptide is removed, there are two linked chains in the insulin molecule (Fig. 1.8c). Thus, insulin is made initially as a larger precursor molecule, pro-insulin. A number of other peptide hormones are synthesized in larger precursor forms which are modified before the hormone is secreted (see the section on peptide and protein synthesis, below).

Some hormones are quite large proteins, for example the glycoprotein hormones from the anterior pituitary which each have two peptide chains. The two gonadotrophins (follicle stimulating hormone and luteinizing hormone) and also thyrotrophin each have two chains, referred to as the $\alpha$- and $\beta$-subunits, not linked by disulphide bridges. The two subunits are synthesized quite separately. The $\alpha$-subunit in each of the three hormones is very similar; but the $\beta$-subunits are different and it is the $\beta$-subunit that confers the biological specificity on the hormone.

STEROID HORMONES

These include the hormones cortisol and aldosterone produced by the adrenal cortex, and the important sex steroids, testosterone (from the testis) and progesterone and oestradiol (from the ovary). The steroid hormones are important in many respects, affecting carbohydrate metabolism, salt and water balance and reproductive function. Small changes in the basic chemical structure cause dramatic changes in the physiological action of this group of hormones.

# HORMONE BIOSYNTHESIS AND SECRETION

An understanding of the secretion and actions of many hormones requires a knowledge of the molecular events at a cellular level. There are two principal types of cell that synthesize either peptide and protein hormones or steroid hormones. The cytological features that distinguish these two types of cell are illustrated in Fig. 1.5. It is useful at this stage to consider some general principles that concern the synthesis and secretion of these two groups of hormones.

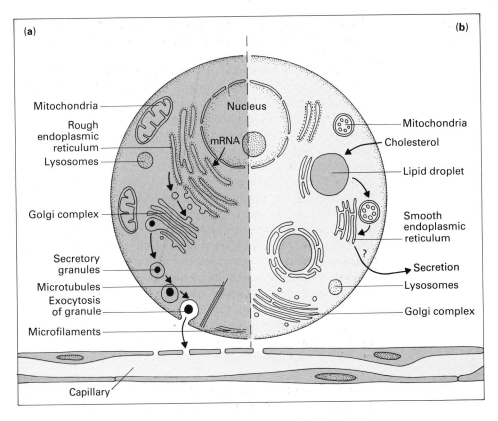

**Fig. 1.5** The cytological features of a peptide hormone synthesizing cell (a), on the left, and a steroid hormone synthesizing cell (b), on the right side.

(a) Before synthesis of the peptide hormone starts, messenger RNA (mRNA) leaves the nucleus and is translated on the ribosomes of the rough endoplasmic reticulum. The nascent protein (hormone) moves to the Golgi complex where it may be further modified and packaged into secretory granules. The granules move to the cell membrane with the involvement of microtubules and actin microfilaments. The granule membrane fuses with the plasma membrane and granule (hormone) release through exocytosis occurs. The hormone then passes through the fenestrations of the capillary into the bloodstream. Lysosomes are involved in the removal of unwanted secretory granules (crinophagy) and cytoplasmic organelles.

(b) Before steroid hormone synthesis, cholestrol enters the cell and is stored as cholesterol esters in the lipid droplets until required. Cholesterol then moves to the mitochondria where it is converted to pregnenolone. Pregnenolone is then transported to the surrounding smooth endoplasmic reticulum where it is transformed by a series of reactions into the appropriate steroid hormone. The mode of egress of the hormone from the cell is not certain.

## Peptides and proteins

### MOLECULAR BIOLOGY OF THE SYNTHESIS RNA AND OF PROTEINS

Protein or peptide hormone synthesis follows the sequence of reactions which have been elucidated since the 1950s. The sequence of events starts with transcription of a gene, proceeds through translation of a messenger RNA (mRNA) and culminates in post-translational modification of the peptide or protein hormone.

In eukaryotic organisms, the essential genetic information is contained in the DNA of the chromosomes within the nucleus. Associated with the DNA in the nuclear chromatin are basic proteins called histones and other proteins called non-histone chromosomal proteins, some of which are likely to have regulatory roles in controlling gene expression. DNA carries genetic information in the form of a code of triplet sequences of nucleotides (bases) within the DNA strands. Before the triplet code may be transcribed to messenger RNA, the DNA containing the genes is attached to the nuclear matrix of the eukaryotic cell. The DNA double-helix is then parted in the region of the gene when it is transcribed by DNA-dependent RNA polymerase to yield messenger RNA (see for example Fig. 1.17, step 5, below).

Each gene consists of a DNA sequence with a central region called the *structural gene*. On either side of the structural region, the gene has important regulatory sequences that define the circumstances under which the DNA segment will be transcribed into RNA (see Fig. 1.6). The number and position of these regulatory sequences vary for individual genes but they tend to follow a common format as outlined in Fig. 1.6. 'Upstream' from the start of transcription, that is on the 5' side of the structural gene, lie those sequences that regulate the binding of RNA polymerase and its associated factors: this is called the *promoter region*. Counting of nucleotides in a gene sequence begins (Fig. 1.6) at the start of the structural gene, which is arbitrarily given the position number of one. The promoter region lies within about 100 bases above the point at which transcription starts. Sequence conservation between different genes led to recognition of the promoter region; this usually included, at about 30 bases before the start of transcription, a sequence similar to the TATA box (a sequence of seven bases found in prokaryotes). Also associated with many genes are elements known as transcription enhancers, and they are found in various positions within or around a gene. These sequences influence when transcription can occur, and they frequently control the tissue specificity of gene expression.

The structural gene itself is made up of *introns* (also known as intervening sequences) and *exons* (for expressed sequence regions; see Fig. 1.6). Transcription of both the introns and exons of the structural gene gives a precursor called pre-mRNA. Post-transcriptional modification eliminates those bases that were the complementary to those of introns in the DNA sequence, and the exon-derived sequences are spliced together to give mature messenger RNA. Two other post-transcriptional events occur to messenger RNA. One of these is the *capping* of the 5' end with

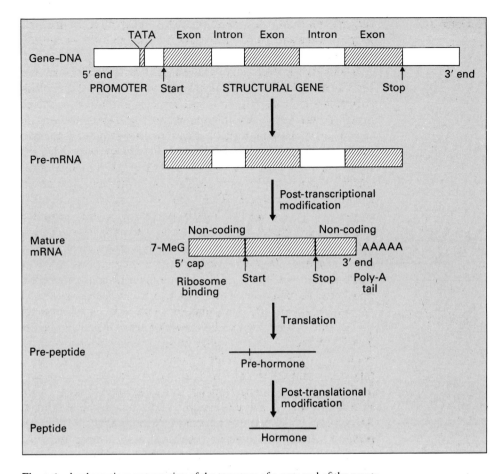

**Fig. 1.6** A schematic representation of the structure of a gene and of the events leading to synthesis of a peptide hormone. The gene consists of double-stranded (ds) DNA. At its 5′ end (the 'upstream' side) is the regulatory region known as the promoter that includes the TATA box. This is followed by a series (variable in number and size) of exons and introns which make up the structural gene. RNA polymerase produces an RNA transcript of the exons and introns in the form of pre-mRNA. Removal of the RNA sequences derived from the introns is followed by splicing together of the the exon-derived sequences. Further post-transcriptional changes include the addition of a 7-methyl guanosine (7-MeG) cap at the 5′ end and a poly-A tail on the 3′ end. When the mature messenger RNA is bound to a ribosome, translation occurs to give a peptide precursor which includes the signal peptide of the prehormone (or pre-prohormone). Post-translational processing (see Fig. 1.8) is needed before the hormone is ready for secretion.

a 7-methyl guanosine residue, and the other involves the addition of a series of adenosine residues (A) to give a poly-A tail at the 3′ end. Messenger RNA moves from the nucleus to the cell cytoplasm for translation of the message into peptide or protein hormones, as described below.

11

Some knowledge of cloning techniques is important to an understanding of current trends in endocrinology, but they can only be discussed briefly here:

In Fig. 1.7 are summarized some of the steps involved in cloning a particular sequence of DNA so that multiple copies of the same sequence can be easily made and then used, for example, to produce relatively large amounts of the 'gene product' in the form of messenger RNA or a protein or peptide hormone in a relatively 'pure' form.

Messenger RNA differs from other forms of RNA such as ribosomal and transfer RNAs. One of the main differences consists of the presence of the 3′ poly-A tail on messenger RNA. This enables messenger RNA to be isolated from disrupted cells using affinity chromatography on columns consisting of polymers of deoxythymidine (oligo-dT). Once messenger RNA has been isolated, the next step preparatory to cloning is to make a complementary DNA strand (called cDNA) using the enzyme reverse transcriptase that yields paired strands of mRNA−cDNA (see Fig. 1.7). Double-stranded complementary DNA (ds cDNA) is made by a series of steps including the action of DNA polymerase I. The ds cDNA sequence may then be incorporated into the DNA of a suitable vector microorganism, as is outlined in the legend to Fig. 1.7.

Plasmids (with circular DNA) and certain λ-phages can be used as vectors to introduce DNA into bacteria, where the vector DNA is replicated by the endogenous bacterial enzymes. The vector DNA is cleaved with an appropriate 'restriction' enzyme that hydrolyses DNA at a specific sequence of nucleotides. The vector DNA and ds cDNA are then joined together (see Fig. 1.7) to form *recombinant DNA*. The re-formed circular DNA from plasmids can be introduced into a bacterium, usually *Escherischia coli*, by artificially making the cell membrane permeable. Alternatively, phage coat-proteins can be added to the λ-vector DNA and the recreated phage is used to infect suitable bacteria. The recombinant DNA is replicated in the host microorganism and the complementary DNA sequence is thus amplified. Those microorganisms that contain the relevant complementary DNA or its gene products (i.e. messenger RNA or protein) are identified and the clones are then isolated.

Modern molecular biology makes possible the isolation of recombinant DNA molecules which contain sequences derived from almost any gene of interest. Culture of the cloned organisms containing these recombinant molecules can yield relatively large quantities of material that can be used for a number of purposes. For example, analysis of the sequence of nucleotides in the complementary DNA makes it possible to deduce the structure of the messenger RNA from which it was prepared: the messenger RNA base sequence in turn gives the amino acid sequence of the peptide. Alternatively, the complementary DNA can be labelled with a radioactive nucleotide and used as a probe to analyse the structure of the gene from which it was derived. 'Genomic

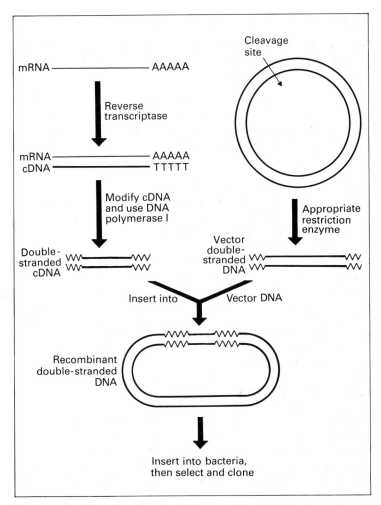

**Fig. 1.7** A schematic résumé of the steps involved in preparation of complementary DNA (cDNA) and its subsequent cloning by use of vector DNA. Messenger RNA is isolated and a complementary DNA copy is then prepared using reverse transcriptase (as shown on the left of the figure). Treatment of the cDNA–mRNA complex follows, to yield a suitable substrate capable of being copied by DNA polymerase I. This enzyme produces double-stranded (ds) cDNA. On the right side of the figure is shown a circular vector DNA that is cleaved at an appropriate position by a restriction enzyme to give linear ds DNA. The ds cDNA is then inserted into the vector DNA, after suitable treatment to ensure that the chain ends will join together to recreate circular ds DNA. The 'recombinant DNA' is then inserted into a bacterium which multipies and amplifies the number of copies of the recombinant DNA. The bacteria that contain the recombinant DNA are then identified. For example, it is possible to include vector gene segments that confer resistance to one or more antibiotics along with the complementary DNA when recombinant DNA is made. The vector-containing bacteria are then grown on medium containing the antibiotics, when only those organisms which carry the recombinant DNA will grow. The bacteria are separated into clones, and the DNA or its products are identified.

libraries' have now been formed that greatly assist in the identification of particular gene sequences. A genomic library is a collection of recombinant molecules that includes all of the DNA sequence of a given species. By use of cDNA probes, information may be gained, for example, about the arrangement of introns and exons in the structural gene. The gene can also be localized on a particular region of a chromosome.

A cDNA probe can be used to show which tissues express a particular messenger RNA, and thus which tissues synthesize a particular hormone. Used quantitatively, the cDNA probe makes it possible to study the control of transcription, and the control of hormone synthesis. It is also possible to introduce complementary DNA into 'expression systems' that are used to manufacture peptide hormones. For this, the complementary DNA has to be incorporated into a suitable vector along with a promoter region active in, for example, *E. coli*. The vector is incorporated into a suitable bacterium which then multiplies. Mammalian expression systems, for example murine cell lines, can also be used. Subsequently, the hormone that is synthesized has to be purified from other components of the host system; it must be free of viral and oncogene (cancer-causing viral gene) contaminants before it can be used in humans. Both human insulin and human growth hormone have been made in this way.

TRANSLATION OF MESSENGER RNA INTO A PEPTIDE HORMONE

Mature messenger RNA is transported from the cell nucleus and is bound to ribosomes that are attached to the endoplasmic reticulum. This is a characteristic feature of protein-synthesizing cells and is called rough endoplasmic reticulum (see Fig. 1.5). The mature messenger RNA has a central region (Fig. 1.6), which is *translated* into protein, with 5′ and 3′ non-translated regions on either side. The 5′ non-translated region contains sequences that are important for the binding of ribosomes made up of ribosomal RNA and protein and factors that affect the efficiencies of translation. Translation of messenger RNA bound to a ribosome begins at the start signal, ATG, which is the triplet base code for the amino acid methionine. Each triplet of bases on the messenger RNA represents a binding site for the specific transfer RNA (tRNA) that contains a triplet base sequence complementary to that of the messenger RNA. As each transfer RNA carrying its specific amino acid binds to the mRNA-ribosome complex it is linked into the growing peptide chain. Peptide synthesis starts at the amino-terminus and proceeds to the carboxy-terminus end, where termination of translation of the messenger RNA ceases at a stop signal such as TGA.

In general, messenger RNA codes for a peptide that is longer than the secreted form of the hormone. The precursor peptide formed (called a prehormone) carries a *signal peptide* extension at the amino-terminus which is lipophilic (literally 'lipid liking'). The endoplasmic reticulum has channel proteins that recognize the signal peptide sequence. These features enable the nascent peptide to cross the endoplasmic reticulum into the cisternal space where the signal peptide is excised by a peptidase to leave the rest of the hormone in the cisternal space. Synthesis of a prehormone can be shown in cell-free translational systems that contain only messenger RNA, ribosomes and other co-factors including transfer RNAs. Under these circumstances, the signal peptide remains attached to the rest of the hormone molecule since there are no cisternal peptidases present. In the case of some hormones, apart from the pre-peptide, there may be another extension of the amino-terminus so that a 'pre-prohormone' is formed.

Other post-translational changes may be needed. As is shown in Fig. 1.8a and c, disulphide bridges are formed in certain proteins within the cisternal space of the endoplasmic reticulum. The newly formed protein then travels through the endoplasmic reticulum, and if it is a glycoprotein, certain carbohydrates may be added at this stage (see Fig. 1.8b and d). From the endoplasmic reticulum the protein or peptide hormone is transferred in vesicles to the Golgi complex, where further carbohydrate additions may occur including the terminal sialic acid residues. The completed protein is then packaged into membrane-bounded vesicles. For certain hormones, it has been shown that specific enzymes are packaged in an inactive form along with the prohormone. In this case, the enzyme is a specific endopeptidase which is capable of cleaving the 'pro-' portion of the protein chain, as in the case of the C-peptide of insulin (Fig. 1.8c).

## STORAGE

Protein or peptide hormone secreting cells store the newly synthesized hormone in small vesicles or secretory granules. These vesicles may be observed under the electron microscope as electron-dense material scattered around the periphery of these cells, just inside the cell membrane. Movement of the vesicles from the Golgi apparatus to a position near the cell membrane appears to be influenced by two types of filamentous structure called microtubules and microfilaments, which are found in all eukaryotic cells so far examined. Microtubules are made up of polymerized protein molecules (tubulin), which form rods of approximately 20 nm in diameter within the cell. Associated with the microtubules are at least three different enzymes, though their functions are at present obscure. The microfilaments are made up of

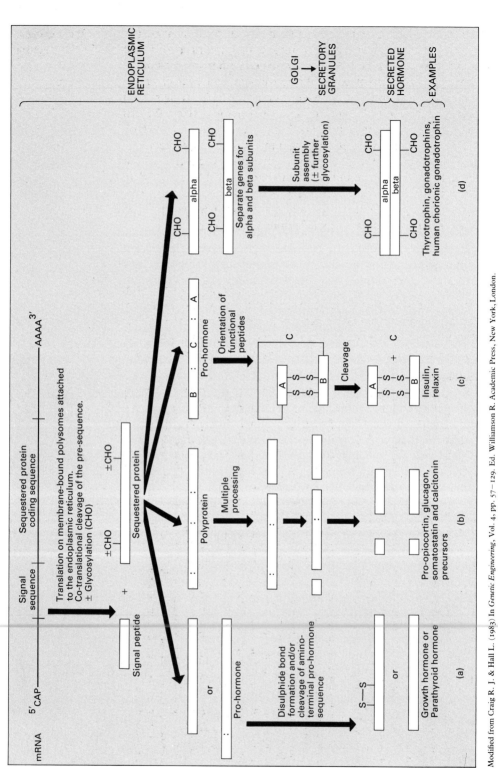

mRNA 5' CAP —— Signal sequence —— Sequestered protein coding sequence —— AAAA 3'

Translation on membrane-bound polysomes attached to the endoplasmic reticulum. Co-translational cleavage of the pre-sequence. ± Glycosylation (CHO)

ENDOPLASMIC RETICULUM

Signal peptide + Sequestered protein ±CHO ±CHO

(a) Pro-hormone — Disulphide bond formation and/or cleavage of amino-terminal pro-hormone sequence → S—S — Growth hormone or Parathyroid hormone

(b) Polyprotein — Multiple processing → Pro-opiocortin, glucagon, somatostatin and calcitonin precursors

(c) B ⋮ C ⋮ A Pro-hormone — Orientation of functional peptides → A S—S—S—S B  C — Cleavage → A S—S—S—S B + C — Insulin, relaxin

(d) CHO alpha CHO / CHO beta CHO — Separate genes for alpha and beta subunits — GOLGI → SECRETORY GRANULES — Subunit assembly (± further glycosylation) → SECRETED HORMONE CHO alpha CHO / CHO beta CHO — Thyrotrophin, gonadotrophins, human chorionic gonadotrophin — EXAMPLES

Modified from Craig R. J. & Hall L. (1983) In *Genetic Engineering*, Vol. 4. pp. 57–129. Ed. Williamson R. Academic Press, New York. London.

the 'muscle-like' protein actin, and are about 5 nm in diameter. Groups of microfilaments are arranged in bundles at different positions within the cell. Actin is associated with myosin subunits, and is probably involved in the movement and control of the positions of subcellular vesicles within the cell. It has been suggested that tubulin acts as the cytoskeleton, giving the cell some degree of rigidity, and also that it provides a framework on which the other cytoskeletal elements, such as microfilaments, are able to control the movement of subcellular organelles within the cell. Both filamentous structures are probably involved in the control of secretion processes, since drugs like colchicine (which disrupts microtubules) and cytochalasin B (which binds to actin microfilaments) block hormone secretion.

SECRETION

Peptide and protein hormones (stored as granules in vesicles at the periphery of the cell) require some stimulus to the cell before the stored prohormone is activated and then released. This stimulus may be hormonal, and in most cases it probably involves a change, for example, in ionic permeability of the cell to $Ca^{2+}$

**Fig. 1.8** Schematic representation of the synthesis of peptide hormones showing some post-translational changes. A signal peptide at the amino-terminal end facilitates movement of a prehormone across intracellular membranes of the endoplasmic reticulum. The signal peptide is removed and the rest of the molecule is sequestered for further processing before it is secreted. Four types of post-translational modification are shown:

(a) Where there is an amino-terminal extension in a prohormone, such as proparathyroid hormone, the extension is removed before secretion. Alternatively, as with growth hormone, the number of amino acids is not changed but intrachain disulphide bonds are created before the hormone is secreted.

(b) A polyprotein yields a number of peptides on specific hydrolysis by endopeptidases, and some of these peptides may be glycosylated. For example, pro-opiocortin (also called pro-opiomelanocortin) can give rise to adrenocorticotrophin plus melanocyte stimulating hormone and β-endorphin; these peptides vary in length and have different biological activities.

(c) Synthesis of highly active molecules such as insulin appears to proceed by folding of the peptide and formation of disulphide bonds. An active molecule is created by specific hydrolytic removal of a connecting (C) peptide and so pro-insulin gives rise to insulin plus C-peptide, which are secreted in equimolar proportions.

(d) Synthesis of the larger protein hormones such as thyrotrophin, the gonadotrophins, luteinizing and follicle stimulating hormones, and also human chorionic gonadotrophin, proceeds from two separate peptides that come together to form the subunits of the protein. These four hormone molecules each have a very similar α-subunit and a hormone-specific β-subunit; both subunits are glycosylated.

ions. The term 'stimulus-secretion coupling' has been used to describe the latter process, in which divalent metal ions are required for interaction between the vesicle membrane, and the plasma membrane for microfilament and microtubule activation, and also for certain enzymes, all of which are probably involved in the secretion process. The specific endopeptidases (or other enzymes) present with the prohormone (or protein) in the storage vesicle are activated during the secretion process, producing the active form of the hormone before it is actually released from the cell.

The mode of secretion from the cell is called exocytosis (Fig. 1.5a). The membrane of an intracellular storage granule fuses with the plasma membrane of the cell which then parts near the point of fusion and the contents of the vesicle are then secreted into extracellular space surrounding the blood vessels. Membrane turnover is increased, and where it has been studied, it appears that the membrane which originally surrounded the vesicle is quickly recycled within the cell and so does not remain a component of the plasma membrane of the cell for long. Large changes in the turnover of membrane phospholipids occur during this period of exocytotic activity, and although particular phospholipids have been shown to be important in different cells, their involvement in the exocytotic process can only be inferred.

## Steroids

### SYNTHESIS

Cholesterol is the natural precursor of all steroid hormones. The biochemical pathway for steroid synthesis starts from acetate, via mevalonate, hydroxymethyl glutaryl CoA and squalene to cholesterol. All the steroid hormone-synthesizing cells of the body, i.e. the adrenal cortex, placenta, testis and ovary, contain intracellular fat droplets in the cytoplasm (Fig. 1.5b). The fat droplets are composed principally of cholesterol esters. This is the primary storage form of hormone precursor, i.e. cholesterol, in these cells. The steroid-secreting cells, unlike the protein and peptide producing cells, do not store hormone in a state ready for secretion, but they synthesize the steroid hormone for secretion as it is required.

The first step in the synthesis of steroid hormones is the hydrolysis of cholesterol esters present in the fat droplets. Cholesterol is then transported from the storage droplets into the mitochondria by a specific membrane carrier-system. Once inside the mitochondrion, the initial reaction is the production of pregnenolone from cholesterol by 'side-chain cleavage' at position C20/C22 under the action of the enzyme, cholesterol desmolase, as is shown in Fig. 1.9. This is an extremely important step in the control of steroid hormone synthesis. The side-chain cleavage reaction occurs in mitochondria and it involves a series of hydroxylations with the cytochrome P-450 system as an electron-acceptor. After removal of the side-chain by cholesterol desmolase, the product, pregnenolone, is transported back out of the mitochondrion to sites in the extensive smooth endoplasmic reticulum

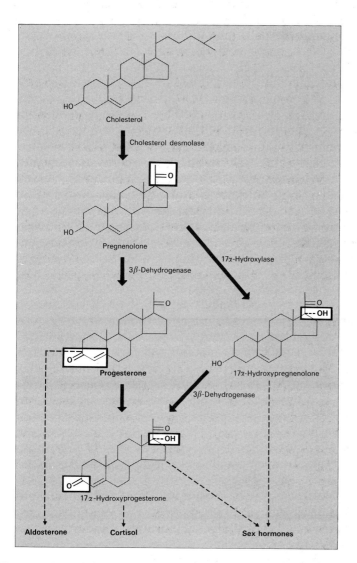

**Fig. 1.9** Cholesterol—the precursor of steroid hormones. The diagram shows the routes by which the principal groups of steroid hormones are synthesized from cholesterol. The enzyme, cholesterol desmolase (the 'side-chain cleavage' enzyme), converts cholesterol to pregnenolone. Then, via progesterone or 17α-hydroxypregnenolone, the principal steroid hormones, aldosterone, cortisol or the sex hormones are synthesized along the routes outlined in chapters 3 and 4, respectively. High-lighting on particular groupings in this and subsequent similar figures indicates the groups which have been most recently modified by the preceding reaction. --- Bonds which are directed beneath the plane of the picture.

found in most steroid synthesizing cells. The smooth endoplasmic reticulum and the mitochondria contain the enzymes required for most of the further transformations of pregnenolone to progesterone and $17\alpha$-hydroxyprogesterone. Subsequently, other compounds are formed depending on cell type, such as the adrenal cortical steroids, and the androgens or oestrogens (the male or female sex hormones, respectively; these are discussed in Chapters 3 and 4).

## TRANSPORT OF HORMONES IN THE BLOOD

Most peptide and protein hormones are hydrophilic, at least on the exterior surface, and they therefore circulate in the bloodstream with little or no association with serum proteins. The more hydrophobic a molecule is, the less likely it is to circulate in the free state, and it therefore associates closely with serum proteins for transport around the body. Thus, there are specific transport proteins in the circulation that bind thyroxine, and many of the steroid hormones. These proteins include thyroxine-binding globulin, cortisol-binding globulin, and sex hormone-binding globulin. Their specificity is so great that minor changes in structure affect binding and, for example, triiodothyronine and aldosterone are only weakly bound to thyroxine-binding globulin and cortisol-binding globulin, respectively. Many hormones may also associate loosely with other circulating proteins, especially albumin. Thyroxine also binds to another protein, known as pre-albumin (so-called because of its faster electrophoretic mobility than albumin).

Hormone bound to protein is in equilibrium with 'free' (or unbound) hormone. The free hormone can diffuse to tissues more readily and so the physiological state usually corresponds more closely with the concentration of the free homone. As a result of changes in the concentration of binding protein the total concentration and the bound concentration of hormone may alter quite markedly with only a small change in the free hormone concentration, and so the physiological status can thus remain unaltered.

## ASSAYS OF HORMONES

Biological assay systems have been essential for the characterization of hormones. In isolating a hormone, it is necessary to have a 'biological end-point' to be sure that the substance being isolated is the one responsible for the biological effect that has been observed. For any hormone, there may be many bioassay systems which have to be carefully characterized, be they *in vivo* or *in vitro*, since factors such as species, strain, sex, age and diet can all alter the responsiveness of the tissue. Even when this source of variation is minimized, there can be considerable variability in the bioassay results and large numbers of animals have to be used to ensure statistical significance of the results. For example, insulin used to be assayed by observing the convulsions produced by the hypoglycaemia that insulin injection into mice produced. It was necessary to use hundreds of mice to compare preparations so that the amount of insulin required to cause convulsions in 50% of the animals could be established as a measure of potency. The route of administration of the hormone (i.e. oral, intravenous or subcutaneous) and the vehicle in which it is given are important because these affect the speed with which the response is produced, and its duration; the timing of the dose and of the measurement also become critical.

The unit of biological activity is defined as that amount of material which will produce a specified biological response. For example, the unit of parathyroid hormone is that which will increase the serum calcium of a 20 kg dog by 0.25 mmol/l. Units of this type are not entirely satisfactory and so reference preparations have been made. These may or may not be pure substances: they are ampouled and a unit may be defined in terms of the contents of an ampoule of an international reference preparation. Since in different species a peptide hormone may differ in amino-acid sequence and since this may affect biological activity, it is desirable to have a reference preparation from the same species as that being studied. In a biological assay the dose—response curve is generally sigmoidal on a linear—log plot, with dose on the horizontal logarithmic axis and the response on the linear—vertical axis: it is necessary to vary the dose so as to get a response on the linear sloping part of this sigmoidal dose—response curve to get a reliable answer (Fig. 1.10).

By using *in vitro* methods, it is often possible to increase sensitivity while avoiding some of the other problems of *in vivo* assays. For example, the number of animals that have to be used to get a precise estimate of potency can sometimes be reduced. Cell membrane preparations and measurement of adenylate cyclase activity (see below) can be employed for *in vitro* assays: the membranes have to be prepared from the natural target tissue of the hormone. Thus thyroid membranes may be used for thyrotrophin assays, liver membranes for glucagon assays and so on. However, it is not possible to measure physiological concentrations of the hormone in this way.

**Binding assays**

Minute amounts of hormone can be measured with this technique if the hormone can be prepared in a labelled (usually radioactive)

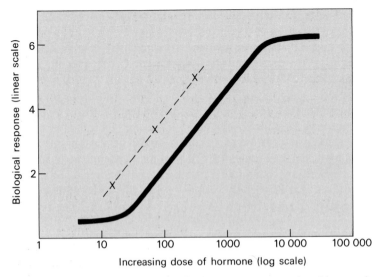

**Fig. 1.10** Schematic representation of a dose−response curve for a bioassay. A dose−response curve is constructed with varying amounts of a reference preparation (dose plotted on log scale). Three different doses of a test material are assayed (shown by crosses joined by a dashed line): for a valid bioassay, the test and reference preparation must give parallel dose−response relationships.

form and if a binding protein with high affinity for the hormone is available. For binding assays of this type, one of two forms of binding protein is commonly used—either an antibody against a hormone or alternatively a natural binding protein, if it exists. If an antibody is used, the method is called a radioimmunoassay, while if a naturally occurring protein is used, it is usually called a competitive protein binding assay. Berson and Yalow developed the first radioimmunoassay in 1959 with antibodies to insulin while, at the same time, Ekins used the natural circulating binding globulin to measure thyroxine.

Antibodies can be prepared against peptide hormones by immunizing animals. Smaller molecules can also be made antigenic by coupling them to larger proteins (usually albumin, though thyroglobulin or poly-lysine have also been used), the small hormone then functions as a hapten. For example, steroids can be coupled to albumin and when animals are immunized with the complex they produce antibodies that react specifically with the steroid. Antibodies are often produced by immunizing guinea-pigs, rabbits or goats, but other species are sometimes used. The immunogen is usually injected in an adjuvant that contains a mixture of oils and dead tubercle bacilli which is known as Freund's adjuvant. The hormone in aqueous solution is emulsified with the adjuvant which was found empirically to improve antibody production by enhancement of the immune response.

A radioimmunoassay can be represented as:

$$H + Ab \underset{k_{-1}}{\overset{k_1}{\rightleftharpoons}} HAb \qquad (1)$$

where H is the hormone, Ab is the antibody and HAb is the hormone−antibody complex. The equilibrium constant ($K$) is obtained from the ratio of the concentrations of the reacting species (represented by the quantities in square brackets):

$$K = \frac{k_1}{k_{-1}} = \frac{[HAb]}{[H][Ab]} \qquad (2)$$

where $k_1$ and $k_{-1}$ are the forward and reverse reaction rate constants. For high sensitivity of the assay it is necessary for $K$ to be high and antibodies with $K = 10^{10}$ l/mole or higher can be obtained which may be used to give highly sensitive assays. The amount of hormone bound is a function of the equilibrium constant $K$, the concentration of antibody, and of course, the concentration of hormone.

After incubation of the hormone and antibody in an assay, the bound and free moieties have to be separated. If radioactively labelled hormone has been added, this can be used to measure the proportion that is free or that which is bound to antibody. These moieties can be separated in one of several ways. For example, dextran-coated charcoal often absorbs a free hormone which can then be separated from bound hormone by centrifugation. Alternatively, the bound hormone can be removed, say, by precipitation with ammonium sulphate, or by use of a second antibody which binds to and precipitates the first antibody.

A schematic representation of an immunoassay calibration curve is shown in Fig. 1.11a. The conditions of the assay have to be optimized to get maximum sensitivity that is often needed to measure physiological concentrations. For this, it is often necessary to have a high specific activity tracer (measured in terms of kbecquerels/$\mu$g or $\mu$curies/$\mu$g) and the hormone is often labelled with iodine-125 so that the mass of tracer added can be minimized. The concentration of antibody has to be optimized, and the antiserum is usually used in high dilution or titre, say 1 in 500000, depending on the affinity of the antibody for the antigen.

A variety of different immunoassay systems are now available. Many use monoclonal antibodies that are produced by selection of a single antibody-producing cell that is then fused with a myeloma or similar cell line that will divide and grow in culture. The antibody secreted may be easily collected from the culture medium, and it is specifically directed against a single epitope, i.e. an antigenic determinant of the antigen molecule: such monoclonal antibodies are therefore highly specific for a particular antigen.

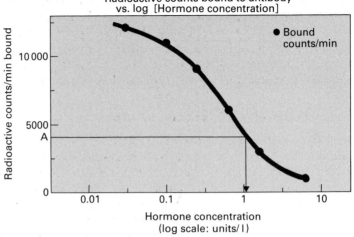

**Fig. 1.11** Radioimmunoassay calibration curves for (**a**) an immunoassay; (**b**) a radioimmunometric assay. Radioactive counts/minute bound to antibody are plotted against the concentration of hormone present in standards. A sample with 'A' radioactive counts/minute bound may then be read off the calibration curve to yield the hormone concentration present in the sample in units/l (where the units could be SI units, e.g. pmol/l, or arbitrary international units/l).

One of a number of variants of the immunoassay is the immunometric assay (Fig. 1.11b). This uses antibodies coated onto a solid surface, such as a plastic tube or microtitre well. The test specimen is added and the antigen is bound to the excess of antibody on the solid phase. A second antibody, directed against another determinant on the antigen is then added. This second antibody may be labelled with an isotope such as iodine-125, an enzyme, or a fluorescent or luminescent agent.

These markers can then be used to measure the amount of antigen bound to the first antibody, which is then proportional to the amount of label bound to the second antibody on the solid phase. The principal advantage of this assay system is that it is capable of measuring concentrations of peptide or protein analytes that cover a concentration range of up to about five orders of magnitude, i.e. $1$ to $10^5$ units/l (see Fig. 1.11b).

### Comparison of bioassays and immunoassays

Peptide hormones can be partially hydrolysed in the body to yield smaller peptides which may still cross-react to a greater or lesser extent with the antiserum in an immunoassay. This usually gives a positive result in an immunoassay, but it often yields a negative result in a bioassay as this material is no longer biologically active. Substances other than proteins, e.g. steroids or drugs, can also be metabolized to inactive or to more active constituents which may or may not cross-react in a particular immunoassay. Bioassay procedures are therefore still very important in carrying out verification and validation of results under circumstances where the above situations might arise, or where the biological potency of the material is actually required.

There are still situations in which satisfactory specific and sensitive immunoassays have not yet been developed, for example, many immunoassays are incapable of differentiating between certain steroid hormones. However, other techniques, such as high-performance liquid chromatography (HPLC), or gas chromatography followed by mass spectrometric analysis (GC/MS), have been employed successfully in conjunction with a relatively non-specific immunoassay, or in some cases in place of the latter technique.

## MECHANISMS OF HORMONE ACTIONS

The *effect* of a hormone can be defined as the observed result of the administration of that hormone to an animal *in vivo* or to a tissue *in vitro*, e.g. the effect of insulin is to lower blood sugar. On the other hand the *mechanism of action* of a hormone is the precise description of the chain of molecular events initiated by the hormone leading eventually to the observed effects on cell metabolism, while the *function* of a hormone is the general role it plays in the economy of the body, e.g. the function of insulin is to regulate carbohydrate metabolism.

For a hormone to regulate cell metabolism, clearly the following conditions must exist:

1 The rate of its release into the bloodstream must be variable and should in turn be controlled by some function of the cellular process that it regulates.

2   The kinds of cell the hormone acts on, i.e. the target-cells, must be able to recognize the hormone as a specific molecule and in some way estimate the concentration of the hormone reaching them so as to produce a graded rather than an all-or-none response.

3   The responsive cells must contain appropriate cell mechanisms for translating the message carried by the hormone so that their own enzyme systems make the appropriate response.

## Specificity of hormone action

The specificity of the response to a particular hormone must be maintained even though it is expressed through a common pathway. The differentiation of some one to two hundred different cell types that occurs during human development is controlled by repression and de-repression of particular genes on the DNA molecules of the fertilized egg and the succession of cells derived from it. One important feature of cell differentiation is the elaboration of specific receptor molecules in the cell membrane or specific structures or proteins in the cell cytoplasm. This is the mechanism whereby the specificity of hormone action is determined within the target cells of the body and it is an essential component of the endocrine control system.

## Hormones acting at the cell surface

Most protein and peptide hormones are fairly large molecules which are water soluble (that is, they are hydrophilic) and so they cannot cross the lipid-containing cell membranes. Therefore they act through receptors on the external surface of the target-cell to induce changes on the inner surface of the cell membrane which in turn lead to alterations in activity within the cell. In some cases these depend on the production of an intracellular messenger. On the basis that the hormone itself is the 'first messenger', the intracellular substance is called the 'second messenger'. The Nobel prize-winning work of Sutherland introduced the concept of a second messenger, in which the importance of cyclic AMP as a mediator of hormone action was shown. Cyclic AMP was found to be capable of inducing a cascade of changes within the cell. In this system, the specificity arises from the structure of the hormone and the specificity of the receptor for the hormone plus, of course, the properties of the target cell itself.

### MEMBRANE RECEPTOR COMPLEXES

The receptors are present in the cell membrane as lipoprotein complexes. Each cell may carry hundreds or thousands of such receptors on its surface. The hormone–receptor interaction involves binding of the hormone, the equilibrium of which may be described by mathematical expressions similar to equations (1) and (2) on page 23. In general, the receptor is linked via a transducer unit that acts as a control point to a catalytic unit which is on the inner surface of the cell. This is shown schematically in Fig. 1.12.

The transducer units bind a nucleotide diphosphate (usually

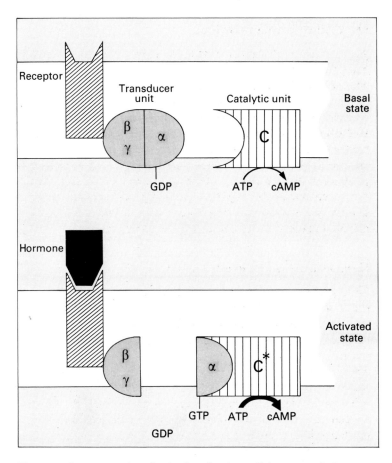

**Fig. 1.12** A representation of activation of an intracellular enzyme by hormone binding to an external membrane receptor. Hormone binds to the external receptor on the cell membrane. The receptor is associated with a transducer unit called the nucleotide regulatory complex (N-complex) which has three components named $\alpha$, $\beta$ and $\gamma$. The name derives from the nucleotide diphosphate (NDP) bound to the complex. On activation, nucleotide triphosphate (NTP) displaces the diphosphate. In the illustration the involvement of guanosine di- and tri-phosphates (GDP and GTP) is shown. The $\alpha$ component of the N-complex dissociates, to bind to and thence activate an enzyme called the catalytic unit (C is altered to C*), probably by inducing a conformational change. Deactivation is achieved when the hormone dissociates from its external receptor; reversal of the intracellular activation occurs when a phosphatase hydrolyses NTP to leave NDP bound to the 'resting' state of the N-complex.

guanosine diphosphate, GDP) in their 'resting' or non-activated states. Interaction between a hormone and its receptor initiates binding of a molecule of guanosine triphosphate (GTP), which displaces the nucleotide diphosphate (GDP) previously bound to the complex. Inactivation occurs by dephosphorylation of the triphosphate to yield the 'resting' state once more. Because of these interactions, the transducer unit is called a *nucleotide regulatory complex*, with the abbreviation 'N-complex' being used, although 'G-complex' is also used in reference to binding of guanosine phosphates.

## Enzyme mediation of hormone action

The catalytic unit is an enzyme. It has been shown that three different types of enzyme are important in the mediation of the actions of various hormones, and these enzymes are adenylate cyclase, phospholipase C and tyrosine kinase. They provide three separate routes by which peptide hormone action at the cell surface may be transmitted within the cell, and each will be considered in turn.

### 1 ADENYLATE CYCLASE AND HORMONE ACTION

The action of many hormones, including adrenaline, glucagon, thyrotrophin and parathyroid hormone, is mediated by adenylate cyclase (Fig. 1.12). This enzyme uses adenosine triphosphate (ATP) as a substrate for the production of adenosine-3', 5'-cyclic monophosphate (cyclic AMP, see Fig. 1.13) and pyrophosphate (PP):

$$\text{ATP} \xrightarrow[\text{cyclase}]{\text{adenylate}} \text{cyclic AMP} + \text{PP}$$

Hormone action on a cell stimulates the enzyme to produce cyclic AMP and hence activate other enzymes as is described below. Once hormone action is complete, cyclic AMP is broken down to adenosine-5'-monophosphate (AMP) by phosphodiesterases present in most cells.

### *The hormone receptor/adenylate cyclase complex*

The hormone receptor is a protein on the outer surface of the cell membrane and adenylate cyclase is present on the inner surface. The hormone signal is transmitted to the enzyme through a nucleotide regulatory complex as outlined above. The N-complex associated with certain hormone receptor/adenylate cyclase systems has been found to be made up of three subunits named alpha, beta and gamma. The N-complex involved in stimulation of the catalytic unit is abbreviated to $N_S$. There is another form, which can predominate over $N_S$ in the cell membrane, and this is an inhibitory nucleotide regulatory complex

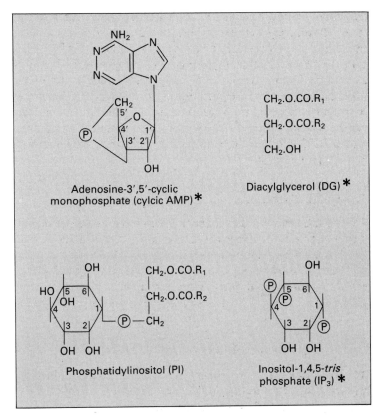

Adenosine-3',5'-cyclic
monophosphate (cylcic AMP) *

Diacylglycerol (DG) *

Phosphatidylinositol (PI)

Inositol-1,4,5-*tris*
phosphate (IP$_3$) *

**Fig. 1.13** Structures of some important metabolic intermediates, including 'second messengers' (which are marked by an asterisk, *), involved in the mechanism of hormone action. The symbol ℗ is the abbreviation for phosphate, $PO_4^-$. Numbers close to the angles of the carbohydrate rings show the chemical numbering convention used to identify substituents attached at these positions. $R_1$ and $R_2$ represent fatty acid chains, e.g. $\cdot (CH_2)_k \cdot CH_3$, where $k$ is variable and there may be 12 or more carbon atoms in the chain and usually there are one or two unsaturated bonds such as $\cdot CH=CH \cdot$ also present; the acyl group is shown as $\cdot CO \cdot R_n$ (where n = 1 or 2).

referred to as $N_I$. The $\beta$-subunit and the $\gamma$-subunit both appear to be similar in each of the two forms of N-complex. However, there are two types of $\alpha$-subunit, called $\alpha_S$ and $\alpha_I$ respectively. The $\beta$ component has a molecular weight of 50−55 000 while the $\gamma$-subunit is much smaller (5000); $\alpha_S$ has a molecular weight of 42 000 and $\alpha_I$ of 39 000.

Partially purified adenylate cyclase has been incorporated into artificial cell membranes made of lipid bilayers. Addition of the $\alpha_S$ subunit can activate adenylate cyclase in this model system. It seems likely therefore that hormonal activation through a receptor induces an association between $\alpha_S$ and adenylate cyclase, with consequent activation of the enzyme and an increase in intracellular cyclic AMP. In the case of the $N_I$-complex, the inhibitory $\alpha_I$ subunit acts either on an adenylate cyclase that has already been stimulated by another hormone, or on adenylate cyclase that still functions in a 'basal' state, to prevent the formation of cyclic AMP.

*Second messenger actions of cyclic AMP within the cell*

Cyclic AMP produced as a result of hormone action serves as a second messenger to transmit the hormone signal into stimulation within the cell. It does this by activation of protein kinases that phosphorylate a variety of proteins, using ATP as a substrate. The cyclic AMP-activated protein kinases have two different subunits, certain of which are found in a molecular arrangement of tetramers with two sets of identical subunits. One of these, the regulatory subunit, can bind cyclic AMP. When this happens, it dissociates from the other subunit, which is the catalytic component that performs the phosphorylation reaction. The protein kinases can phosphorylate other enzymes, a process which can either activate or deactivate the enzyme. A number of examples of these actions are discussed further, particularly in Chapter 7.

The hormone signal is terminated by dissociation of the hormone from its receptor, following which the cyclic AMP is destroyed by phosphodiesterases and the catalytic and regulatory subunits of the protein kinase reassociate.

## 2 PHOSPHOLIPASE C AND HORMONE ACTION

A number of hormones including thyrotrophin releasing hormone, angiotensin II and vasopressin can modulate the activity of phospholipase C. This enzyme catalyses the reaction:

$$PIP_2 \xrightarrow{\text{Phospholipase C}} DG + IP_3$$

where, $PIP_2$ is phosphatidylinositol-4,5-*bis*phosphate, DG is diacylglycerol and $IP_3$ is inositol-1,4,5-*tris*phosphate.

The structure of the two products was shown in Fig. 1.13. Diacylglycerol (DG) and inositol-1,4,5-*tris*phosphate ($IP_3$) act as intracellular second messengers. Diacylglycerol acts on cell-membrane associated protein kinase C that results in protein or enzyme phosphorylation within the cell, while $IP_3$ acts primarily to mobilize calcium within the cell.

Changes in calcium flux have long been known to be important in the activity of a variety of cells, for example in muscle contraction and in exocytotic secretion from exocrine glands. Changes in intracellular calcium have also been shown to be important in endocrine cells, for example in the pituitary. In 1975 Michell recognized that many hormones and neurotransmitters that appeared to use calcium as an intracellular signal also caused changes in the metabolism of the membrane phospholipid, phosphatidylinositol (PI). The sequence of metabolic reactions involved in

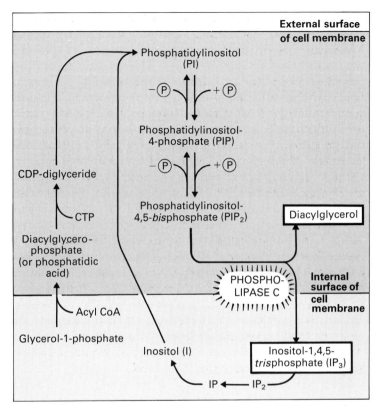

**Fig. 1.14** Metabolism of phosphatidylinositol. Glycerol-1-phosphate is
esterified by acylCoA (i.e. coenzyme A activated fatty acids) to yield
diacylglycerophosphate (or phosphatidic acid). Enzymatic incorporation of
cytosine triphosphate (CTP) yields cytosine diphosphodiacylglyceride (CDP-
diglyceride) that is then combined with inositol (I) to form phosphatidylinositol
(PI). Further phosphorylation takes place to yield phosphotidylinositol phosphates PIP and $PIP_2$. The phosphate group, $PO_4^-$, is represented by the symbol
Ⓟ. These phosphorylation/dephosphorylation reactions are reversible and they
take place in the lipid matrix of the cell membrane. Phospholipase C hydroloysis
yields diacylglycerol (DG) in the lipid membrane matrix, while $IP_3$ appears in
the cell cytosol. $IP_3$ may then be dephosphorylated to yield inositol once more.

the metabolism of glycerol, inositol and its phosphate derivatives
is shown in Fig. 1.14.

*The hormone receptor/phospholipase C complex.* When a hormone
binds to a receptor on the cell surface, transmission of the signal
to the enzyme catalytic unit, phospholipase C, appears to be
transduced by way of a nucleotide regulatory complex (called
$N_p$) in a manner analogous to that of the adenylate cyclase
system.

*Second messenger actions within the cell*

*Inositol-1,4,5-trisphosphate (IP₃).* Hormone-stimulated break-
down of phosphatidylinositol *bis*phosphate ($PIP_2$) rapidly produces

31

inositol*tris*phosphate (IP$_3$) that is released into the cytosol. Inositol-1,4,5-*tris*phosphate can mobilize intracellular calcium ions in the cytosol, and the endoplasmic reticulum is probably the principal source (see Fig. 1.15). The free calcium ion concentration, i.e. that not bound to intracellular proteins or lipids, within unstimulated cells is about 0.1 $\mu$mole/l. When the cell is stimulated the free calcium ion concentration may rise by a factor of 10-fold locally within the cytoplasm. The extracellular calcium ion concentration is approximately 1 mmol/l, and the substantial electrochemical gradient that results is opposed by the plasma membrane and by calcium pumps within the membrane. There are several trans-locase or pump systems which drive calcium ions out of the cell, notably a calcium-activated ATPase and a $Na^+/Ca^{2+}$ ion-exchanger. Growth factors can also induce a phospho-inositol response that leads to an increase in intracellular calcium and diacylglycerol that activate protein kinase C. This yields an increase in intracellular pH by a stimulation of the $Na^+/H^+$ antiport (see Fig. 1.15) that decreases the hydrogen ion concentration within the cell. Relatively small pH and ionic changes can have large effects on enzymes and metabolic reactions within the cell.

Calcium ions can act on several enzymes such as phospholipase A$_2$ and a number of protein kinase systems within the cell (see Chapter 7). Calcium ion activation of phospholipase A$_2$ liberates arachidonate from phospholipids, and this can generate a range of potent local tissue activators such as leucotrienes, the prostaglandins and the thromboxanes. Some of the effects of changes in intracellular calcium ion concentration are mediated through calmodulin. This is a protein that has four calcium binding sites; little calcium is bound to calmodulin at the basal calcium ion concentration, but binding becomes significant when the calcium ion concentration rises. The binding of calcium to calmodulin causes conformational changes that permit the protein to interact with enzymes, including calmodulin-dependent protein kinases, adenylate cyclase, cyclic nucleotide phosphodiesterase and $Ca^{2+}$-ATPase. A decrease in the intracellular calcium ion concentration reverses the action by dissociation of calmodulin from its acceptor enzyme.

*Diacylglycerol (DG).* Protein kinase C is usually present in a relatively inactive state within the cell and diacylglycerol increases its activity. Protein kinase C is a calcium and phosphatidyl serine dependent enzyme and diacylglycerol dramatically increases the affinity of this enzyme for calcium ions. The activity of protein kinase C is greatly enhanced when both effectors (i.e. diacylglycerol and $Ca^{2+}$) are present together. In some cases, calcium may be responsible for initiation of the physiological response, after which the calcium ion concentration within the cell will rapidly return to the basal levels. In these circumstances,

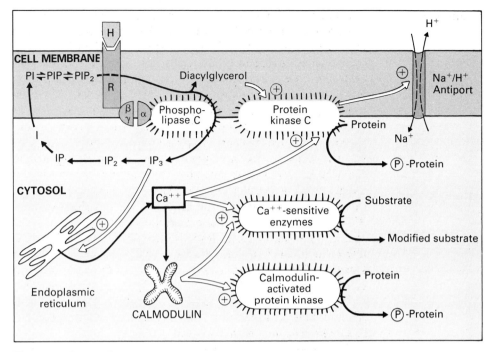

**Fig. 1.15** *Hormonal stimulation of phospholipid turnover and calcium metabolism within the cell.* Metabolism of phosphatidylinositol (see Fig. 1.14) is shown in an abbreviated form on the left of this figure, with the phospholipids (PI, PIP, $PIP_2$) present in the membrane and the inositol phosphates (IP, $IP_2$, $IP_3$) in the cell cytoplasm. Hormone action stimulates phospholipase C, which then hydrolyses phosphatidyl*bis*phosphate ($PIP_2$) to yield diacylglycerol (DG) and inositol*tris*phosphate ($IP_3$). Inositol*tris*phosphate is involved in mobilizing calcium from the intracellular stores, particularly the endoplasmic reticulum, while diacylglycerol activates protein kinase C and also increases the enzyme's affinity for calcium ions, which causes further stimulation of the enzyme. The effects of the hormone action on these enzyme systems are to stimulate the phosphorylation of proteins and enzymes, and hence alter intracellular metabolism (see Chapter 7). The $Na^+/H^+$ antiport is also stimulated by action of some growth factors to decrease the intracellular hydrogen ion concentration and hence raise the intracellular pH; this can affect a variety of enzymes and intracellular reactions.

diacylglycerol activation of protein kinase C may be responsible for maintenance of longer term cellular activity.

3  TYROSINE KINASE AND HORMONE ACTION

The actions of insulin and of epidermal growth factor depend on their ability to activate tyrosine kinase. This enzyme is present in the cell membrane, and it is responsible for catalysing the phosphorylation of tyrosyl residues in proteins:

$$\text{ATP} + \text{Tyrosyl} \cdot \text{protein} \xrightarrow[\text{kinase}]{\text{tyrosine}} \text{Phosphotyrosyl} \cdot \text{protein} + \text{ADP}$$

Thus, insulin action stimulates the activity of a protein kinase

33

which is different from the protein kinases referred to in the previous two sections. Tyrosine kinase phosphorylates the phenolic hydroxyl group of tyrosyl residues, while the other protein kinases phosphorylate hydroxyl groups of serine and threonine. The action of tyrosine kinase may affect that of protein kinase and so the two pathways could interact.

*The hormone receptor/tyrosine kinase complex*
The insulin receptor complex has been isolated and characterized. It is a glycoprotein which exists as a tetramer made up of two

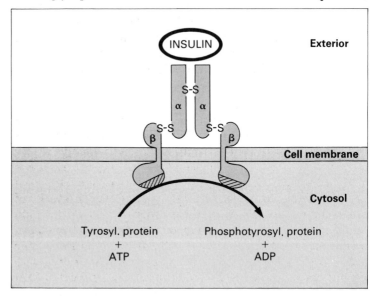

**Fig. 1.16** Possible structure of the insulin receptor, which is an integral membrane glycoprotein (about 350 000 average relative molecular weight). The receptor is composed of two α-subunits which carry the majority of the carbohydrate units (molecular weight about 130 000, 720 amino acid residues) linked to each other and to the two β-subunits (molecular weight about 90 000, 620 amino acids) by disulphide bonds. The receptor is translated from a single messenger RNA, with the α-subunit followed by the β; then, after disulphide bridge formation, a short sequence of amino acids is cleaved by protease action to separate the two subunits. Insulin binding takes place predominantly to the α-subunit, as has been shown by affinity-labelling techniques with $^{125}$I-labelled insulin. The amino-terminus of the first third of the β-subunit lies on the extracellular side of the cell membrane. A narrow bridge of about 23 hydrophobic amino acids is likely to span the membrane to the intracellular carboxy-terminal two-thirds of the subunit. An ATP binding site is located 49 amino acids from the membrane, and the tyrosine kinase domain (hatched) is located in this region of the receptor. Insulin binding to the receptor activates this protein (tyrosine) kinase which then phosphorylates tyrosyl residues on a number of proteins (designated 'tyrosyl.protein' in this figure). Tyrosine kinase is unusual in that it phosphorylates the phenolic hydroxyl group on the tyrosyl side chain, rather than the hydroxyl group of serine or threonine which are phosphorylated by most other protein kinases. The receptor for epidermal growth factor is analogous to half the insulin receptor and has an one alpha and one beta chain.

$\alpha$-chains and two $\beta$-chains. The $\alpha$- and $\beta$-chains are derived from a single glycosylated precursor of molecular weight 190000, and the amino acid sequence has been determined indirectly from the nucleotide sequence of a cDNA. The receptor (see Fig. 1.16) has a molecular weight of about 350000, and comprises two sets of disulphide-linked $\alpha$- and $\beta$-subunits that are also joined by disulphide bonds. The $\alpha$-chain has 720 residues and carries the insulin binding-site; it is on the outer surface of the cell membrane. The $\beta$-chain of 620 amino acid residues has a sequence of 23 hydrophobic amino acids that is long enough to span the cell membrane. Tyrosine kinase activity is found on that portion of the $\beta$-chain that lies on the cytoplasmic side of the membrane. Insulin binding to the external receptor probably alters the conformation of the receptor, which in turn activates the tyrosine kinase on the inner cell surface.

*Binding to the insulin receptor*
A study of the kinetics of insulin binding to its receptor indicates that there is a decrease in affinity of the receptor for hormone at high insulin concentrations. Examination of the insulin receptor model shown in Fig. 1.16 suggests how this may occur. At low or normal insulin concentrations, where it is presumed that only a single binding site on each receptor is occupied, the affinity of insulin for its receptor is high and actions of insulin are fully expressed within the cell. Binding of one molecule of insulin to the first site will probably alter the affinity of the second site for insulin binding. When the insulin concentration increases to saturate one binding site of the receptor, then occupancy of the second binding site would further alter the conformation of the receptor and thus suppress the response of the tyrosine kinase, and hence of the cell, to insulin. The process is referred to as 'down regulation' of the receptor. The phenomenon of down regulation is also seen at high hormone concentrations with a number of other hormone receptors. The receptor site on the outside may be internalized when it has insulin bound to it and so new receptors must be produced to replace those that have been used.

*Actions of insulin*
Insulin controls virtually every aspect of growth and metabolism by affecting the transport of metabolites and intracellular metabolic pathways of most, if not all, of the different cell-types within the body. Some of the major metabolic reactions that are influenced by insulin are discussed in Chapter 7 in relation to carbohydrate metabolism: insulin action affects calcium-sensitive enzymes and protein kinase activities. However, it is important to remember that insulin has major actions in controlling fatty acid and amino acid metabolism too. There is some evidence

that insulin also has an action in increasing protein synthesis in some cells. Another important action of insulin is to alter the permeability of cell membranes of a variety of tissues, such as those of the intestine, muscle and adipose. Insulin stimulates the uptake of carbohydrates and amino acids into these tissues in a selective manner, such that only certain sugars (e.g. glucose or galactose) or amino acids (e.g. alanine) are taken up. The cell membrane carries a specific carrier system for each of these metabolites that requires energy in the form of ATP and that exhibits saturable kinetics: this is called an insulin-sensitive 'active transport' mechanism.

## Hormones acting on the nucleus: steroid and thyroid hormones

The steroid and thyroid hormones have very different actions on target-cells, but they are similar in that they both exert their effects by acting on the nucleus. Both groups of hormone are relatively hydrophobic and they act on a wider spectrum of target-cells, in general, than do the peptide and protein hormones. They exert their effects at nuclear receptor sites, and as a consequence of this, there is a relatively long lag-period of 30 to 60 minutes or longer between the time of exposure of the target-cell to the hormone and the onset of a biological response.

### STEROID HORMONES

The steroid hormone group includes the oestrogens, progestogens, androgens, mineralocorticoids, glucocorticoids and the active form of vitamin D3. These hormones cross the target-cell membranes to reach the nucleus where they are bound to specific receptor proteins (see Fig. 1.17). Originally, using broken-cell fractions, it seemed that steroid hormones were transported through the cytoplasm on specific binding proteins; however, these cytosol steroid-binding proteins may have originated from the nucleus during disruption of the cells.

#### *Steroid hormone receptors*

A single cell can contain separate receptor proteins that are each specific for different steroid hormones. For example, distinct oestrogen, progesterone and glucocorticoid hormone receptors are all present in human breast tumour tissue. The steroid receptor-proteins have characteristic structural features, and they are made up of subunits of molecular weights greater than 65 000. The subunits carry two separate domains, one that binds steroid hormone and one that binds to DNA. There may be up to 100 000 glucocorticoid receptors per liver cell, each with four identical subunits joined non-covalently. The uterine

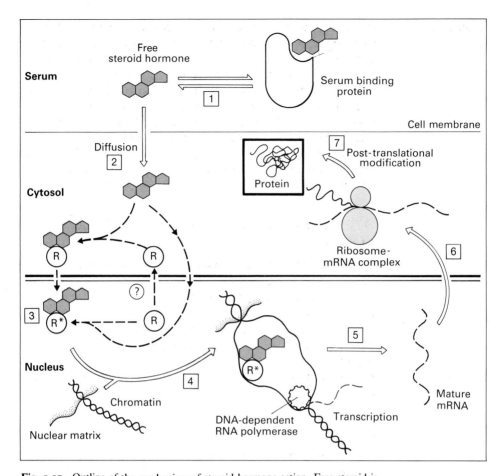

**Fig. 1.17** Outline of the mechanism of steroid hormone action. Free steroid is in equilibrium ①  with that bound to serum binding-proteins, and it diffuses ② across the target-cell membrane. Binding to the steroid hormone receptor-protein Ⓡ may occur in the cell cytoplasm or more probably in the cell nucleus. The hormone−receptor complex ③ interacts with chromatin that is attached to the nuclear-matrix structures. Associated with DNA double-helical strands in the chromatin are histone and non-histone proteins that regulate the transcription of information coded in the DNA. The hormone−receptor complex binds ④ to a receptor site on the regulatory region of one DNA strand associated with a particular gene. This affects the promoter region (see Figs 1.6 and 1.18) which then permits DNA-dependent RNA polymerase to start transcription of the triplet base code by separation of the two strands of DNA to yield a specific messenger RNA ⑤. Post-transcriptional modification and splicing of the exon sequences follows, and messenger RNA passes out ⑥ of the nucleus. Peptides and proteins are formed by translation of the message on ribosomes attached to the endoplasmic reticulum. Finally, modification of the protein occurs to give the final gene product (see p. 94).

oestrogen receptor is present at a lower concentration (about 10 000 per cell), and it has two subunits. The progesterone receptor has two different subunits; both the A- and B-subunits can bind progesterone, but only the A-subunit carries the DNA

37

binding site. These receptor proteins are important to the action of steroid hormones in the nucleus.

*Receptor−nuclear interactions*

Steroid hormones regulate transcription of specific genes by induction or suppression and so direct the amount of messenger RNA produced for particular proteins. The glucocorticoids induce the messenger RNA for a number of proteins, for example for tyrosine aminotransferase in hepatocytes (see also p. 94). Similarly, the production of progesterone-receptor protein is initiated by the action of oestrogen on the uterine endometrium.

The steroid−receptor complex binds to DNA, and the receptor is thus the transducer that transfers the hormone signal to the regulatable gene. It is likely that these regulatory proteins are part of a larger class of nuclear regulatory proteins that control expression of genetic information. Upstream from the structural gene and its promoter region (i.e. towards the 5′ end of DNA; see Fig. 1.6) lies the regulatory site that contains the steroid hormone−receptor binding site (see Fig. 1.18). There is a conserved nucleotide sequence of nine bases at around 140 bases before the start of the structural gene that is present in all steroid hormone-regulated genes. Nearer the gene is the promoter region that was described in Fig. 1.6. These regions are critical to the control and expression of steroid hormone action on its target-cells.

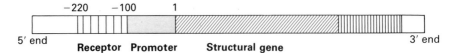

5′ end    **Receptor   Promoter**    **Structural gene**    3′ end

−220    −100    1

**Fig. 1.18** Diagram of a steroid hormone-controlled gene segment. The receptor region and promoter region both carry sequences of bases which are conserved in different genes and in different species. Steroid hormone binding to the receptor region is shown in Fig. 1.17, and the approximate positions of the control segments are shown in relation to the start of the structural gene over which they exert an influence.

DNA-dependent RNA polymerase action is controlled by the promoter region, and this in turn is subject to the action of the steroid hormone−receptor complex at the regulatory site on the DNA strand. The messenger RNA produced by the transcription process is then further processed by splicing together in the nucleus of the exon sequences as was discussed earlier. Final expression of steroid hormone action is the synthesis of specific proteins and enzymes within the cell (see Fig. 1.17).

THYROID HORMONES

Unlike the entry of steroid hormones into the cell, which is apparently by passive diffusion, the thyroid hormones are actively transported by a specific carrier mechanism. The thyroid hormones have an action on most cells of the body, and this could be a mechanism whereby the cell controls its demand for these hormones. There has been no clear evidence to suggest the presence of cytosol binding proteins for the thyroid hormones in target cells. The thyroid hormones stimulate DNA-dependent RNA polymerase activity and this is discussed further in Chapter 5. In general, there is a switch to the intracellular formation of catabolic enzymes that result in increased cellular activity.

## CONTROL OF THE ENDOCRINE SYSTEM

The endocrine system is an essential part of a refined and relatively complex control system which has developed, through successive stages of evolutionary advancement, to varying degrees of sophistication in the many different classes of the animal kingdom. Hormones provide a mechanism by which the body can relay chemical signals throughout the hierarchy of different cell types perfused by the bloodstream, and which in their combined form go to make up the animal.

Homeostatic (self-regulating) control systems are common features of engineering and electronic design, and the basic principles of such systems also apply to biological systems. Since the primary role of the endocrine system is one of control, it is useful to consider the possible mechanisms available for control. In the following discussion, the hormone will be considered to be the signal, and the target-cell will yield the response to this signal (see Fig. 1.19).

### SIMPLE CONTROL

An elementary control system is one in which the signal itself is limited, either in magnitude (i.e. amplitude) or duration (i.e. frequency): thus, only enough signal or hormone is produced at a time to induce a transient response. Certain neural impulses are of this type; a refinement which is introduced, to discriminate a positive signal from background 'noise', is to ensure that the target-cell cannot or does not respond below a certain threshold level of the signal. An example of this is the pulsatile release of gonadotrophin releasing hormone from the hypothalamus.

### NEGATIVE FEEDBACK

This is probably the commonest form of control in biological as well as other systems. In essence, the signal produces a response which feeds back on the signal generator to decrease the level of signal. Examples are found in metabolic reaction sequences where the product of a reaction sequence will feed back and inhibit its own production when the concentration builds up to a certain

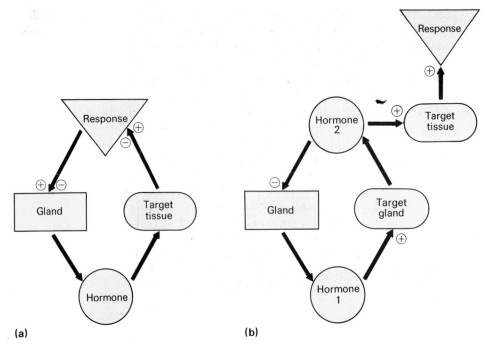

(a)

(b)

**Fig. 1.19** Two outline schemes for control of hormone action.

(a) The gland releases a hormone which acts on target tissue to either stimulate (+) or inhibit (−) a response. The response itself may either inhibit or stimulate the original gland to decrease or increase supply of the original hormone.

(b) The gland produces a hormone (1) which acts on a second gland. The latter target is stimulated to produce a second hormone (2) which then acts on target tissues to induce a response. In addition, the second hormone is capable of controlling release of the first hormone by feedback inhibition (−).

level (e.g. histidine synthesis). In order to regulate hormone release by this mechanism, the hormone must act on its target-cell to produce as a response a substance which is capable of entering the bloodstream and acting on the releasing cell to inhibit or modulate production of the original stimulator. Thus, many of the hormones of the anterior pituitary which are trophic or stimulating hormones, and which act on *other* endocrine glands such as the thyroid, adrenal cortex or gonads to simulate production of other hormones, are controlled by negative feedback: the resulting thyroid or steroid hormones then act on the pituitary to decrease the amount of the respective trophic hormone being released.

POSITIVE FEEDBACK

As the name suggests, this is a system in which the signal generator is stimulated by the response which it induces. In engineering terms this is an intrinsically unstable control system, but there are specific biological systems where such a 'control' system can be of benefit. Control, used in the positive feedback situation, refers to a continued generation of the signal, as cessation of the stimulus only occurs when the system inducing the response cannot function any longer: in this case, the positive feedback has led to termination of the event. Examples of such a positive feedback system are relatively rare, but two situations involving the peptide hormone oxytocin are worth describing briefly. During childbirth or parturition, the stretch receptors in the distended vagina send neurological signals to the brain where oxytocin release from the posterior pituitary is stimulated. This hormone is carried in the blood and acts at the uterus to cause it to contract, which in turn activates the cervical receptors to stimulate more oxytocin release: delivery terminates the positive feedback. In a similar manner, suckling causes stimulation of the nipple receptors which result in increased oxytocin release with a corresponding increase in the milk-ejection reflex; removal of the stimulus terminates the response which is the release of oxytocin.

INHIBITORY CONTROL

Certain hormones either have a very general action on a variety of target-cells (e.g. growth hormone) or do not produce a specific product which is released into the bloodstream (e.g. prolactin, which stimulates milk synthesis in the breast). These hormones can be controlled by an inhibitory hormone which prevents their release, and it is only when these inhibitory hormones or factors are suppressed (for example, by neurological or other factors), that release of these hormones is permitted.

METABOLIC CONTROL

To some extent, this is an extension of negative feedback. Certain hormones have to be converted to an active form in order to act; for example, testosterone to dihydrotestosterone in the testis, and thyroxine to triiodothyronine for expression of thyroid hormone action in almost all cell types. This control is probably regulated locally by the levels of the product, or active hormone to which the precursor hormone is converted.

ENDOCRINE DISORDERS

In any complex regulatory system, it is likely that disordered function will have important consequences, and the endocrine system is no exception. Underproduction or overproduction of hormones can occur. For example, lack of growth hormone in children causes dwarfism while excess of the hormone leads to gigantism. The effects of overproduction of growth hormone in adults in whom the epiphyses have fused are rather different and lead to a condition called acromegaly. Many clinical disorders were recognized before the endocrine disturbance was understood, and it was only after further study that the underlying causes have been revealed. For example, as outlined at the beginning of the chapter, Addison described the effects of disease of the adrenal cortex in which there is a lack of cortisol and aldosterone. Because of the decrease in circulating cortisol there is a compensatory overproduction of adrenocorticotrophin by the anterior pituitary. Apart from stimulating cortisol production, this pituitary hormone at high concentrations can stimulate melanocytes in the skin to produce melatonin; this explains the over-pigmentation which is one of the features of Addison's disease. Thus, attempted correction of a deficiency of one hormone by overproduction of another can have important consequences. In other conditions, disordered synthesis, such as that of a steroid hormone, may occur when a particular enzyme is missing (arising from a genetic defect). The consequences of this can arise in part from the lack of that steroid and in part from an accumulation of other precursor steroids that build up as a result of the enzyme deficiency. One of the commonest endocrine diseases is diabetes mellitus. This can be due to lack of secretion of insulin from the $\beta$-cells of the Islets of Langerhans in the pancreas. The same clinical disease can, however, be caused not by lack of insulin secretion but by resistance to its actions i.e. a receptor disorder.

These examples show that studies of the endocrine system can explain the underlying cause of a disorder, just as study of an endocrine disorder itself can demonstrate the normal control function of the endocrine system in regulation of the tissues of the body.

## Endocrine rhythms

Most, if not all, organized bodily activities show periodic rhythmic or cyclic changes. Ultimate control of these rhythms probably arises from the nervous system, and some brain areas have been identified as centres for such regulation, e.g. the suprachiasmatic nucleus in the hypothalamus. Some rhythms controlled by these endogenous mechanisms appear to be independent of environmental change. Others are co-ordinated and are said to be 'entrained' by external (exogenous) cues such as the 24 hour light−dark cycle. These external cues are called 'zeitgebers', literally, time-givers.

Rhythms based on the 24 hour cycle are called 'circadian' (circa = about; dies = day). Those with a shorter period are termed 'ultradian', and those with a period longer than 24 hours are termed 'infradian', e.g. the 28 day menstrual cycle in women or seasonal reproductive periods in animals. Many hormone functions show a circadian rhythm. For example, cortisol secretion is maximal between 4 and 8 am; while growth hormone and prolactin are maximally secreted about one hour after an individual has gone to sleep. Hormonal rhythmicity also changes during the life cycle of an individual: in puberty, gonado-trophins are secreted in relatively large amounts and the con-centrations are maximal at night, whereas in sexually mature individuals they are secreted in small, pulsatile amounts throughout the 24 hour period.

From a practical point of view, a knowledge of the rhythmicity of hormone secretion is clearly very important. Sampling the blood concentration of a hormone for clincial or experimental reasons must take into account the variability of hormone levels throughout the day and night, otherwise such measurements are not useful in providing diagnostic or other scientific information.

## SUMMARY

In summary, this chapter describes the general mechanisms of action of hormones at their target-cell receptors as well as chemical classification of these hormones. Many peptide and protein hormones, as well as adrenaline, act by binding to a specific receptor on the cell surface to stimulate production of the second messenger, cyclic AMP, which acts by modulating a variety of protein kinases within the cell. Hormones such as thyrotrophin releasing hormone, vasopressin and angiotensin II can activate phospholipase C that gives rise to the alternate second messengers, inositol-1,4,5-*tris*phosphate and diacylglycerol. These two sub-stances mobilize intracellular calcium and activate protein kinase C, which in turn affect the activities of other protein kinase and calcium-dependent enzymes within the cell. Insulin acts at a cell-surface receptor to stimulate tyrosine kinase. Insulin alters the permeability of certain cell membranes to carbohydrates and amino acids, as well as modulating their metabolism and also that of fatty acids. Growth hormone and prolactin alter cellular transcription and translation by some mechanism which remains to be elucidated. Steroid hormones and triiodothyronine act (by different mechanisms) at the cell nucleus. Advances in under-standing the endocrinological control processes have been possible only because bioassay systems, and more recently immunoassay methods, have been developed which permit measurements of minute concentrations of these hormones. Subsequent chapters will discuss specific aspects of each of the endocrine organs in detail, and it will therefore be assumed that the general mech-anisms described above have been assimilated.

# FURTHER READING

CRAPO L. (1986) *Hormones: the messengers of life*. W. H. Freeman, San Francisco.

POISNER A. M. & TRIFARO J. M. (Eds.) *The Secretory Process*: Vol. 1 (1982), The Secretory Granule; Vol. 2 (1985), The electrophysiology of the Secretory Cell. Elsevier Biomedical, Amsterdam.

PUTNEY J. (Ed.) (1985) *Receptor Biochemistry and Methodology*: Vol. 17, Phosphoinositides and Receptor Mechanisms. Alan Liss, New York.

O'RIORDAN J. L. H. (Ed.) (1985) *Recent Advances in Endocrinology and Metabolism*, Vols. 1 & 2. Churchill Livingstone, Edinburgh.

RUBIN R. P. (1982) *Calcium and Cellular Secretion*. Plenum Press, New York.

SIBLEY D. R. *et al.* (1983) Regulation of transmembrane signalling by receptor phosphorylation. *Cell* 48, 913–922.

WALLIS M., HOWELL S. L., & TAYLOR K. W. (1985) *The Biochemistry of Polypeptide Hormones*. John Wiley & Sons, Chichester.

WILLIAMS R. H. (Ed.) (1985) *A Textbook of Endocrinology* 7th edn. W. B. Saunders, Philadelphia.

DARNELL J., LODISH H. & BALTIMORE D. (1986) *Molecular Cell Biology*, p. 1187. Scientific American Books.

# 2 The hypothalamus and pituitary

The existence of the pituitary gland has been known for at least 2000 years. According to Aristotle the pituitary was the organ through which one of the four essential humors of the body, the phlegm or pituita, passed from the brain into the body. In the 19th century Rathke studied the development of the pituitary (hypophysis) and showed that it consisted of two distinct parts, namely the anterior pituitary (or adenohypophysis) and the posterior pituitary (or neurohypophysis). Pierre Marie described the association between acromegaly (a condition characterized by the increased growth of the extremities) and pituitary tumours. In 1909 Cushing was the first to remove part of the pituitary of an acromegalic patient and he noticed an improvement in the condition. Evans and Long showed in animals that injections of crude extracts of the anterior pituitary caused increased growth and even gigantism. These studies led, eventually, to the isolation of growth hormone. Other functions of the pituitary were also discovered; for example, its effects on lactation (through prolactin), and the gland was shown to regulate the function of the thyroid (through thyrotrophin), the adrenals (through adrenocorticotrophin) and the gonads (through luteinizing hormone and follicle stimulating hormone). In recognition of the importance of the hormones which are secreted by the anterior pituitary it was suggested that the pituitary could be considered as the 'conductor of the endocrine orchestra', though this view has now to be modified since the pituitary is itself regulated by the nervous system via the hypothalamus.

The second part of the pituitary, the neurohypophysis, secretes two hormones, vasopressin and oxytocin; these are released from the posterior pituitary by neurones whose cell bodies are in the hypothalamus. The anterior pituitary does not have any neuronal connections with the hypothalamus even though it is in fact under hypothalamic control: this control occurs through a system of portal veins, the existence of which was discovered in 1930 by Popa and Fielding. Subsequently, it was shown by Wislocki that the blood flows downwards from the hypothalamus to the pituitary. From these observations, Harris developed the concept of the control of the adenohypophysis by humoral factors produced in the hypothalamus and carried to the anterior pituitary in the portal vessels. This led to the award of the Nobel Prize to Schally and Guillemin, who independently isolated and established the structure of some of those so-called 'releasing hormones'.

## MORPHOLOGY OF THE MAMMALIAN HYPOTHALAMO-HYPOPHYSEAL SYSTEM

### DEVELOPMENT

The hypothalamo-hypophyseal system is derived from two ecto-dermal components. One of these is Rathke's pouch, which is a dorsal outgrowth of the buccal cavity developing just in front of the buccal membrane. Rathke's pouch detaches itself and de-velops into the anterior pituitary. The second ectodermal com-ponent, the infundibulum, develops as a downgrowth from the neurectoderm forming the floor of the third ventricle immediately caudal to the future optic chiasma. This eventually develops into the pituitary stalk and the posterior pituitary. The remainder of this ventral neurectoderm, as far back as the mammillary bodies, forms the median eminence while in its lateral walls the hypo-thalamic nuclei differentiate and form the sides of the third ventricle.

### ANATOMY

In the adult, the pituitary lies in a bony cavity, the sella turcica or the pituitary fossa, in the sphenoid bone. The human adult pituitary weighs about 0.5 g, but this can increase during preg-nancy to 1.0 g with the anterior pituitary accounting for about three-quarters of its weight. The pituitary is connected to the hypothalamus by the stalk (Fig. 2.1) which carries axons to the neurohypophysis and blood vessels to both parts. The pituitary gland is anatomically closely related to a number of other im-portant structures. Superiorly there is the optic chiasma, which lies just anterior to the pituitary stalk; anteriorly and below is the sphenoid air sinus; while laterally is the cavernous venous sinus, through which run the third, fourth and sixth cranial nerves.

The arterial supply of the hypothalamo-hypophyseal system comes from the inferior and superior hypophyseal arteries. The former supplies the posterior lobe, while the anterior and pos-terior branches of the superior hypophyseal artery supply the median eminence and the pituitary stalk. These branches form a capillary plexus in the external layer of the median eminence and the upper part of the pituitary stalk. From this primary plexus arise the long and short hypophyseal portal veins, which run the length of the pituitary stalk and enter the anterior pituitary to form a secondary plexus of sinusoidal capillaries. Eighty to ninety per cent of the nutrient blood supply reaches the adenohypophysis

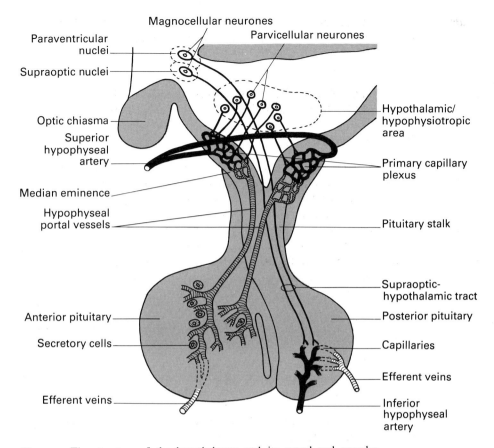

**Fig. 2.1** The structure of the hypothalamus and its neural and vascular connections with the pituitary. The blood supply to the median eminence consists of the superior hypophyseal artery whose branches form the primary capillary plexus in the median eminence. From the plexus arise the hypophyseal portal vessels which terminate in the anterior pituitary and supply its secretory cells. Efferent veins drain the anterior pituitary into dural sinuses. The posterior pituitary has a direct systemic supply from the inferior hypophyseal artery. Note that the axons from the parvicellular neurones of the hypothalamic/hypophysiotropic area (shown in white) terminate close to the primary capillary plexus. The axons of the magnocellular neurones of the supraoptic and paraventricular nuclei run down the pituitary stalk as the supraoptic-hypothalamic tract and terminate close to the capillaries supplying the posterior pituitary. The optic chiasma is also shown.

by means of the long portal vessels with the balance being supplied by the short portal vessels. Blood flows from the primary capillary plexus in the median eminence down the portal veins to the sinusoidal vessels in the anterior pituitary. Anatomical and physiological studies strongly suggest that there may also be a reverse flow of hypothalamic and pituitary peptides along the pituitary stalk and back to the brain: this may account for their presence in the spinal fluid. Venous blood from the pituitary stalk and the pituitary gland drains by a number of veins into the adjacent cavernous sinus.

There are two groups of nuclei in the hypothalamus with neuro-endocrine functions. One is composed of the paired supraoptic and paraventricular nuclei in the anterior hypothalamus; the other group is referred to collectively as the hypothalamic-hypophysiotrophic nuclei (Fig. 2.1). The function of the posterior pituitary is dependent on the former group while that of the anterior pituitary is dependent on the latter group.

*The supraoptic and paraventricular nuclei*

The posterior pituitary (or neurohypophysis) consists of nerve fibres whose terminals abut on capillaries. These fibres arise from the neurones of the paired supraoptic and paraventricular nuclei in the anterior part of the hypothalamus. The neurones are large, pyriform and characterized by the presence of cyto-plasmic secretory droplets which stain intensely with Gomori's chrome haematoxylin phloxin stain. The neurones making up this anterior group of hypothalamic nuclei are referred to collect-ively as the magnocellular neurosecretory system because of their large size. The magnocellular neurones of the supraoptic and paraventricular nuclei are the cells of origin of the hormones stored in, and secreted from, the posterior pituitary; namely vasopressin and oxytocin. Under the electron microscope the neurones can be seen to contain membrane-bound secretory granules, 120–200 nm in diameter. The newly synthesized hormone is packaged in the granules with a larger protein, neurophysin. The granules are eventually transported down their fibres to the terminals of the axons at a rate of 8 mm/hr. When the neurones are stimulated, the granules are released by exocytosis and their contents diffuse into the adjacent, fenestrated, capillaries. Stimulation of release of these two hormones, e.g. by either dehydration or suckling, leads to the disappearance of stainable neurosecretory material from the magnocellular neurones. Immunocytochemical studies show that neuronal perikarya staining for either vasopressin or oxytocin are scattered through both the supraoptic and the paraventricular nuclei. In addition to the nerve fibres projecting down to the posterior pituitary, some vasopressin-positive fibres have been shown to terminate in the external layer of the median eminence. The presence of the associated storage and transported proteins, the neurophysins, has also been demonstrated immunocytochemically in neuronal perikarya and their axons.

*Hypothalamic-hypophysiotropic nuclei*

These are found principally in the lateral wall of the third ventricle: there is functional overlap between morphologically distinguishable nuclei in the hypothalamic-hypophysiotropic area (Fig. 2.1). The neurones in this region are smaller and neuro-secretory droplets cannot be demonstrated in them with Gomori's stain: they are referred to as the parvicellular neurosecretory system. While the neurones of the supraoptic hypothalamic tract run through the median eminence on their way to the posterior pituitary, the nerve fibres of the parvicellular system of the hypothalamus terminate in the external or palisade layer of the median eminence, in close proximity to the capillaries of its primary plexus. These nerve terminals contain small dense-cored vesicles, 80–120 nm in diameter, which presumably represent the storage form of the 'releasing hormones' that control the secretion of the hormones of the anterior pituitary. Indeed, some releasing hormones such as those that stimulate corticotrophin and growth hormone release can be demonstrated in this region by immunohistochemical techniques. It is believed that the discharge of these releasing hormones involves exocytosis and that they diffuse into the adjacent capillaries of the primary plexus. The boundaries of the hypothalamic nuclei, from which these neurones arise, outline the hypophysiotropic area, though these are less easily defined than the supraoptic and paraventricular nuclei.

*Innervation of neurosecretory neurones*
The hypothalamus receives nerve fibres directly or indirectly from virtually all areas of the brain and so its activity must, in part, be regulated by higher centres. This complex neural input reflects the centrality of the hypothalamus as a regulatory centre for many vital functions. Hypothalamic peptidergic neurones are capable by themselves of sustaining a certain degree of autonomous function, as indicated by experiments in which the hypothalamo-pituitary complex has been surgically disconnected from the rest of the brain. In such experiments the basal secretions of growth hormone, follicle stimulating hormone and luteinizing hormone are largely unchanged and release of adrenocorticotrophin in response to insulin-induced hypoglycaemia or stress is unaffected. However, superimposed on this autonomy are inputs to these neurones both from within the hypothalamus and from other parts of the brain such as the septum, hippocampus, anterior thalamus, amygdala, pyriform cortex and midbrain. Of major importance in the control of the neurosecretory cells of the hypothalamus are pathways which release noradrenaline, adrenaline, dopamine, serotonin and acetylcholine. Mono-aminergic nerve terminals have been demonstrated synapsing on hypothalamic peptidergic neurones and on their axons in the median eminence near the perivascular space adjacent to the primary capillary plexus. Peptide neurotransmitters or neuromodulators, for example opioid peptides, substance P and bombesin, are likely to be involved in the modulation of hypothalamic releasing-hormone secretion; some of these opioid peptides have been shown to exert effects on the secretion of most pituitary hormones.

49

The secretory cells of the anterior pituitary are arranged in clumps, or in branching cords of cells separated by the sinusoidal capillaries, arising from the hypophyseal portal vessels. They are held together in a reticular fibre framework (Fig. 2.1). Using traditional light microscope techniques, the cells of the anterior pituitary can be classified as chromophobes (poorly stained) and the chromophils (well stained) which are further subdivided into those that stain with acid dyes (acidophils) and those that stain with basic dyes (basophils). Electron microscopy has revealed that the cells of the anterior pituitary possess all the characteristics of protein-secreting cells, i.e. they have a prominent rough endoplasmic reticulum, Golgi complex and secretory storage granules. Hormone is released by exocytosis of the granules and then diffusion occurs through the perivascular space to the blood vessels. The chromophobe cells are sparsely granulated while the chromophils are richly granulated. Using immunocytochemical stains for particular hormones, acidophils can be divided into two subgroups, the somatotrophs which secrete growth hormone and the mammotrophs which produce prolactin. The basophils, by similar criteria, can be divided into three populations of cells, the thyrotrophs producing thyrotrophin (thyroid stimulating hormone), the gonadotrophs producing luteinizing hormone and follicle stimulating hormone, and the corticotrophs producing adrenocorticotrophin. It is now generally agreed that most chromophobes are quiescent forms of the several kinds of chromophils. In addition there are some undifferentiated cells, and in some species (but not man) there are melanotrophs that produce melanocyte stimulating hormone.

## FUNCTIONAL RELATIONSHIPS OF THE HYPOTHALAMUS AND ANTERIOR PITUITARY

The neuroendocrine role of the hypothalamus was initially studied by observing the effects of ablation or electrical stimulation. Lesions in the hypothalamus and median eminence could produce atrophy of various endocrine glands leading, for example, to disruption of the menstrual cycle and production of female sex hormones. It was also shown that it was possible to interrupt selectively the secretion of one or more of the pituitary hormones. In early studies it was shown that electrical stimulation of the anterior hypothalamus could evoke ovulation and subsequently it became clear that electrical stimulation could also evoke secretion of other anterior pituitary hormones, for example, of the thyroid gland (Fig. 2.2). Experiments of this type have been used to localize function in different areas of the hypothalamus.

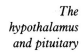

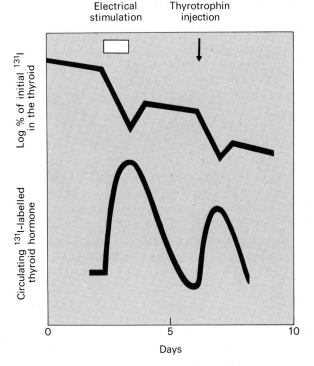

Fig 2.2 Stimulation of the hypothalamus, through implanted electrodes, increases the release of thyroid hormones; this was shown in animals that had been given radioactive iodine to label the thyroxine. When the hypothalamus is stimulated, there is a decrease in the radioactivity in the thyroid and an increase in radioactivity in circulating thyroid hormone. The effect could be mimicked by injection of thyrotrophin. The explanation of these findings is that the hypothalamic stimulation causes release of thyrotrophin releasing hormone and this in turn stimulates the release of thyrotrophin from the anterior pituitary. Finally, thyrotrophin stimulates thyroid hormone release from the thyroid gland.

## Neurohumoral control of the anterior pituitary

RELEASING FACTORS

Since there is little, if any, secretomotor innervation of the adenohypophysis, the possibility of neurohumoral control was developed by Harris who recognized the functional significance of the fact that blood reaching the anterior pituitary gland had first to traverse the primary capillary plexus located in the median eminence (Fig. 2.1). While earlier experiments on the effects of transection of the pituitary stalk had been equivocal, Harris showed that the portal vessels were capable of rapid regeneration and that if an impermeable barrier was placed between the cut ends of the stalk, then the effects of disruption of pituitary function, such as gonadal failure, thyroid inactivity, adrenal insufficiency and failure of growth in the young, could be consistently observed. In addition it was shown that pituitaries grafted under the renal capsule or in the eye had little ability to restore target organ function in hypophysectomized animals, but pituitaries placed under the median eminence (so that they became revascularized by the portal vessels) were functionally active. Evidence of this type led to formulation of the hypothesis that a neurohumoral substance released from nerve endings in the median eminence could enter capillaries of the hypothalamic-pituitary portal circulation and be carried into the sinusoids of the anterior lobe to regulate the secretion of the appropriate trophic hormone (Fig. 2.3).

Subsequently, extracts of the hypothalamus and the median eminence were shown to contain substances capable of stimulating anterior pituitary activity. In 1955 a crude extract from the neurohypophysis was shown to be capable of stimulating the release of adrenocorticotrophin and was named corticotrophin releasing hormone (CRH). However, since the neurohypophyseal hormone, vasopressin, could also evoke the release of adrenocorticotrophin, there was some controversy regarding the existence of a specific corticotrophin releasing factor. It was not until about a quarter of a century later, in 1981, that the structure

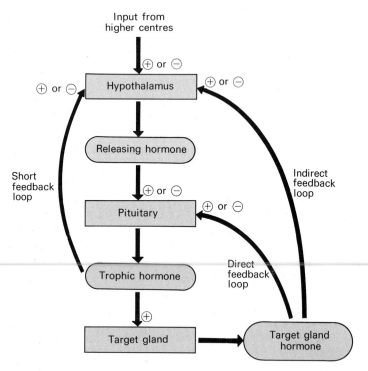

**Fig. 2.3** A schematic representation of the interactions between higher centres, the hypothalamus, the pituitary and peripheral endocrine glands, showing feedback regulation. The controlling factors can be stimulatory (+) or inhibitory (−).

of a corticotrophin releasing hormone was established. However, the earlier demonstration that the corticotrophin releasing hormone must exist led to an intensified search for other factors. It should be noted that the acceptance of a compound as a new releasing or inhibiting factor requires the fulfilment of several criteria. For example, a substance having the principal activity should be extractable from the hypothalamus and it should be capable of influencing the secretion of an anterior pituitary hormone by direct action on the gland, either *in vitro* or *in vivo*.

*Isolation of releasing hormones*

Hypothalamic extracts containing substances that could release adrenocorticotrophin, follicle stimulating hormone, luteinizing hormone and thyrotrophin, and that could either inhibit or release growth hormone and prolactin, were eventually isolated. In the 1960s a thyrotrophin releasing factor was purified independently by Schally and Guillemin. For these studies it was necessary to use the hypothalami of over 2 million sheep; about 1 ng (3 pmol) of the most highly purified preparation could stimulate the release of thyrotrophin. The structure of this compound was difficult to establish because, although it is only a tripeptide, the amino-terminus is blocked by the formation of a pyroglutamyl ring and the carboxy-terminal proline is blocked by an amide group. Once it had been isolated, and its structure determined, it was reasonable to refer to it, not as 'thyrotrophin releasing *factor*', but as 'thyrotrophin releasing *hormone*' (TRH). It should be noted, however, that the bioassay systems used to follow the isolation of a particular substance may have led to an oversimplified view of the function of the compound, since it is known that thyrotrophin releasing hormone can also stimulate the release of prolactin, and it may also have other actions on the neural system.

Gonadotrophin releasing hormone (GnRH) causes the release of both luteinizing hormone and follicle stimulating hormone from the pituitary, and although it is possible that there might be two separate hypothalamic factors controlling the release of each of the two gonadotrophins, there is no good evidence to support this suggestion. Isolation and characterization of what was called luteinizing hormone releasing hormone (LHRH) showed it to be a decapeptide which also has a pyroglutamyl amino-terminal residue and an amide group at the carboxy-terminus; the hormone is now more generally referred to as gonadotrophin releasing hormone (GnRH) because it can stimulate release of follicle stimulating hormone as well.

Another hypothalamic hormone which has been fully characterized structurally has inhibitory properties and is somatostatin (growth hormone release inhibiting hormone—GHRIH). Somatostatin, however, is not confined to the hypothalamus but is found in other parts of the brain and spinal cord, and also occurs in the pancreatic islet delta cells (see Chapter 7). When administered experimentally, it can be shown to inhibit the secretion of a wide variety of hormones, including gastrin, vaso-active intestinal peptide (VIP), glucagon and insulin.

The primary structure of human hypothalamic growth hormone releasing hormone (also called somatocrinin) has been determined. Biologically active peptides were purified from human pancreatic tumours that were associated with excessive pituitary growth hormone secretion. Three molecules were characterized, with the largest having 44 amino acids and the two others comprising sequences 1−37 and 1−40 of the larger molecule, but their relative physiological significance is uncertain. Extensive structural homology of somatocrinin isolated from bovine, porcine and murine hypothalamic tissue has been found with the human pancreatic peptide. All these peptides are potent stimulators of human pituitary growth hormone secretion.

Corticotrophin releasing hormone was purified from sheep hypothalami and its sequence shows it to have 41 amino acids and a molecular weight of about 5000. It is the largest releasing hormone so far identified. It has a corticotrophin releasing activity 30−50 times more potent than vasopressin; this activity is calcium ion dependent and is inhibited by corticosteroids.

The presence of other hypothalamic hormones have been postulated including one that can inhibit prolactin secretion. Inhibitory control of prolactin secretion by the hypothalamus is demonstrated by the fact that hypothalamic lesions, stalk transection, and transplantation of the pituitary, all result in enhanced prolactin secretion. In addition, hypothalamic extracts can inhibit prolactin secretion by mammotrophs *in vitro*. Dopamine, which is a potent inhibitor of the secretion of prolactin *in vitro*, is present in the hypothalamus and in the portal blood, and it may be the physiological prolactin inhibiting factor. However, it has been shown that a carboxy-terminal region of the precursor of human placental gonadotrophin releasing hormone inhibits prolactin and stimulates gonadotrophin secretion from the anterior pituitary cells *in vitro*. This peptide has been called 'gonadotrophin releasing hormone associated peptide' (GAP), but its physiological relationship to dopaminergic control has still to be established.

It seems likely that there is also a prolactin releasing factor, in addition to thyrotrophin releasing hormone which, as was indicated above, has a powerful effect on prolactin secretion. One candidate for such a role is vasoactive intestinal peptide (VIP) which has been found in the hypothalamus and in the portal blood. This peptide is a potent stimulator of prolactin release, and passive immunization of animals against vasoactive intestinal peptide causes a decrease in prolactin secretion.

*Assay of releasing hormones*

While it might be desirable to measure the release of the hypothalamic factors directly, this is often difficult as these compounds are rapidly degraded. Although measurable amounts of some of these factors are found in the peripheral circulation (e.g. somatostatin, corticotrophin releasing hormone, somatocrinin), it is unclear whether they derive from hypothalamic or other tissue sources. Bioassay systems have been devised for all the known hypothalamic hormones. *In vivo* their effects may be detected either by measuring changes in the relevant pituitary hormone (e.g. by immunoassay of thyrotrophin) or through the secondary effect on a target gland (e.g. by observing the release of thyroid hormones). *In vitro* systems can also be used; in these, pituitary glands or isolated pituitary cells are either superfused or dispersed in tissue culture, and the hormones released from the pituitary cells in response to the releasing hormone are then measured by specific immunoassays.

*Mechanism of action of releasing hormones*

To act on the pituitary, the hypothalamic hormones bind to specific receptors on the plasma membrane of the target-cell. It is known that pituitary hormone secretion is dependent, to a large extent, on intracellular calcium ions. Thus, depolarizing concentrations of potassium ions and other substances that promote calcium ion entry cause an increase in pituitary hormone release, while substances that limit calcium ion entry are inhibitory. The hypothalamic releasing hormones appear to fall into two categories, at least as far as their mechanism of action is concerned. On the one hand, thyrotrophin and gonadotrophin releasing hormones stimulate phospholipase C and phosphoinositide metabolism (see Chapter 1) which leads to the production of the two second messengers, inositol-1,4,5-*tris*phosphate and diacylglycerol (see Fig. 1.15). Inositol *tris*phosphate causes the release of intracellular calcium ions that leads to an acute secretory response which, at least in the case of thyrotrophin releasing hormone, does not require influx of calcium ions from the extracellular milieu. The subsequently sustained release is likely to be dependent on the increase in intracellular calcium ion concentration and of calcium and diacylglycerol activation of protein kinase C. Effects of these two releasing hormones on pituitary cyclic AMP accumulation probably arise indirectly from effects of protein kinase C on adenylate cyclase.

The stimulatory action of the other group of releasing hormones, including corticotrophin and growth hormone releasing hormones and vasoactive intestinal peptide, are mediated through activation of adenylate cyclase. Their actions appear to be expressed through the stimulatory nucleotide regulatory complex

55

$N_S$ (see Chapter 1), and cyclic AMP may well have effects on calcium ion influx by modulation of membrane ion channels.

The mechanism of action of inhibitory factors is not as well understood. Although dopamine is known to inhibit adenylate cyclase by the $N_I$ nucleotide regulatory complex it can also inhibit prolactin secretion in the face of raised intracellular cyclic AMP concentrations. This suggests that a different inhibitory mechanism may be involved: both dopamine and somatostatin cause a lowering of the intracellular concentration of calcium, but their mechanism of action is uncertain.

HORMONE CONTROL OF ANTERIOR PITUITARY ACTIVITY

Regulation of the release of hormones by the anterior pituitary is a complex process, with a number of interacting factors. The secretion of a number of pituitary hormones is modulated by a direct negative feedback, exerted by hormones secreted by the target endocrine gland of a particular pituitary hormone (Fig. 2.3). Thus an increase in the secretion of hormone from a target gland generally leads to a decrease in the secretion of the pituitary hormone. Less common is a direct positive feedback; this is likely, however, to be the mechanism whereby sustained high levels of oestrogen produced by the ovary induce a sudden rise in the secretion of luteinizing hormone in the middle of the menstrual cycle (see Chapter 4). Positive feedback loops are, however, unstable, unless there are other regulatory factors.

Feedback control can also occur via the hypothalamus and this regulation again may be positive or negative. The effect on the hypothalamus may be direct or indirect in controlling the secretion of either releasing or inhibitory neurohormones. The third type of control system that may be present is the short-loop feedback in which the pituitary hormone regulates its own secretion, either directly on the cell of origin of the hormone or indirectly via the appropriate hypothalamic neurones. These are all closed-loop control systems but in addition there may be other important modulating factors. For example, stress, exercise and temperature changes produce open-loop neural transients which can regulate the secretion of hypothalamic hormones. Regulatory influences of this type may be especially important in the control of secretion of growth hormone and prolactin, which affect a variety of target-cells throughout the body rather than having a distinct target gland that is capable of secreting a hormone that can inhibit release of the pituitary hormone.

Most anterior pituitary hormones exhibit a circadian rhythm that is superimposed on a pattern of pulsatile release controlled by the pulsed secretion of their releasing hormones. The physiological relevance of pulsatile release may be related to the phenomenon of 'down regulation' or desensitization of target-cell receptors. This occurs when the receptors are continuously stimulated, and leads to decreased target-cell responses to the same or higher hormone concentrations: intermittent stimulation protects against this target-cell desensitization. However, it must be appreciated that the neural events which control pulsatility are at present poorly understood.

The pineal gland has been described as a neuroendocrine transducer. In the cells of the pineal, 5-hydroxytryptamine is converted into melatonin by the action of the enzyme *N*-acetyltransferase. This enzyme is under neural control by noradrenergic post-ganglionic fibres from the superior cervical ganglion. Melatonin release exibits a circadian rhythm with a nocturnal peak that is entrained to light/dark cycles, i.e. photoperiodicity. The pineal in lower vertebrates is photosensitive. However, this is not the case in mammals, where neural connections between the retina and pineal are responsible for periodicity. Although the functions of the pineal in mammals is unclear, melatonin exerts an inhibitory influence over gonadal function by means of a central action upon release of growth hormone releasing hormone.

## Hormones of the anterior pituitary

GROWTH HORMONE (GH, also called somatotrophin)

As its name implies, this hormone stimulates growth and in terms of weight this is the major hormone of the anterior pituitary.

*Structure and synthesis*
Growth hormone has been isolated from many vertebrate species and is a protein whose amino acid sequence is species specific. The importance of this is that only human growth hormone is effective in man. The primary structure of human growth hormone was first reported by Li in 1969, though the incorrect assignment of certain amino acid residues was subsequently corrected by Niall in 1972. Human growth hormone is a protein with 191 amino acids. It is synthesized as a larger prehormone from which the signal peptide is removed before the hormone is secreted, and two disulphide bonds are formed within the single peptide chain. Human growth hormone can be extracted from human pituitaries but they are not a good source of the hormone which has therefore also been made by genetic engineering techniques. The first step was to prepare complementary DNA (cDNA, see Fig. 1.7) for human growth hormone, starting with messenger RNA from human pituitaries. The complementary DNA was incorporated in the circular DNA of plasmid pBR 322

which was then introduced into the bacterium *E. coli*, with which it was reproduced. From this complementary DNA for pre-growth hormone, a fragment was prepared consisting of 551 base-pairs that coded for amino acids 24 to 191 of human growth hormone. The original complementary DNA was then cleaved with the restriction enzyme HaeIII: in this way, the regions coding for both the presequence and for the first 23 amino-terminal amino acids were removed. The portion of complementary DNA coding for the amino-terminal sequence 1−23 was then put back as a chemically synthesized oligonucleotide containing the necessary sequence of bases. The synthetic oligonucleotide and the larger fragment of the native complementary DNA were incorporated into the DNA of the vector phGH107, along with a double-promoter sequence and a ribosome binding site; this recombinant plasmid was inserted into *E. coli* K12. This plasmid confers tetracycline resistance on the infected *E. coli*. Therefore, bacteria that are not infected by the plasmid are killed when grown in medium containing tetracycline, and those that are resistant grow and produce human growth hormone. The synthetic oligonucleotide that had been made chemically began at its 5′ end with the 'start' signal ATG. Because of this, the peptide produced had a methionine residue at the amino-terminus, followed by the 191 amino acids of human growth hormone. The methionyl-growth hormone was separated from bacterial proteins and it was shown to have the same amino acid sequence and disulphide bonds as native human growth hormone. Human growth hormone can also now be made in mammalian expression systems and it can be made without the extra methionine residue.

*Assay*
As has been found with other hormones, the isolation of growth hormone and an understanding of its physiology was dependent on the development of suitable assay systems. Although several bioassay techniques have been developed, they are all time-consuming and relatively insensitive. The most commonly used is the tibial assay in which the growth hormone-induced increase in width of the proximal epiphysis of the tibia is measured in hypophysectomized rats. Radioimmunoassay techniques are now used routinely for the assessment of growth hormone concentrations and have virtually replaced bioassay techniques for the routine assessment of growth hormone concentrations in patient sera and for physiological studies on growth hormone secretion.

*Effects of growth hormone*
Unlike most of the pituitary hormones, growth hormone does not have a single target gland: instead it can influence a variety of tissues. It promotes growth of bone, soft tissue and viscera. This is particularly important in young, growing animals, though

growth hormone seems to be relatively unimportant in the fetus and in the neonate. Growth of long bones occurs at the epiphyseal plates where there are actively proliferating cartilage cells. This effect ceases once the epiphyses of the long bones have fused. In addition, growth hormone has physiological actions which antagonize insulin action, and so in many respects the actions of these two hormones are opposite. High concentrations of growth hormone administered over prolonged periods are capable of causing a reduction in binding of insulin to its target-cell receptors and these, in turn, produce a fall in glucose transport into cells, with reduced glucose catabolism. After a meal, growth hormone causes an increased uptake of amino acids into muscle cells, and at longer time-intervals there is also an effect on lipid metabolism with the free fatty acids produced providing an energy source for muscle tissue. Receptors for growth hormone exist in the plasma membranes of several cell types. By some mechanism which remains to be elucidated, growth hormone can modulate DNA transcription and RNA translation within the cell; this effect is not dependent upon the activation of adenylate cyclase.

*Mechanism of action of growth hormone—somatomedins*
Some of the effects of growth hormone result from a direct action; these include the increased uptake of amino acids into muscle cells by stimulating membrane transport. However, other effects (including stimulation of growth) are mediated indirectly. The first of these indirect effects to be recognized was the stimulation of uptake of sulphate into cartilage. It was found that growth hormone could stimulate this *in vivo* but not in tissue culture. This effect is mediated through what was referred to as 'sulphation factor': this is now known to be a polypeptide growth factor called somatomedin C. This growth factor has a molecular weight of 7649 and the amino acid sequence has been established demonstrating its identity with insulin-like growth factor-1 (IGF-1) and its close homology with insulin-like growth factor-2 (IGF-2). These growth factors have a structure which is somewhat similar to that of pro-insulin. Somatomedin C is produced by a direct action of growth hormone on the targest tissues where it acts as a local hormone. It has insulin-like activities, for example, on fat cells. In addition to effects on sulphate incorporation into cartilage, somatomedins can stimulate $^{14}$C-leucine incorporation into glycosoaminoglycans in cartilage, $^{14}$C-proline into collagen and $^{3}$H-thymidine into DNA in cartilage cells and fibroblasts.

*Secretion and episodic release*
The basal concentration of growth hormone in plasma is below 1 mIU/l but it can fluctuate rapidly with peaks up to 60 mIU/l resulting from pulsatile release of hormone (see Fig. 2.7); bursts of hormone secretion are most frequent in adolescents, and

account for the greatly increased total daily secretion in this age group. When secretion stops the hormone disappears quite rapidly from the circulation with a half-life of less than 30 minutes.

### Control of growth hormone release

Control of growth hormone secretion from the pituitary is mediated by the interactions of growth hormone releasing hormone and somatostatin. A feedback role for somatomedin C (IGF-1) directly at the pituitary and also a short-loop feedback effect of growth hormone itself on the hypothalamus has been proposed. Release of growth hormone releasing hormone and somatostatin are under the control of the central nervous system so that stresses (e.g. exercise, excitement, cold, anaesthesia, surgery and haemorrhage) can all produce a rapid increase in the concentration of growth hormone in serum. The most significant and consistent changes in growth hormone secretion are associated with sleep, and bursts of secretion occur every 1−2 hours during deep sleep (see Fig. 2.7). The association of this secretion of growth hormone with sleep is a close one, so that if the onset of sleep is delayed, then the enhanced release of growth hormone is also delayed.

Since growth hormone affects carbohydrate, protein and fat metabolism, it might be expected that metabolic products also influence growth hormone secretion and this is indeed the case. Thus, an oral glucose load rapidly suppresses the secretion of growth hormone (Fig. 2.4). Conversely, hypoglycaemia induced by insulin injection triggers a release of growth hormone in response to this stress condition, and it may be used as a test of growth homone secretion. Infusions of certain amino acids, particularly arginine, can also stimulate growth hormone release, while elevated free fatty acid concentrations suppress it.

*Other factors.* The secretion of growth hormone is also modulated by other hormones. Glucocorticoids suppress growth hormone secretion while oestrogens may sensitize the pituitary to the action of growth hormone releasing hormone; therefore, basal and stimulated growth hormone concentrations are slightly higher in women. Noradrenaline, dopamine and serotonin are also implicated in modifying growth hormone secretion.

### PROLACTIN

### Structure and assay

The structure of human prolactin is very similar to that of growth hormone and for a long time it was believed that the human pituitary, unlike the pituitary of many animals, did not contain prolactin. However, human prolactin has now been isolated and its structure determined, revealing many structural similarities

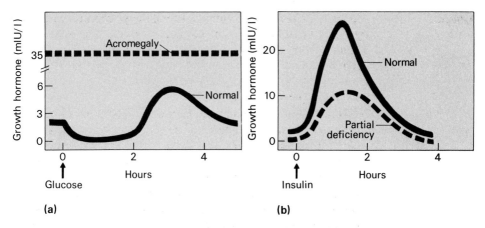

**Fig. 2.4** Dynamic tests of the regulation of the release of growth hormone.

(a) Administration of glucose normally suppresses growth hormone release though subsequently there is enhancement as blood sugar falls; in contrast, in acromegalic subjects, release of growth hormone is not suppressed by administration of glucose, and so the excessive secretion of growth hormone continues.

(b) Injection of insulin, by reducing blood sugar, increases the release of growth hormone in normal subjects. This response is lacking in patients with complete hypopituitarism but in those with partial deficiency there may be a reduced response.

mIU/l refers to the concentration of growth hormone in milli-international units per litre.

with the primary structure of human growth hormone. Bioassays of prolactin have usually been based either on its proliferative action on the mucosal epithelium of a pigeon's crop, or on its mammogenic (lactogenic) effect in mammals. As *in vivo* assays of the lactogenic effect on mammary gland activity are unsatisfactory, tissue cultures of mammary explants are generally used. The stimulatory effect of prolactin is usually measured either histologically or biochemically. Immunoassays for prolactin have made it possible to measure circulating prolactin and so study its secretion.

*Effects of prolactin*
The most obvious and perhaps main action of prolactin is to stimulate lactation. It acts on the prepared breast to stimulate growth and support the secretion of milk. The mammary gland is rudimentary in young girls but in the adolescent, oestrogen, growth hormone and adrenal steroids act together to stimulate the growth of the duct system. Alveolar growth is stimulated by oestrogen, progesterone, growth hormone, adrenal steroids and prolactin. Insulin and thyroid hormones are also necessary for mammary gland development. Following childbirth, prolactin and the adrenal steroids are both essential for the initiation and maintenance of lactation. Hypophysectomy in experimental animals results in the immediate cessation of milk secretion

61

whereas adrenalectomy only leads to a gradual reduction in milk secretion. Prolactin interacts with receptors in the mammary gland and subsequently, without involving the adenylate cyclase system, increases transcription and ultimately translation of messenger RNA which results in the synthesis of certain enzymes (e.g. galactosyl transferase) and milk proteins (e.g. casein and $\alpha$-lactalbumin).

*Other effects.* Prolactin has effects on the ovaries and testes in mammals (see Chapter 4), and in non-mammals it has important effects on salt and water balance and in controlling behaviour—for example, in birds it induces nest building activity.

*Control of secretion*

The normal concentration of prolactin in human serum is below 400 mIU/l. It is rapidly cleared from the circulation with a half-life in plasma of less than 30 minutes. Secretion is probably largely controlled by hypothalamic inhibitory and releasing factors. Dopamine is probably the main inhibitory factor while thyrotrophin releasing hormone, oestrogens and vasoactive intestinal peptide (VIP) can stimulate prolactin secretion. Prolactin is released episodically; like growth hormone the highest concentration is found at night and it is dependent on sleep. However, the most profound changes in the serum concentration of prolactin occur during pregnancy and lactation. The concentration of prolactin increases progressively, up to 10-fold, through pregnancy and remains elevated during lactation and is stimulated by suckling. The secretion rate declines during the later stages of lactation. As with most of the other hormones of the anterior pituitary, stress (e.g. surgery, myocardial infarction and repeated venepuncture) stimulates prolactin release. Pharmacological agents can also be used to stimulate the release of prolactin; for example, administration of L-$\alpha$-methyl dopa (which inhibits dopamine synthesis) results in increased circulating concentrations of prolactin and can induce lactation. The dopamine agonists, such as the precursor of dopamine, L-dopa, and the ergot derivative bromocriptine, both inhibit prolactin release. Many of the drugs used in the treatment of psychological disorders and many anti-emetics stimulate the secretion of prolactin because of their dopamine antagonist properties and so induce lactation: thus galactorrhoea can be an important side-effect of such treatment.

ADRENOCORTICOTROPHIN (ADRENOCORTICOTROPHIC HORMONE; CORTICOTROPHIN: ACTH) AND RELATED PEPTIDES

*Structure*

Adrenocorticotrophin is a peptide with 39 amino acid residues arranged in a single chain with a molecular weight of 4500.

The amino acid residues 1−24 are common to all the species that have been studied so far, though species specific variations have been found in the section comprising residues 25−39. Adrenocorticotrophin is one of a family of related peptide hormones that are derived (Fig. 2.5) from a larger precursor glycoprotein of molecular weight 31 000, known as pro-opiomelanocortin (POMC). Other products are the melanocyte stimulating hormones α-, β-, and γ-MSH, lipotrophin molecules and β-endorphin. The pituitaries of several species, but not man, contain two melanocyte stimulators: α- and β-MSH; the former has 13 amino acids which are identical with the first 13 residues of adrenocorticotrophin. Lipotrophin was originally given its name because it was thought mistakenly to have fat mobilizing

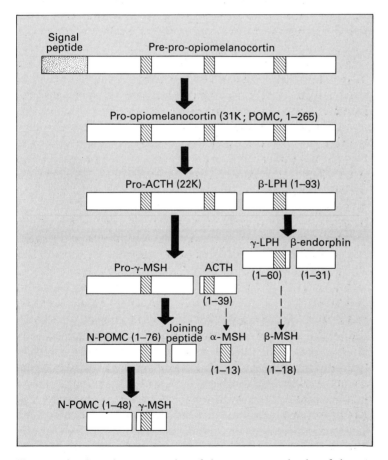

**Fig. 2.5** A schematic representation of the precursor molecules of the pro-opiomelanocortin family of peptides. Smaller peptides are derived from precursor molecules by specific peptidase actions. Hatched areas represent melanocyte stimulating hormone (MSH) structural units. ACTH is adrenocorticotrophin, LPH is lipotrophic hormone and N-POMC is the amino-terminal sequence of pro-opiomelanocortin (POMC). The number of amino acids in each peptide unit is shown in parentheses.

activity. There are two lipotrophin molecules ($\beta$-lipotrophin with 93 residues and $\gamma$-lipotrophin with 60 residues). Beta-endorphin is derived from $\beta$-lipotrophin; the name endorphin is derived from the *end*ogenous m*orphine*-like activities of this group of peptides. They have now been found in many tissues and may have a role in inhibiting signals to the brain arising from extreme stress or pain. Met-enkephalin is a smaller peptide that contains the amino acid sequence identical with positions 61–65 of $\beta$-endorphin: however, met-enkephalin is normally formed from another parent protein (see pp. 113–115 and Fig. 3.13).

*Assays*
Bioassays have played an important part in studies of the secretion of adrenocorticotrophin into the circulation, since the actions of the hormone on the adrenal gland can be relatively easily measured. Hypophysectomized animals are usually used for this purpose since the basal secretion from their adrenal glands is low. The output of steroids can be measured directly, but an indirect method has also been employed in which the depletion of the ascorbic acid content of the adrenal cortex, which accompanies steroidogenesis, is measured. Dispersed adrenal cells or slices of the adrenal gland in tissue culture have also been used in bioassays.

Radioimmunoassays have been developed, some of which are directed against the amino-terminal region (which is the part of adrenocorticotrophin important for biological activity) and some of which are specific for the carboxy-terminal region of the molecule which contains the species specific but biologically inactive portion of the molecule. Now, highly sensitive two-site immunoradiometric (IRMA) assays are available that will measure only intact adrenocorticotrophin (1–39).

*Effects on the adrenal cortex*
The actions of adrenocorticotrophin are largely confined to the adrenal cortex (see Chapter 3); it stimulates steroid synthesis, especially the synthesis of cortisol, by increasing the conversion of cholesterol to pregnenolone in the zona fasiculata and reticularis. Administration of adrenocorticotrophin also results in an increase in adrenal blood flow and of cortical cell protein synthesis. If the administration is prolonged, adrenal hypertrophy results. Adrenocorticotrophin can have effects outside the adrenal gland; thus, when present in large excess it produces darkening of the skin, a result of the melanocyte stimulating hormone sequence in adrenocorticotrophin which stimulates melanin synthesis in melanocytes.

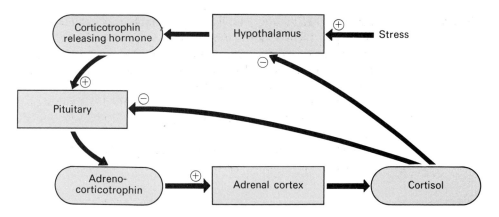

**Fig. 2.6** A schematic representation of the regulation of the production of cortisol from the adrenal cortex and of feedback regulation to the hypothalamus and pituitary.

*Control of secretion*

Control of the secretion of adrenocorticotrophin is thought to be largely under the influence of hypothalamic corticotrophin releasing hormone (CRH), the secretion of which is in turn determined by blood cortisol acting by negative feedback at the hypothalamic level and by neural inputs from other brain centres (Fig. 2.6). The 41 amino acid residue corticotrophin releasing hormone isolated in the early 1980s seems to provide the major part of the hypothalamic activity that releases adrenocorticotrophin. However, it may only be a part of a 'corticotrophin releasing factor complex', which includes other peptides such as vasopressin that potentiates the action of corticotrophin releasing hormone (1−41) *in vitro*. In addition, cortisol also acts directly on the pituitary corticotrophs, and administration of glucocorticoids inhibits pituitary adrenocorticotrophin release in response to exogenously administered corticotrophin releasing hormone. The most characteristic feature of adrenocorticotrophin secretion is its circadian rhythm which is related to the light/dark cycle: the concentration of adrenocorticotrophin is lowest around midnight; it then increases until the time of rising, and thereafter slowly declines. As with growth hormone, adrenocorticotrophin release is episodic and is stimulated by stress such as pain, fear, fever or hypoglycaemia; the latter is a useful clinical test of pituitary reserves of adrenocorticotrophin.

THYROTROPHIN (THYROID STIMULATING HORMONE, TSH)

*Structure*

Thyrotrophin is composed of two subunits ($\alpha$ and $\beta$) both of which contain carbohydrate moieties. The molecular weight is about 28 000 and varies slightly in different species. It should be noted that the structure of the $\alpha$-subunit is similar for thyrotrophin, luteinizing hormone and follicle stimulating hormone. However, the $\beta$-subunit in each of these three hormones is different and it is this chain which confers hormonal specificity. It has been possible to produce $\alpha$- and $\beta$-subunit hybrids; for example, with the $\alpha$-subunit derived from thyrotrophin and the $\beta$-subunit from luteinizing hormone. Thyrotrophin is synthesized and secreted by specific basophil cells of the anterior pituitary called thyrotrophs.

*Assays*

The concentration of thyrotrophin was often unmeasurable in normal subjects by older radioimmunoassay techniques. With sensitive immunometric assays, however, it is now possible to define both the upper and lower limits of the normal basal range for thyrotrophin concentration, which is about 0.4 to 5 mIU/l. Thyrotrophin disappears from the circulation with a half-life of about 15 minutes. Several bioassay techniques have been developed for thyrotrophin which depend on stimulation of iodide uptake by the thyroid gland or the release of hormones from the thyroid gland (see Chapter 5). Equivalent *in vitro* bioassays have also been developed; for example, the stimulation of adenylate cyclase in the thyroid gland or the acute release of thyroid hormones are used as the response to thyrotrophin in such assays.

*Control of secretion*

Negative feedback control involving the hypothalamic–pituitary–thyroid axis was the first of these endocrine control systems to be demonstrated. Thyrotrophin releasing hormone stimulates the synthesis and release of thyrotrophin by the pituitary thyrotrophs. In turn, thyrotrophin stimulates hormonogenesis in the thyroid gland and release of the thyroid hormones, thyroxine and triiodothyronine, which exert negative feedback on the pituitary to decrease the secretion of thyrotrophin. It is not yet clear whether thyroid hormones also act on the hypothalamus itself. The basal secretion of thyrotrophin is dependent on the tonic release of thyrotrophin releasing hormone by the hypothalamus. Focal hypothalamic lesions or transection of the pituitary stalk result in deficiency of thyrotrophin and subsequent hypothyroidism. Acute exposure to cold results in a temporary increase in thyrotrophin secretion. The set point for regulation of the secretion of thyrotrophin appears to be determined by the level of thyrotrophin releasing hormone secreted by the hypothalamus. However, it is likely that the primary site for negative feedback control by thyroid hormones is at the level of the pituitary, where increased concentrations of thyroid hormone decrease the effectiveness of thyrotrophin releasing hormone action on the pituitary and hence inhibit thyrotrophin secretion. While thyrotrophin releasing hormone acts rapidly via cyclic AMP to increase secretion of thyrotrophin, there is a long period before the inhibitory effect of thyroid hormone is observed.

GONADOTROPHINS: LUTEINIZING HORMONE (LH)
AND FOLLICLE STIMULATING HORMONE (FSH)

These hormones are secreted by the basophilic cells of the anterior pituitary called gonadotrophs. Their actions will be considered in greater detail in Chapter 4, but in brief, luteinizing hormone acts in females to induce ovulation and then maintain the secretory functions of the corpus luteum. In males, luteinizing hormone acts by stimulating the Leydig cells of the testes to produce testosterone. Follicle stimulating hormone in women acts to stimulate the development of ovarian follicles (which accounts for its name), while in males it stimulates spermatogenesis and the production of androgen-binding protein (ABP). Pituitary secretion of luteinizing hormone and of follicle stimulating hormone is inhibited by high concentrations of gonadal steroids (i.e. androgens or oestrogens) but there is another regulatory factor which also inhibits follicle stimulating hormone production; this is a peptide called inhibin which is secreted by the gonads. Castration causes a marked rise in luteinizing hormone and follicle stimulating hormone synthesis and secretion. Conversely, administration of androgens or oestrogens (the male and female gonadal steroids, respectively) results in lower concentrations of gonadotrophins in plasma. Paradoxically, however, there can also be a positive feedback effect by sustained high concentrations of oestrogen which leads to the sudden rise in luteinizing hormone release seen just before ovulation occurs. Luteinizing hormone secretion is pulsatile, with pulses occurring about every 90 minutes. This pulsatile pattern is important to the action of this hormone, and important changes may occur in some pathological conditions that are not detected by measurement of random basal levels of luteinizing hormone.

## Inappropriate production of anterior pituitary hormones

OVERSECRETION OF PITUITARY HORMONES

Oversecretion is usually due to a benign tumour, known as an adenoma. While these tumours do not produce secondary deposits elsewhere in the body and are usually small, they may grow and become locally invasive and some of the symptoms of a pituitary tumour therefore arise from its local expansion. These symptoms can best be understood by consideration of the anatomy of the pituitary gland. Since the pituitary gland lies in the pituitary fossa at the base of the skull, enlargement of the tumour will press on the walls of the fossa and may cause headaches. If the tumour extends upwards it may begin to press on the optic chiasm which will give rise to loss of the temporal fields of vision—that is, bitemporal hemianopia. Less commonly, it may also extend sideways and invade the cavernous sinus and damage the oculomotor nerves and give rise to a drooping of the eyelid and loss of eye movements on the affected side. Finally, if it extends downwards and forwards and enters the sphenoid sinus, the tumour may grow into the nasopharynx, and lead to loss of cerebrospinal fluid (CSF) which may come out through the patient's nose, a condition called CSF-rhinorrhoea.

Radiological examination of the skull in lateral view will show changes in the outline of the anterior wall, floor or the posterior wall of the pituitary fossa. The extent and localization of the upwards expansion of the tumour can often be crudely assessed by measuring the visual fields, but for more precise examination of the extent of the tumour, computerized tomography on the newer generation of scanners allows accurate delineation of the size and shape of the tumour and of its relationship with vital structures such as the optic chiasma, pituitary stalk or cavernous sinus. It is even possible with this technique to demonstrate microadenomas that are small and entirely within the pituitary fossa. Invasive procedures, such as air encephalography and arteriography are now rarely needed and are only used where there is some doubt about the diagnosis. For an air encephalogram, a lumbar puncture is performed, some cerebrospinal fluid is taken which is then replaced by air. The air moves upwards to provide an outline of the pituitary fossa and the ventricles when they are viewed radiographically. It is then possible to see whether there is a risk of the tumour pressing on the optic chiasma before any changes in the visual fields occur.

Tumours secreting excessive amounts of growth hormone, prolactin or adrenocorticotrophin are not uncommon. Secretion of lipotrophin parallels that of adrenocorticotrophin (see Fig. 2.5). Thyrotrophin and gonadotrophins are rarely produced in excess and some pituitary tumours do not appear to secrete any known pituitary hormone, although they may still contain numerous secretory granules on electron microscopy.

*Effects of growth hormone secreting tumours (gigantism, acromegaly)*
If a patient develops a growth hormone secreting pituitary tumour before puberty, then growth will be excessive, gigantism will result and the patient may grow to be 7 feet tall. More commonly, the tumour develops after the epiphyses have fused and growth of the long bones is no longer possible. Under these circumstances the condition known as acromegaly will develop

(the term acromegaly describes enlargement of the extremities). Patients will have large hands and feet, with thickening of the bones and very considerable thickening of soft tissues. The lower jaw may become very prominent, while soft tissue thickening may affect the nose, the forehead, the tongue and the chin. Excessive sweating and headaches are other common clinical features, and large tumours may present with loss of visual field. Occasionally, these patients complain of a change in their facial appearance, but this is usually very slow and insidious in onset and in the majority of cases the presence of acromegaly is noted only when the patient attends a physician for some other reason. When acromegaly is suspected, it may be useful to ask, for example, whether rings on the fingers have had to be enlarged or whether the patient's shoe size has changed. An excess of growth hormone leads to resistance to insulin and therefore the patients may present with symptoms of diabetes mellitus; even if symptoms have not yet developed, there may be abnormal glucose tolerance of a diabetic pattern (see Chapter 7). If acromegaly progresses, then, as well as leading to facial disfigurement, it may be associated with complications such as enlargement of the heart because of hypertrophy of cardiac muscle, which in part may be attributable to hypertension, causing increased workload on the organ. In addition, diabetes mellitus may cause further complications.

The diagnosis of acromegaly is usually confirmed now by measurement of growth hormone in serum. In normal subjects, growth hormone is usually not detectable in serum, i.e. $< 1\,\mathrm{mIU/l}$. However, as the circulating concentration of growth hormone is influenced by a number of factors including stress, starvation and exercise, it is necessary to perform measurements on samples taken in a basal state after a night's sleep and an overnight fast. Anxious patients may have high serum concentrations of growth hormone without necessarily having acromegaly. Conversely, some patients with active acromegaly have random (i.e. non-fasting) serum growth hormone concentrations in the range ocassionally seen in normal individuals, that is $10-20\,\mathrm{mIU/l}$. In such situations, it is helpful to differentiate between these states by observing whether growth hormone secretion can be suppressed. The most convenient test is to give glucose orally because it is a very effective suppressor of growth hormone secretion (Fig. 2.4). If the level is raised because of stress, it will normally be reduced to normal after an oral glucose load: on the other hand, if the patient has acromegaly, glucose will not suppress the secretion of growth hormone. Computer-assisted tomographic scanning of the pituitary will reveal the adenoma, which may frequently show extrasellar extension.

If severe acromegaly develops in a young patient, treatment is required, but if mild acromegaly is found in an elderly person treatment is sometimes not necessary, although troublesome symptoms such as headache or sweating may still be relieved by appropriate treatment of their acromegaly. The choice of treatment will depend on anatomical considerations. Thus, if the tumour has a large upwards extension, then an operation from above (i.e. the 'trans-frontal' approach) will be needed. However, many tumours may now be approached from below, i.e. the trans-sphenoidal approach, even in the presence of some supra-sellar extension; this avoids the need for intracranial surgery. In some cases radiotherapy is helpful, particularly where complete tumour resection is not possible. Medical treatment with the dopamine agonist bromocriptine is possible since it sometimes suppresses growth hormone release in acromegalics and it may also shrink the tumour, although in normal subjects bromocriptine raises growth hormone levels. Theoretically it would also be possible to treat acromegalic patients with somatostatin and a long-acting preparation of this peptide is currently undergoing therapeutic evaluation.

*Effects of adrenocorticotrophin secreting tumours: Cushing's disease*
Production of excessive amounts of adrenocorticotrophin will produce the condition known as Cushing's disease (see Chapter 3). It is appropriate at this stage to distinguish briefly between 'Cushing's disease' and 'Cushing's syndrome'. The latter is a general term applied to abnormalities resulting from a chronic excess of glucocorticoids, while 'Cushing's disease' is a more specific term in which hypercortisolism arises from inappropriate adrenocorticotrophin secretion from the pituitary. The results of trans-sphenoidal surgery suggest that the majority of cases with bilateral adrenal cortical hyperplasia have a small adrenocorticotrophin secreting tumour of the pituitary. Because these pituitary tumours are very small, usually no abnormality is seen on an x-ray of the skull, and sometimes the adenoma may not be clearly visible even using computer-assisted tomography. Many patients with Cushing's disease were treated by removal of their adrenal glands. Whilst this certainly cures the Cushing's syndrome, the pituitary tumour remains. Following removal of the adrenal glands, the feedback suppression of steroids on the tumour is lost and the pituitary tumour may begin to grow and secrete more adrenocorticotrophin. Another action of the hormone then becomes apparent, with an increase in skin pigmentation owing to the melanocyte-stimulating activity of the amino-terminus of adrenocorticotrophin (see p. 63); this is called Nelson's syndrome and surgical removal of the pituitary tumour may then be necessary. The primary treatment of choice for Cushing's disease is thus trans-sphenoidal removal of the micro-adenoma, where possible, and not adrenalectomy.

At one time many pituitary tumours were thought to be non-secretory and were known as 'functionless' pituitary tumours; but when it became possible to measure human prolactin by immunoassay, it was found that approximately three-quarters of these apparently non-functioning tumours were actually secreting prolactin. This condition is more common in women than in men and these patients generally present with a disturbance of sexual function. In women there may be interference of the menstrual cycle with amenorrhoea (see Chapter 4), while in men overproduction of prolactin causes impotence. These symptoms seem to result from an inhibition of the action of gonadotrophins on the gonads as a result of the high concentration of prolactin, although the pulsatile secretion of luteinizing hormone may also be impaired. As a consequence, the concentration of circulating oestrogens falls in women, while in men the concentration of testosterone may decline, although it may still remain in the normal range. It might be expected that a negative feedback mechanism at the hypothalamic–pituitary level would compensate and thus increase gonadotrophin production. This does not occur and basal concentrations of the gonadotrophins remain approximately normal although their pulsatile release may be reduced. This indicates that prolactin has, in addition, some effect on the feedback control of gonadotrophin output. In women the overproduction of prolactin may also lead to the secretion of milk (called galactorrhoea). The presence of a prolactinoma can readily be diagnosed by measuring the concentration of prolactin in the circulation, but it should also be noted that some drugs used in psychiatric therapy, e.g. chlorpromazine and anti-emetics such as metaclopramide or prochlorperazine, can stimulate the release of prolactin. Treatment of prolactinomas with bromocriptine, or with similar dopamine agonists, readily supresses prolactin secretion and usually results in shrinkage of the tumour. Surgical removal of a prolactinoma is sometimes necessary, in cases resistant to or intolerant of bromocriptine, but this treatment does not always reduce serum prolactin concentrations to the normal range.

### 'Functionless' pituitary adenomas

Other tumours in the region of the pituitary or its stalk may cause hyperprolactinaemia by preventing delivery of hypothalamic prolactin inhibitory factors. Non-functioning pituitary tumours may present with pressure effects such as headaches or loss of visual field. Such patients may also have hypopituitarism and/or hyperprolactinaemia. In contrast to the treatment of prolactinomas (i.e. adenomas of the mammotrophs), medical therapy does not result in a decrease in tumour size: surgery and radiotherapy, either alone or in combination, are usually required, and hormone replacement therapy may also be required as is described below.

Reduced pituitary function, i.e. 'hypopituitarism', can result from hypothalamic disease. Interference with the action of releasing hormones arises from damage to the pituitary stalk which prevents the passage of releasing hormones to the pituitary as was mentioned in the previous paragraph. Hypopituitarism is more commonly due to a disturbance of the pituitary gland itself, since disorders of the hypothalamus, such as tumours in this area, are uncommon. However, if a tumour of the hypothalamus does develop it may produce a combined picture of failure of the entire pituitary, affecting both anterior and posterior pituitary functions. Destruction of the pituitary gland itself, resulting from a large tumour, surgery, haemorrhage into the gland or thrombosis of its blood vessels, also leads to hypopituitarism. When the pituitary is progressively destroyed, its hormones may not all be lost at the same time. If pituitary function declines gradually, gonadotrophin and growth hormone secretion often fail before the secretion of adrenocorticotrophin and thyrotrophin decline. The hyperplastic pituitary of pregnancy seems to be particularly susceptible to hypotension resulting from postpartum haemorrhage. The compromised pituitary blood flow results in anterior pituitary infarction and the first manifestation of damage to the pituitary will then be failure of the onset of lactation.

*The effects of deficiency of anterior pituitary hormones*
The symptoms of pituitary failure are the result of reduced function of the various target organs. If there is simultaneously a deficiency of all the hormones of the anterior pituitary, the picture of 'panhypopituitarism' results. Lack of adrenocorticotrophic hormone causes failure of secretion of cortisol from the adrenal cortex, although the adrenal can still release aldosterone. The lack of cortisol (see Chapter 3) causes a non-specific lack of health and well being, with a reduced response to stress, and convalescence from minor illnesses takes longer than normal. Deficiency of thyrotrophin leads to reduced secretion of thyroid hormones and causes hypothyroidism (myxoedema) (see Chapter 5). Deficiency of gonadotrophins leads to loss of libido and to amenorrhoea in women, and a loss of potency in men (see Chapter 4). Deficiency of growth hormone does not seem to have any effect once growth has been completed, but in a young person lack of growth hormone causes dwarfism. Total absence of prolactin is rare probably because it is under inhibitory control by hypo-

thalamic factors, and a partial deficiency seems to have little effect. Occasionally there is an isolated defect of a single, or sometimes two, hormones of the pituitary. For example, some children have an isolated deficiency of growth hormone and this causes short stature; it usually arises from lack of growth hormone releasing hormone. Fig. 2.7 illustrates the normal pattern of release of growth hormone from the pituitary and the effects of partial and complete deficiency of this hormone. Treatment of growth hormone deficiency requires regular injections of human hormone: the response to this is shown in Fig. 2.8. Isolated deficiency of gonadotrophin can occur and is usually caused by a lack of gonadotrophin releasing hormone because these patients will often respond to injections of this substance.

Support for a diagnosis of hypopituitarism can be obtained most easily by measurement of the production of hormones from target glands. Thus, adrenocorticotrophin production will be reflected by the serum concentration of cortisol; blood samples are taken at 8 a.m. and midnight, and the concentration should

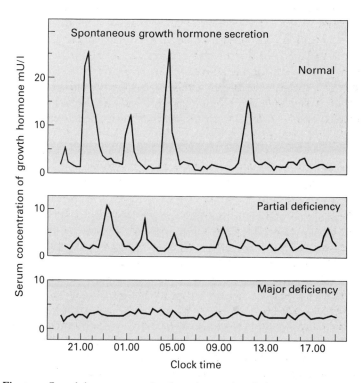

Fig. 2.7  Growth hormone secretion from the anterior pituitary gland in normal and deficient humans. Pulsatile release is evident in the normal individual in the upper panel, and occurs especially during deep sleep. These features diminish in partial growth hormone deficiency (middle panel), and they are absent in complete deficiency.

73

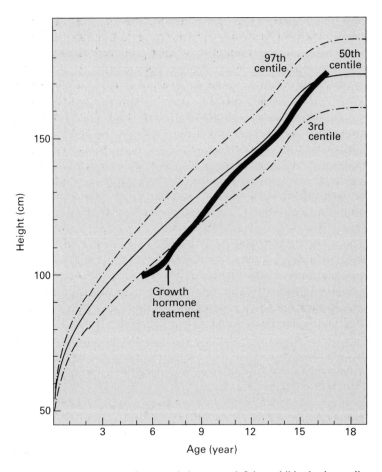

**Fig. 2.8** The response of a growth hormone deficient child: the heavy line shows the child's growth pattern before and during treatment. The other lines show the growth curves for normal children and the treated child which approaches the middle of the normal range (on the 50th centile).

normally be high in the morning and low in the evening. Similarly, the production of thyrotrophin will be reflected by the serum concentration of thyroid hormones. In each of these cases, however, the possibility that the deficiency is due to primary disease of the target organ has to be considered. Gonadotrophin production may be assessed from a patient's history; if a woman is having normal menstrual periods, it is virtually certain that she is producing gonadotrophin. If a patient suffers from amenorrhoea, it may be caused by gonadotrophin deficiency resulting from pituitary disease or another cause. In men loss of libido and impotence may be due to a hormonal defect, although commonly it is due to psychological factors. Measurement of peripheral circulating concentrations of testosterone is used in an indirect assessment of gonadotrophin production.

Assay of the hormones released by the anterior pituitary can be useful in investigation of hypopituitarism. For example, measurement of growth hormone concentrations in peripheral blood may indicate whether it is being produced, though this is not very satisfactory since even in normal subjects it is often undetectable. For this reason it is necessary to use a stimulation test to assess pituitary function. The most effective of these tests is the insulin-induced hypoglycaemia test which almost invariably produces an increase in growth hormone concentration in peripheral blood in a normal person (Fig. 2.4), but not in a patient with hypopituitarism. This stress test is also very useful because it stimulates the release of corticotrophin releasing hormone by the hypothalamus, and thus adrenocorticotrophin production from the pituitary and cortisol production from the adrenal cortex. Partial loss of pituitary function may occur, with loss of growth hormone production but with preservation of the cortisol response. It is important to assess the pituitary reserve of adrenocorticotrophin because this is an indication of the patient's ability to respond to stress; for example, during intercurrent illness or surgical operation. Administration of synthetic releasing hormones for thyrotrophin, gonadotrophin, corticotrophin or growth hormone may also give useful information about the respective pituitary hormone reserves.

*Treatment of hypopituitarism*

It is not practicable to give a patient frequent injections of adrenocorticotrophin or thyrotrophin; instead it is usual to give tablets of cortisol or thyroxine to replace the secretions of the respective target glands. Growth hormone replacement is only important if the condition develops before growth is completed and the epiphyseal plates have not fused. Human growth hormone has to be given by injection and it is needed because growth hormone from animals does not act in human beings. Human growth hormone was difficult to obtain since it had to be extracted from pituitary glands obtained at autopsy. Each pituitary from a cadaver contains about 7 mg of growth hormone (about 20 IU) but it took the extracts of several hundred pituitaries to treat a child until puberty. There has been concern that some preparations of human growth hormone might be contaminated with a 'slow virus' that causes a fatal disease that presents with dementia and is known as Jacob Creutzfeld's disease. Thus, the availability of synthetic human growth hormone by molecular biology techniques outlined earlier in this chapter represents a major contribution both to the supply of the hormone and to patient safety.

Gonadotrophins are available in a variety of forms for therapy (see Chapter 4). In the male, human chorionic gonadotrophin is used in place of luteinizing hormone; this leads to increased production of testosterone and some testicular enlargement in the prepubertal patient but comparatively poor spermatogenesis. To induce fertility by stimulation of spermatogenesis it is necessary to give injections of follicle stimulating hormone or human menopausal gonadotrophin extracted from urine; the latter preparation has a considerable follicle stimulating hormone activity. Alternatively, injection of gonadotrophin releasing hormone provides a successful therapeutic alternative for patients with isolated deficiency of this peptide. If spermatogenesis is not important, then treatment with testosterone alone can result in the development of secondary sex characteristics and a restoration of sexual potency. In women, development of secondary sex characteristics and regular uterine bleeding can be produced by cyclical administration of oestrogens, or of oestrogens together with progestogens as used in oral contraceptives. In addition, if ovulation is required (see Chapter 4), injection of follicle stimulating hormone (or human menopausal gonadotrophin) is necessary for follicle maturation and it has to be followed by injections of luteinizing hormone (as human chorionic gonadotrophin) to secure follicle rupture and release of the ovum; again, pulsatile gonadotrophin releasing hormone therapy has been used with some success. Prolactin replacement is not necessary.

## FUNCTIONS OF THE POSTERIOR PITUITARY GLAND (NEUROHYPOPHYSIS)

### Oxytocin and vasopressin

The two hormones released from the posterior pituitary are oxytocin and vasopressin. Between 1895 and 1915 the major effects of neurohypophyseal extracts were established. For some time there was controversy as to whether the rise in blood pressure (vasopressor activity), the contraction of the uterus (oxytocic effect), the expression of milk (galactokinetic effect) and the reduction of urine flow (antidiuretic action) could all be attributed to a single hormone. It was thought there might be a peptide of molecular weight of about 30 000 reponsible for all these effects. However, through the work of du Vigneaud, two hormones were isolated and their structure determined: oxytocin in 1953 and vasopressin (or antidiuretic hormone, ADH) in 1957. Oxytocin and vasopressin have molecular weights of approximately 1000 and are nonapeptides with the disulphide bond of cystine linking positions 1 and 6 to give a ring structure that is essential for biological activity (see Fig. 1.4).

*In vivo*, precursor molecules exist. They consist of a neuro-hypophyseal hormone plus a neurophysin: that for vasopressin contains neurophysin I which is a glycopeptide while that for oxytocin contains neurophysin II which is a polypeptide that does not contain carbohydrates. The neurophysins have molecular weights of around 10000 and although several neuro-physins may be extracted it appears that there are only two major peptides, the others being breakdown products. The amino acid sequences of the neurophysins have been determined but so far no biological action has been found for them.

Synthesis of the precursor molecules occurs in the nerve cells of the supraoptic and paraventricular nuclei, on the rough endo-plasmic reticulum. They are then transferred to the Golgi com-plex and packaged into granules, 120–200 nm in diameter. The neurosecretory granules now move down the axons through the stalk to the posterior pituitary at a rate of approximately 8 mm/hr which is faster than the rate of normal axoplasmic flow. The precursor possesses no biological activity; the hormone only appears as the granules are being transported and it is thought that the hormone, together with its associated neurophysin, is liberated by proteolysis from the larger precursor molecule.

NEUROSECRETORY CELLS OF THE SUPRAOPTIC AND
PARAVENTRICULAR NUCLEI

The neurosecretory cells of the neurohypophysis are neurones that can generate and conduct action potentials. Their axons terminate in the posterior pituitary where they abut on to capil-laries, the endothelial cells of which are separated from the nerve endings by a perivascular space and two basement membranes. Specialized glial cells, the pituicytes, lie between the axon term-inals. Release of the hormones occurs by exocytosis and neurophysin is released with the hormones. The paraventricular and supraoptic nuclei are controlled by other neurones richly innervated by ascending catecholamine pathways. Most are derived from medullary noradrenergic cell neurones, although cholinergic and opioid pathways also innervate these two nuclei. Noradrenergic and cholinergic pathways have generally been found to be stimulatory, while dopamine and opioid peptides are inhibitory.

The hormones of the posterior pituitary circulate in blood largely in an unbound form and so are removed rapidly from the circulation with a half-life of about 5 minutes. The kidney acts as the main site of clearance of the hormones.

CONTROL OF VASOPRESSIN SECRETION

The main physiological stimulus for the release of vasopressin is an increase in the osmotic pressure in the circulating blood. Vasopressin causes retention of water by the kidney which re-duces plasma osmolality. This in turn acts as a negative feedback signal on the hypothalamic osmoreceptors which then suppress the activity of the magnocellular neurones which secrete vaso-pressin. The effect of osmolality on vasopressin release was

77

clearly demonstrated by Verney; he showed in 1942 that infusion of hypertonic saline into trained, conscious dogs caused a 2% increase in the osmolality of plasma leading to inhibition of water diuresis. The inhibitory response could be mimicked by infusion of posterior pituitary lobe extract. Verney postulated that vasopressin release was mediated by osmoreceptors located in the anterior hypothalamus. It has been suggested that the magnocellular neurones themselves are osmosensitive. An alternative explanation is that there may be sodium receptors in the vicinity of the third ventricle. The organum vasculosum of the lamina terminalis have been postulated as the anatomical site of Verney's osmoreceptors.

In addition, there are a number of non-osmotic factors which may stimulate vasopressin release. For example, a fall in blood volume of 8% or more stimulates vasopressin release. In addition, alterations in blood volume also change the relationship between osmolality and the release of vasopressin. The fact that haemorrhage is a potent stimulus for the release of vasopressin could be important since at high concentrations the hormone has a vasoconstrictor effect. The response depend on baroreceptors located in the carotid sinus and the aortic area, and on plasma volume receptors present in the left atrium. In addition, reduction in $Pa_{O_2}$ and an increase in $Pa_{CO_2}$ stimulate the release of vasopressin. A number of hormones, including angiotensin II, adrenaline, cortisol, and sex steroids (oestrogen and progesterone) may also regulate the release of vasopressin. The effects of sex steroids may explain the fluid retention which can occur in the latter part of the menstrual cycle.

As with other hypothalamic hormones, the central nervous system plays an important part in the regulation of the release of these hormones. Pain and trauma associated with surgery cause a marked increase in the circulating concentration of vasopressin, as do nausea and vomiting. Psychogenic stimuli may also be effective in releasing these neurohypophyseal hormones. The activity of the neurohypophyseal system is also influenced by environmental temperature; a rise in temperature stimulates vasopressin release before there is any change in plasma osmolality.

ACTIONS OF VASOPRESSIN

Vasopressin, in the concentrations which normally circulate, has its chief action in the kidney (Fig. 2.9) where it reduces the flow of urine and leads the latter to become more concentrated. It acts on the final section of the distal convoluted tubule and on the collecting ducts to increase their permeability to water and hence its reabsorption, since the renal interstitium has a high osmolality. Because the kidney is such a complex organ, much of our knowledge of vasopressin action has come from observations

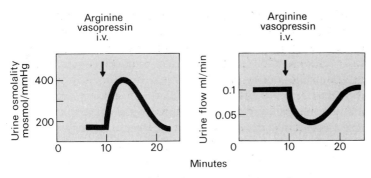

**Fig. 2.9** Administration of vasopressin reduces urine flow and leads to excretion of more concentrated urine (i.e. urine with higher osmolality).

on amphibian bladder membranes, although more recently single mammalian nephrons have been used. Vasopressin binds to the peritubular surface of the collecting ducts but produces its effect on the luminal membranes. Water leaves the cells partly via the lateral membranes and enters the lateral intracellular spaces. The intracellular messenger for vasopressin action on the kidney is cyclic AMP; vasopressin-sensitive adenylate cyclase has been demonstrated in the collecting duct and part of the distal convoluted tubule. The mechanism of action of vasopressin on the smooth muscle of arterioles, however, does not seem to involve cyclic AMP. Its action on blood vessels has been known for some time to be of pharmacological importance, and vasopressin or its analogues have been used to obtain haemostasis, for example, when there is severe bleeding from the gastrointestinal tract, or postpartum haemorrhage. Measurements of cardiac output and total peripheral resistance in the conscious state show that physiological concentrations of vasopressin can exert potent vasoconstrictor actions.

Four other actions of vasopressin are of some interest; these are its glycogenolytic activity in the liver, its effects on the coagulation of blood (by increasing fibrinolysis and factor VIII), its effects on conditioned learning (which it improves) in rats and a contribution to the control of adrenocorticotrophin secretion. The latter two effects have led to speculation that it may be a transmitter in the central nervous system.

CONTROL OF OXYTOCIN SECRETION

Oxytocin circulates in very low concentrations and is normally undetectable in the blood but it is elevated during parturition, lactation and also during mating. During parturition the concentration of oxytocin rises to peak values at the time of delivery of the fetus and expulsion of the placenta. Vaginal stimulation is an important factor controlling its release, though other factors

79

such as the fall of progesterone and the increase of oestrogen concentration may play a part. If a balloon is inflated in the vagina, oxytocin is released; this response is known as Fergusson's reflex. A positive feedback mechanism thus operates when a fetus moves down the birth canal. Under the influence of muscular contraction produced by oxytocin, there is vaginal distension which stimulates still further secretion of oxytocin. Stimulation of the nipple also causes release of oxytocin during suckling and this leads to ejection of milk. Even the sight and sound of an infant can stimulate milk ejection, but stress inhibits the release of oxytocin and so reduces the flow of milk.

ACTIONS OF OXYTOCIN

Oxytocin has two sites of action, namely the uterus and the mammary gland. By increasing the contraction of the uterus, it aids in the expulsion of the fetus and the placenta. In addition to a possible role in regulating the release of oxytocin, ovarian steroid hormones may influence its action by altering uterine sensitivity; progesterone appears to block and oestrogen appears to potentiate the response of the uterus to oxytocin. In some species, oxytocin has been shown to be produced by the corpus luteum of the ovary where it can enhance luteolysis directly or by means of prostaglandin production from the uterus. In the mammary gland, the myoepithelial cells surrounding the alveoli and ducts contract to expel milk from the alveoli and are sensitive to oxytocin. Oxytocin may also increase excretion of sodium; both oxytocin and vasopressin have been shown to act synergistically to promote sodium removal.

## Disordered secretion of the posterior pituitary

DEFICIENT SECRETION

Diabetes insipidus occurs when vasopressin secretion is reduced or absent. The term diabetes insipidus stems from the days when physicians used to taste the urine and contrasted it with the condition of diabetes mellitus in which the urine has a sweet taste. Patients with diabetes insipidus pass extremely large volumes of up to 20 litres of urine in 24 hours; this is of low specific gravity and low osmolality. This condition has to be distinguished from one caused by failure of the kidneys to respond to vasopressin; this is called nephrogenic diabetes insipidus. Increased passage of dilute urine can also result from a psychological disturbance (psychogenic polydipsia) in which the patient drinks inappropriately large volumes of water. Administration of drugs such as lithium carbonate can produce polyuria, by an action on the kidney. Pituitary diabetes insipidus is most commonly produced by damage to the neurohypophyseal system. It can occur as a result of head injury or the growth of a tumour and is sometimes called central diabetes insipidus, as opposed to nephrogenic diabetes insipidus which is of renal origin and may be a rare inherited condition. Isolated diabetes insipidus may also occur in the absence of any visible structural lesion, and in some of these cases it may be caused by an autoimmune process which destroys the vasopressin neurones. Polyuria which follows destruction of the neurohypophysis may be transient, since some recovery of function may occur with release of vasopressin from the ends of the neurones.

A patient with diabetes insipidus is unable to reduce the flow of urine when deprived of water, and the plasma osmolality consequently rises. If a vasopressin radioimmunoassay is available, diagnosis is best confirmed by monitoring hormone concentrations after an infusion of hypertonic saline. Alternatively, a water deprivation test may be used. Because of the inability to concentrate urine, the flow of dilute urine continues and the patient loses weight. If body weight falls by 5% during the course of the deprivation test, the test must be terminated and the patient allowed to drink, to avoid dangerous dehydration. During a water deprivation test the osmolality of urine specimens of a patient with diabetes insipidus will not differ by more than 50 mosmol/kg. In a normal subject the plasma osmolality ranges from 275 to 295 mosmol/kg while the range of urine osmolality is wide, from 40 to 1000 mosmol/kg. After water deprivation, the urine osmolality will normally rise, to exceed 800 mosmol/kg while the plasma osmolality remains below 295 mosmol/kg. In contrast, the urine of patients with diabetes insipidus will be less concentrated than plasma, and the osmolality of plasma will rise above 300 mosmol/kg. Patients with nephrogenic diabetes insipidus will not respond to vasopressin. Therefore they can be distinguished by administration of exogenous vasopressin or a synthetic analogue at the end of a water deprivation test.

Vasopressin deficiency used to be treated with injections of pitressin tannate in oil, but these injections are painful. Synthetic forms of vasopressin are available, one of which is lysine vasopressin, but this is short-acting. The form of vasopressin now most commonly used is a synthetic analogue, 1-desamino-8-D-arginine vasopressin (DDAVP). The lack of an amino group at the amino terminus of this synthetic peptide and the presence of a dextro-, as opposed to the normal laevo-, residue at position 8 leads to resistance to destruction by amino- and carboxy-peptidases. This synthetic peptide can be absorbed from the nasal mucosa and so is sprayed into the nose of patients being treated for diabetes insipidus. Partial deficiency of vasopressin can be treated by drugs such as chlorpropamide which potentiates the action of vasopressin on the kidney.

If vasopressin or a synthetic analogue is used in the treatment of diabetes insipidus there is a risk of water intoxication developing. The hormone causes retention of water and the patient will complain of headache and may become drowsy. Oedema does not develop, but the concentration of sodium in plasma will be low in patients with water intoxication.

OVERPRODUCTION OF VASOPRESSIN

Inappropriate secretion of vasopressin can occur in some circumstances. An excessive release from the pituitary may be induced by drugs or abnormalities in the physiological control mechanism, as may be seen in pulmonary disease or in certain disorders of the central nervous system. Ectopic production of vasopressin can also occur in patients with tumours, for example, in some types of cancer of the lung. This inappropriate release of vasopressin leads to water retention and the urine becomes more concentrated than plasma, even though plasma sodium may fall below 110 mmol/l; there is continued loss of sodium but renal and adrenal function otherwise remain normal. However, the symptoms of water intoxication may develop and the patient may become irritable, drowsy and then develop nausea and vomiting, followed by convulsions, stupor and coma. The logical treatment of this condition is to restrict fluid intake, though a temporary improvement can be achieved by infusion of hypertonic saline. In the future, treatment of inappropriate secretion may well involve vasopressin analogues which have been developed to competitively inhibit vasopressin's antidiuretic effect.

## SUMMARY

The pituitary gland has been termed the 'conductor of the endocrine orchestra'. However, control of the release of the pituitary hormones is mediated by either positive or more commonly negative feedback, so it is unlikely that the pituitary gland exerts more than a permissive, even though rather extensive, control over the endocrine system. Most of the hormones of the anterior pituitary are regulated by releasing hormones (or factors) secreted from the hypothalamus into the adenohypophyseal portal vasculature. Most of the pituitary hormones themselves are in turn controlled by negative feedback inhibition: the pituitary hormones in the circulation interact with their target tissues which, if they are endocrine glands, are stimulated to secrete further hormones that feed back to inhibit release of the pituitary hormones. For example, certain steroid hormones inhibit selectively adrenocorticotrophin, luteinizing hormone and follicle stimulating hormone secretion, and the thyroid hormones control thyrotrophin release. Where the target tissue does not produce a hormone, as in the case of growth hormone or prolactin, then release from the pituitary is controlled by inhibitors. Prolactin is under inhibitory control by dopamine, but both releasing and inhibiting hormones from the hypothalamus (as well as inhibition by glucose) control growth hormone release. The two neurohypophyseal hormones, oxytocin and vasopressin, are synthesized in the supraoptic and paraventricular nuclei and are stored in granules at the end of nerve fibres in the posterior pituitary. Oxytocin is released in response to peripheral stimuli of the cervical stretch receptors or of suckling stimulus at the breast. In a similar fashion, vasopressin (antidiuretic hormone) release is stimulated by changes in the activity of hypothalamic osmoreceptors. Some of the more detailed mechanisms of regulation of each of the endocrine organs by the pituitary hormones are given in the following chapters.

## FURTHER READING

BENNET G. W. & WHITEHEAD S. A. (1983) *Mammalian Neuroendocrinology.* Croom Helm, London.
BROOK C. (1985) *Clinical Paediatric Endocrinology* 2nd edn. Blackwell Scientific Publications, Oxford.
FORSLING M. L. & GROSSMAN A. (1986) *Neuroendocrinology: A Clinical Text.* Croom Helm, London.
HUMBEL B. E. (1984) Insulin-like Growth Factors, Somatomedins and Multiplication-Stimulating Activity. In *Hormonal Proteins and Peptides,* Vol. XII, Ed. Li C. H. Academic Press, New York.

# 3　The adrenal gland

The presence of the adrenal glands was noted in 1563 by Bartholomaeus Eustachius who called them 'the glandulae renibus incubentes'. In the 17th century they were commonly called the 'suprarenal capsules' and it was not until the latter part of the 19th century that the term 'adrenal' came to be used. In 1805 Cuvier described the differences between the two main parts of the adrenal gland and, subsequently, the terms cortex and medulla were introduced, referring to the outer and inner parts respectively. Little was known of the function of the adrenal gland until in 1855 Thomas Addison published his classical monograph entitled *The Constitutional and Local Effects of Disease of the Suprarenal Capsule*. He vividly described the effects of adrenal insufficiency, with the unusual association of increased pigmentation of the skin and progressive fatigue. It was only later that Brown-Sequard showed that removal of the adrenal glands was fatal: it had not been easy to show this because of the technical difficulty in many animal species of removing all adrenal tissue. Following the demonstration that the adrenal was essential to life, there was a debate as to whether the cortex or medulla was more important. In 1894 Oliver and Schaffer extracted a substance from the medulla which could raise blood pressure. The pressor agent was adrenaline (epinephrine) which was isolated, and chemically characterized and synthesized between 1900 and 1904. Much later, in 1948, another catecholamine, noradrenaline, was isolated. Demonstration of the properties of adrenaline made it seem that the medulla was more important than the cortex. However, it was eventually shown that the converse is true and patients dying of Addison's disease were successfully treated with extracts of the adrenal cortex.

The adrenal cortex secretes hormones (corticosteroids) which, among other actions, affect carbohydrate metabolism and electrolyte balance; these two groups of effects are referred to as glucocorticoid and mineralocorticoid activities, respectively. For many years it was not clear whether or not these two functions were regulated by a single substance. In the 1930s it was generally thought that there was probably a single important steroid hormone secreted by the adrenal cortex (i.e. a Unitary Theory). However, largely due to the work of Reichstein and Kendall, a large number of steroids were extracted from the adrenal gland and chemically characterized. These included cortisol (originally called Compound F) and 11-deoxycortisol (Compound S) as well as deoxycorticosterone. Subsequently many steroids were chemically synthesized, including cortisone which can be converted in the liver to cortisol which is an important steroid that is secreted by the cortex. Cortisone *in vivo* was found to have the ability to suppress an inflammatory reaction and because of this was used in the treatment of rheumatoid arthritis. It is a glucocorticoid, but when given in large doses it was found also to have a sodium retaining effect, that is, mineralocorticoid activity as well. Thus, the 'Unitary Theory' that there was a single important adrenal steroid hormone gained support again, for a while, and it seemed likely that cortisol was the important hormone. Then another important steroid, namely aldosterone, was identified.

The original steroids extracted from the adrenal cortex were obtained from a crystalline fraction. There was, however, another portion, the amorphous fraction, and it was from this that, in 1952, Simpson and Tait in London, in collaboration with Reichstein in Switzerland, isolated and characterized aldosterone which was found to have most potent mineralocorticoid effects. In man aldosterone and cortisol are the two most important adrenal steroid hormones. Aldosterone is particularly important as a mineralocorticoid but cortisol can also be important in this context because, although its potency as a mineralocorticoid is much lower than that of aldosterone, its secretion rate is much higher and thus it can contribute to the maintenance of electrolyte balance (see p. 97). It may be noted, however, that the pattern of steroid secretion differs in various species, so that, for example, in the rat corticosterone rather than cortisol is the major glucocorticoid. In addition, the adrenals are also capable of synthesizing some sex hormones in small amounts.

## MORPHOLOGY

### ANATOMY

The two adrenal glands are small, triangular in shape and bilaterally positioned on the superior poles of the kidneys. Their total weight in humans is between 8 and 12 g depending on age and they are usually heavier in females than in males. The cortex makes up 80−90% of the gland and has a yellow colour due to its content of lipid; the inner part, the medulla, is reddish-brown and makes up 10−20% of the gland.

### CYTOLOGY OF THE CORTEX

There are three morphologically distinguishable zones within the adrenal cortex; the glomerulosa, the fasciculata and the reticularis

(Fig. 3.1). This zonation is functionally important because aldosterone comes from the zona glomerulosa while cortisol comes from the zonae fasciculata and reticularis.

The outer zone, the zona glomerulosa, lies under the capsule and makes up 5−10% of the cortex. In man its cells are closely packed and form small, ill-defined clumps, but in other species the cells are arranged in a continuous layer. The glomerulosa cells possess the general characteristics of steroid-producing cells; there is relatively little rough endoplasmic reticulum but abundant smooth endoplasmic reticulum, arranged in anastomosing tubules, 40−70 nm in diameter. Some lipid droplets are present and

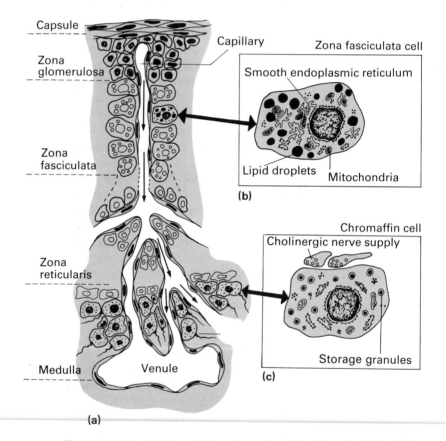

**Fig. 3.1** (a) A section through the cortex and medulla of the adrenal gland. The capsule surrounds the gland and capillaries run through the cortex and empty into a medullary venule. The three zones of the cortex are shown: the thin, outer zona glomerulosa; the thick central, zona fasciculata; and the inner zona reticularis. The medulla consists of chromaffin cells and cholinergic nerve supply.

(b) The cytology of a zona fasciculata cell. Note the large number of lipid droplets, and extensive smooth endoplasmic reticulum associated with mitochondria.

(c) The cytology of a medullary chromaffin cell. Note the numerous membrane bound storage granules of catecholamine and the synaptic terminals of its cholinergic nerve supply (see also Fig. 3.12).

the mitochondria of these cells are usually round or elongated and possess lamellate cristae.

The middle cortical zone, the zona fasciculata, forms about 75% of the volume of the adrenal cortex. Its cells are larger than those in the zona glomerulosa and are arranged in long cords disposed radially with respect to the medulla; the cords are separated by the straight cortical capillaries. Fasciculata cells are characterized by an abundance of smooth endoplasmic reticulum and lipid droplets containing cholesterol esters; the cells also contain large amounts of ascorbic acid. The mitochondria are large and usually spherical in shape; small parallel stacks of rough endoplasmic reticulum are present in continuity with the smooth endoplasmic reticulum.

In the zona reticularis there is an anastomosing network of short cords of cells with interdigitating capillaries. The cells of the zona reticularis have characteristic features. Under the light microscope their acidophilic properties reveal two kinds of cell, one a deeply staining, compact cell and the other a less intensely stained, clear cell; these tinctorial differences probably reflect differing physiological states. Ultrastructurally, there is a less extensive smooth endoplasmic reticulum, and fewer lipid droplets than in the zona fasciculata with more lysosomes and larger lipofuscin granules, which increase in number with age. The mitochondria tend to be more elongated and have both short and long tubular cristae. Cell contacts between cortical cells in all the zones involve desmosomes, but in the zona fasciculata and reticularis large and numerous gap junctions are found, functionally coupling the cortical cells.

CYTOLOGY OF THE MEDULLARY CHROMAFFIN TISSUE

Histologically, the medulla is composed of chromaffin cells, named from their capacity to show a brown coloration when exposed to an aqueous solution of potassium dichromate; this is thought to be due to the oxidation of catecholamines to a brown pigmented polymer.

Chromaffin cells tend to be columnar in shape and are arranged in anastomosing epithelioid cords separated by vascular spaces. The cells tend to be polarized with their long axes at right angles to the adjacent fenestrated capillaries.

Ultrastructurally, the most prominent feature of the cells is the abundance of membrane-bound, electron-dense granules, 150−400 nm in diameter. These granules are thought to be the storage site of the catecholamines, noradrenaline and adrenaline.

The cells also contain elongate mitochondria, rough endoplasmic reticulum, and a Golgi complex where the granule matrix appears to be packaged. Each chromaffin cell is innervated by a cholinergic, preganglionic sympathetic neurone.

*The paraganglia.* These are small groups of chromaffin cells which are histologically similar to those of the adrenal medulla, and which also have the same embryological origin. Similar chromaffin granules are found in these cells, which electron microscopic evidence indicates contain noradrenaline. The paraganglia are widely scattered in the retropleural and retroperitoneal tissues, some being associated with sympathetic ganglia and others with parasympathetic nerves. Whether or not they release catecholamines into the circulation in normal circumstances is uncertain. They are, however, occasionally the site of growth of a tumour, a phaeochromocytoma which can secrete into the general circulation.

### BLOOD AND NERVE SUPPLY

The blood supply of the adrenal gland (Fig. 3.2) is derived from a circle of different arteries arising from the superior, middle and inferior adrenal arteries. The small vessels from these trunks pierce the capsule and break up into a plexus. From this, three kinds of vessel arise, the capsular vessels, the cortical vessels and the medullary arterioles. The cortical vessels descend from the

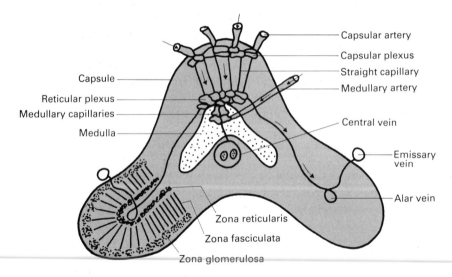

**Fig. 3.2** A section through the centre of the human adrenal gland showing the capsule, the cortex and its three zones; zona glomerulosa, zona fasciculata and zona reticularis; and the central medulla. Also shown is the gland's blood supply. Arteries pierce the capsule and form a capsular plexus. From this arise the straight capillaries which run between the columns of zona fasciculata cells and eventually anastomose to form the reticular plexus of capillaries in the zona reticularis. These in turn empty into the medullary capillaries, which eventually fuse to form venules that run into the large central vein. Note that some cortical blood can escape via the alar veins into the emissary vein. The medulla also has a direct arterial supply which runs from the capsular arteries directly to the medullary capillaries.

capsular plexus and form the capillary bed which supplies the cortical parenchyma. The straight capillaries between the fasciculata finally anastomose in the zona reticularis and then empty into the medullary vascular bed. The medullary arterioles penetrate the cortex and supply the medullary tissue directly. Thus, the medulla has a double blood supply, a systemic one via the long medullary arterioles and a secondary one derived from the cortical capillaries, which may be likened to a portal system. Medullary venules collect the blood which empties into the central vein. This originates in the tail of the gland and is surrounded by a cuff of cortical tissue where it indents the medulla from below in the body of the gland. Heavy, longitudinal muscle columns of the central vein, by shortening and swelling, can obstruct the smaller veins entering it. Overflow of blood then occurs by an alternative route, the alar veins at the wings of the gland, which also drain the zona reticularis plexus. Emissary veins between the alar veins and others running along the surface of the gland serve as an additional regulator of blood flow. The central vein of the right adrenal empties into the inferior vena cava while on the left side it drains into the left renal vein. Thus, much of the blood the medulla receives is rich in the corticoid hormones which are necessary for the production of adrenaline. Further, the hormones of the adrenal can be stored in its vascular channels to be released in spurts as the muscle of the central vein contracts or relaxes.

The innervation of the gland is derived from the splanchnic nerves which arise from lateral horn preganglionic sympathetic neurones at spinal cord levels $T_8-T_{11}$. Some of these pre-ganglionic fibres synapse with postganglionic sympathetic neurones in the coeliac ganglion, the fibres of which innervate the blood vessels in the adrenal. Other preganglionic splanchnic fibres enter the medulla, ramify among the tissue and end in cholinergic synapses on the chromaffin cells, which are the equivalent of postganglionic neurones. However, the cells of the adrenal cortex do not have a secretomotor innervation.

DEVELOPMENT

Embryologically the adrenal is derived from two components (Fig. 3.3), ectodermal neural crest cells which form the medulla, and mesodermal cells which give rise to the cortex.

*Medulla*
In the human, during the fifth week of development, cells originating from the neural crest migrate from each side of the neural tube towards the dorsal aorta where they position themselves laterally and just posterior to it. Most of these cells form a bilateral chain of segmentally arranged sympathetic ganglia but

89

Chapter 3

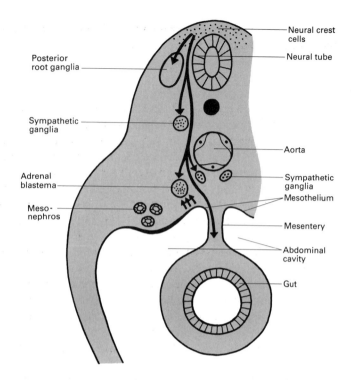

**Fig. 3.3** The development of the adrenal gland. The cortex is derived from the mesothelium lining the body cavity. The cells invade ( ↑ ↑ ↑ ) the underlying stroma and form a compact mass, the adrenal blastema. Neural crest cells migrate ventrally; some give rise to posterior root ganglia and sympathetic ganglia while others invade the adrenal blastema and form the medulla of the gland. Note also the neural tube, aorta, mesonephros, mesentery and gut.

some of the neural crest cells, called phaeochromaffinoblasts, invade the medial aspect of the developing adrenal cortex, position themselves in its centre and eventually become the adrenal medulla. These cells do not form nerve processes although they are the equivalent of postganglionic neurones. They differentiate into two kinds of chromaffin cells which synthesize and secrete noradrenaline and adrenaline, respectively. During fetal life the chromaffin cells secrete only noradrenaline but just before birth some cells begin to synthesize adrenaline.

The evidence for the neural crest origin of the chromaffin tissue is based in part on studies involving $^3$H-thymidine labelling of chick neural crest cells transplanted from one embryo into a host embryo and their eventual localization by radioautography in the centre of the newly formed gland. There is also evidence from the experiments of Le Douarin, in which quail neural crest tissue (whose cells can be easily distinguished from host cells by their distinctive nuclear chromatic mass) was grafted into host chick embryos, where their subsequent localization in the centre of the gland could be observed.

*Cortex*

The adrenal cortex originates from mesothelial cells located at the cranial ends of the mesonephros; these lie between the root of the mesentery and the developing urogenital ridge. During the fifth week of development these cells proliferate and invade the underlying retroperitoneal mesenchyme. They form an acidophilic mass of cells which are penetrated on their medial aspect by the phaeochromaffinoblasts at about the seventh week of development. The mesothelial-derived cells form the primitive fetal cortex. In the human, a second wave of mesothelial-derived cells proliferate, surround the fetal cortex and eventually form the cortex of the adult gland. Mesenchymal cells which surround the fetal cortex differentiate into fibroblasts and lay down the collagenous capsule. The blood and nerve supplies of the gland also develop during this period. At the end of fetal life the adrenal gland is about 20 times bigger relative to other organs than it is in the adult and is large even compared with the kidney.

Postnatally, the fetal cortex regresses and it has usually disappeared by the end of the first year of life, being replaced by the mature cortex. The glands decrease in weight by a third during the first weeks after birth and do not regain their original birth weight until the end of the third year of life. Complete absence of both glands is rare, as is the existence of true accessory glands, consisting of both cortex and medulla. However, ectopic adrenal cortical tissue alone occurs frequently, as do patches of medullary tissue. These isolated groups of cells may be found in the adult spleen, or retroperitoneally; for example, below the kidneys, along the aorta, in the pelvis or associated with gonadal structures. Functionally ectopic adrenal tissue, whether of cortical or medullary origin, is of no significance unless it becomes hyperplastic or malignant—then its location may become very important.

Zonation of the cortex begins during late fetal life. The zona glomerulosa and zona fasciculata are present at birth but the reticularis is not obvious until the end of the sixth year. Differentiation of the cells in the cortex and the development of function in the fetus appear to be under the control of adrenocorticotrophin, secreted by the fetal pituitary gland. Thus the adrenal gland of rats or rabbits does not develop or grow normally if the fetal pituitary or hypothalamus has been removed surgically *in utero*, or if secretion of adrenocorticotrophin in the fetus has been suppressed by continuous infusion of cortisol. Similarly, the adrenals are small in the anencephalic (i.e. brainless) human fetus, because little or no corticotrophin releasing factor is released from the grossly malformed or absent hypothalamus.

*Role of the fetal cortex. In vitro* studies of primate adrenals and estimation of steroids in umbilical venous blood showed that the fetal adrenal is capable of steroid production at an early stage of gestation. Glucocorticoids in the fetus are involved in a number of important processes:

1  Production of surfactant from type II cells of the alveoli of the lung—a lack of which leads to the respiratory distress syndrome in newborn infants.

2  Development of hypothalamic function and of the thyroid—pituitary axis.

3  The sequential changes of placental structure and in the ionic composition of amniotic and allantoic fluids during development.

4  They are most important in the initiation of the endocrine changes of the fetus and mother which are responsible for parturition.

5  The development of hepatic enzymes, including those involved in gluconeogenesis.

6  Induction of thymic involution.

The fetal adrenal gland makes dehydro*epi*androsterone and androstenedione that also provides the substrate for oestrogen synthesis by the placenta (see Fig. 4.8).


# FUNCTION OF THE ADRENAL CORTEX

The division of the cortex into separate layers as described above is very important since the zones produce different steroids (e.g. aldosterone is only produced in the zona glomerulosa). This can be shown when the zones are separated; for example, when the capsule is stripped off taking with it the zona glomerulosa and leaving the zona fasciculata and the zona reticularis behind. The zonal production of steroids can also be studied in isolated cell preparations, made by treating adrenal tissue with collagenase to disperse the cortical cells.


## Function of the zonae fasciculata and reticularis

These two areas of the adrenal cortex are important for the production of cortisol, which is the most important hormone with glucocorticoid activity in man, though corticosterone is also produced. The pathway of synthesis of cortisol is shown in Fig.

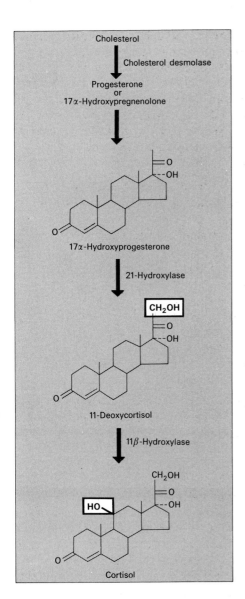

**Fig. 3.4** The pathway of synthesis of cortisol in the zonae fasciculata and reticularis.

3.4. In the adrenal cortex there is relatively little storage of hormone and active synthesis is required when the need for hormone increases.

EFFECTS OF CORTISOL

*Changes in carbohydrate, fat and protein metabolism*
The metabolic effects of cortisol vary with the target tissue: in muscle, adipose and lymphoid tissue it is catabolic but in liver it stimulates the synthesis and storage of glycogen. These effects

93

are opposite to those of insulin (see Chapter 7). Cortisol increases the concentration of glucose in blood by stimulating gluconeogenesis in the liver and decreasing, to a lesser extent, the utilization of glucose in other tissues. The increased blood glucose is available for the production of glycogen and is important in maintaining liver glycogen during prolonged fasting. The increase in liver glycogen after administration of corticosteroids provides the basis of a useful bioassay of glucocorticoid activity.

These effects on metabolism are produced by entry of cortisol into cells causing an increased synthesis of many enzymes via an action in the nucleus (see pp. 36–38). In liver, pyruvate carboxylase activity increases within 6 hours and glucose-6-phosphatase and fructose-1,6-diphosphatase increase in 3–6 days of administration of cortisol. All of these enzymes are involved in gluconeogenesis which depends on the availability of a source of amino acids which are derived from protein catabolism in many tissues including muscle and skin; stimulation of protein catabolism is another characteristic feature of the action of cortisol. Moreover, cortisone (which is converted to cortisol) has been shown to activate certain hepatic enzymes which are involved in the metabolism of amino acids; these enzymes include tyrosine transaminase which catalyses the transfer of amino groups from tyrosine and phenylalanine and tryptophan to glutamate. Enzymes of the urea cycle are also induced by cortisol acting on the liver. At the same time the energy required for gluconeogenesis is obtained from the breakdown of fats, the release of fatty acids and inhibition of the synthesis of new fat molecules in adipose tissue (see Chapter 7).

*Anti-inflammatory effects*
In addition to its effects on metabolism cortisol acts on the body's defence mechanisms, where it suppresses tissue response to injury and has an anti-inflammatory action. Cortisol in moderately high concentrations leads to a reduction in the size of lymph nodes and involution of the thymus. It reduces the number of lymphocytes in blood and so decreases antibody production which yields an immunosuppressive effect. These effects can be useful therapeutically but they also reduce resistance to infection.

*Other effects*
Although cortisol is predominantly a glucocorticoid, it does have mineralocorticoid effects as has already been mentioned; it can help to maintain extracellular fluid volume and prevent the shift of water into cells and it can help maintain tissue perfusion which may be particularly important during stress. Cortisol can have a number of other effects, many of which only become apparent if it is present in excess. It sensitizes arterioles to the action of noradrenaline and has permissive effects on the actions

of noradrenaline on carbohydrate metabolism. In addition it can stimulate secretion of acid by the stomach and increase activity in the central nervous system to produce euphoria or even mania.

SECRETION OF CORTISOL

*Regulation*
The anterior pituitary, through secretion of adrenocorticotrophin, controls the activity of the zona fasciculata/reticularis. Adrenocorticotrophin stimulates the production of cortisol by increasing the activity of cholesterol desmolase, the rate limiting step in cortisol synthesis (see Fig. 3.4). If a small pulse of adrenocorticotrophin is administered to an experimental animal, glucocorticoid production increases within 5 minutes and then wanes over the next 10 minutes. However, if the stimulation is continued over a longer period of time, then cytoplasmic lipid droplets and ascorbic acid in the fasciculata cells decrease and eventually the zona fasciculata and zona reticularis will increase in thickness. In this period the clear cells of the fasciculata appear to change into the compact cells of the zona reticularis because they become depleted of fat. While this is happening adrenocorticotrophin appears to have little effect on the zona glomerulosa.

In hypophysectomized animals the lack of adrenocorticotrophin leads to shrinkage of the zona fasciculata and zona reticularis to less than half their original thickness. The cells lose lipid droplets, the smooth endoplasmic reticulum dwindles and the concentration of ascorbic acid in the cells falls (for reasons which are not clear). These cytoplasmic changes, of course, are accompanied by a reduction in glucocorticoid output. These changes in the cortical region of the adrenal clearly illustrate the 'trophic' nature of the actions of adrenocorticotrophin, modulating the structure and function of the zonae fasciculata and reticularis. The control of steroid production in the zona fasciculata is largely determined by changes in the concentration of adrenocorticotrophin in plasma, and the secretion of this trophic hormone is in turn regulated by corticotrophin releasing hormone as described in Chapter 2. Thus removal of the pituitary leads to an almost complete abolition of cortisol synthesis.

*Negative feedback of cortisol on secretion of adrenocorticotrophin*
The end product of the action of adrenocorticotrophin, namely cortisol, has a direct inhibitory action on the pituitary (see Fig. 2.6). It also exerts a negative feedback action on the hypothalamus, to inhibit the release of corticotrophin releasing hormone. The secretion of corticotrophin releasing hormone can be stimulated by emotion, stress and trauma. There is also a

circadian rhythm of hypothalamic/pituitary activity operating during the sleep/wake cycle. As a result the concentration of cortisol in plasma of man is minimal around midnight and rises to a maximum between 6 to 8 a.m., thereafter falling slowly during the day. In contrast, in nocturnal animals such as the rat, the peak concentration is found in the evening rather than during the day. Superimposed on these trends is an episodic pattern of release with fluctuations lasting for periods of several minutes. Since the adrenal–pituitary feedback system is not very well 'damped', large swings in the concentrations of adrenocorticotrophin and cortisol in the circulation can readily occur. However, if the system is suppressed for a long time by the administration of exogenous steroid, then it can take many months for the synthesis and release of adrenocorticotrophin, and hence of cortisol, to be restored.

*Measurement of secretion rate*
It will be appreciated that the importance of a hormone in controlling a given process will depend not only on the biological activity of that hormone, but on its secretion rate (Fig. 3.5). *In vitro* this can be measured when isolated adrenal glands are incubated. In experimental animals the secretion rate can be established *in vivo* by collecting the venous effluent from the adrenal gland over a period of time and measuring the amount of hormone in that blood. In man it is also possible to estimate the secretion rate, this time by using isotope dilution methods, since most natural steroids have a biological half-life in the circulation of between 1 and 2 hours and since many of them are excreted as unique metabolites in urine. If a particular steroid is excreted in the urine as a unique metabolite, then the amount by which an administered radioactively labelled tracer steroid is diluted by endogenously produced steroid can be calculated. For this purpose urine has to be collected until excretion of the labelled, exclusive metabolite is completed, which may take a few days. The metabolite is then extracted from the urine and the specific radioactivity is measured (i.e. the ratio of the radioactive counts per unit mass). From this information the amount of steroid secreted can be calculated. Alternatively, a radioactively labelled steroid can be infused at a constant rate and when equilibrium is achieved the secretion rate may be calculated; it is equal to the product of the *metabolic clearance rate* (see below) and the endogenous plasma steroid hormone concentration. In exactly the same way that renal clearance is defined as the volume of blood which is irreversibly cleared of a substance in unit time, so the *metabolic clearance rate* of a hormone is that volume of blood which is completely and irreversibly cleared of hormone in unit time and it represents the sum of all the individual clearance rates of different organs. The effects of metabolism and excretion of the hormone are included in the calculation of clearance rate.

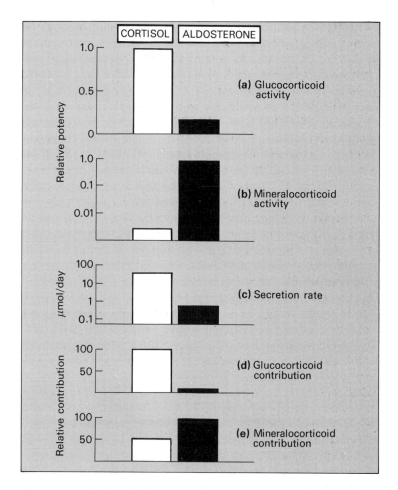

**Fig. 3.5** A comparison of cortisol and of aldosterone.

(a) Glucocorticoid activity was measured as ability to increase glycogen in the liver: cortisol is very potent in this assay.

(b) Mineralocorticoid effects were measured in terms of the ability to reduce the ratio of the excretion of sodium to the excretion of potassium in urine; aldosterone is much more potent.

(c) Since the rate of secretion of cortisol is much higher, it can have significant mineralocorticoid effects (see **d** and **e**).

On a weight basis, it might seem that cortisol has limited mineralocorticoid importance as compared with aldosterone (Fig. 3.5b). However, when account is taken of cortisol's secretion rate, which is 100 times greater than that of aldosterone (Fig. 3.5c), and its 1000 times greater concentration in plasma, then its mineralocorticoid contribution is substantial compared with that of aldosterone. Therefore, it may have a much greater importance than is generally realized in regulating mineral metabolism. In man 70–90% of the mineralocorticoid effects of the venous effluent from the adrenal gland is attributable to secretion of aldosterone, but the rest is largely attributable to the effects of cortisol. However, cortisol is not the major factor in the controlling system for regulation of sodium, potassium and extracellular fluid volume, since its secretion does not vary with sodium intake.

*Transport of circulating cortisol*

In plasma there is a specific corticosteroid-binding globulin (transcortin) which is a glycoprotein of molecular weight 52 000 synthesized in liver. About 80% of the circulating cortisol is bound to this protein: serum albumin can bind some 15% of the circulating cortisol. If the concentration of cortisol is increased so that the specific binding sites are saturated, then much of the surplus is carried by albumin. Transcortin-bound cortisol is protected from metabolism and inactivation in liver. Transcortin has a much lower affinity for aldosterone (the circulating concentration of which is about one thousandth of that of cortisol). If the concentration of the binding proteins is elevated, then the total concentration of the hormone in plasma will be increased; this happens in pregnancy and in women taking a contraceptive pill. However, once a new equilibrium has been established, the concentration of 'free' hormone will be restored. Thus it is necessary to take account of the concentration of binding globulin when considering the physiological significance of a total steroid concentration determined in plasma.

EFFECTS OF OVERPRODUCTION OF CORTISOL

Overproduction of cortisol results in a characteristic clinical picture called Cushing's syndrome. One feature of this is obesity, which has a typical distribution affecting especially the face and the trunk. In contrast, peripherally, because of muscle wasting, the limbs seem thin, and the patient can complain of difficulty in climbing stairs. In addition, the skin may atrophy and develop characteristic purple striae, and as a result of weakness of blood vessels there will be spontaneous bruising. These changes are attributable to overproduction of cortisol (see Table 3.1) but in addition there may be evidence, in female patients, of virilization because of overproduction of male sex hormones which causes increased growth of hair (hirsutism), for example, on the face. Glucose tolerance is impaired and overproduction of glucocorticoids may cause diabetes mellitus. There may be an increase in the total white cell count but relatively few lymphocytes are present in the blood.

Continuous overproduction of steroids leads to loss of the normal circadian rhythm of cortisol production, so that the concentration of cortisol in the evening does not fall and is similar to the concentration in the morning. Clinically, it is important to decide whether the overproduction of glucocorticoids is due primarily to disease of the adrenal cortex. This is Cushing's

**Table 3.1** Changes due to increased glucocorticoid activity.

| Basic action | Effects in excess (Cushing's syndrome) |
|---|---|
| 1 Increased glucogenesis and hepatic glycogenesis and increased catabolism of protein | Diabetes mellitus<br>Muscle wasting; easily bruised thin skin; thin (osteoporotic) bones that easily fracture |
| 2 Increase and redistribution of body fat | Central obesity, 'moon faces', 'buffalo' hump, relatively thin limbs |
| 3 Involution of lymphatic and thymic tissue and reduced inflammatory response | Susceptibility to infection |
| 4 Increased secretion of acid by the stomach | Predisposition to gastric ulcer |
| 5 Suppression of release of adrenocorticotrophin | Adrenal cortical insufficiency with hypotension, following removal of source of excess steroid |
| 6 $Na^+$ retention: redistribution of body fluids | Hypertension |

syndrome, which can be due to a benign adenoma or to the development of a malignant tumour, a carcinoma. If the disorder is due to a primary change in the adrenal, then the treatment is removal of the abnormal adrenal tissue. If, however, the overactivity of the adrenal cortex is because it is overstimulated, as a result of overproduction of adrenocorticotrophin (Cushing's disease), then it may be more appropriate to operate on the pituitary where there may be a small tumour. Differentiation between a primary disorder of the adrenal, and secondary overactivity of the adrenal cortex because of a pituitary lesion, is best made by measuring the concentration of adrenocorticotrophin. If the pituitary is normal, then the high concentrations of cortisol will suppress the release of adrenocorticotrophin and its concentration in the plasma will be low. If, on the other hand, there is overproduction of adrenocorticotrophin, then obviously its concentration in plasma will be inappropriate to the concentration of cortisol. It is of interest to note that peptides like adrenocorticotrophin can be made in tissues other than the pituitary, for example, in a patient having an undifferentiated carcinoma in the lung causing very high concentrations of adrenocorticotrophin and fragments of the peptide in the circulation.

In Cushing's syndrome the plasma concentration of sodium and potassium is usually normal; the urinary excretion of cortisol is raised. There may, however, be electrolyte disturbances with a fall in the plasma potassium (hypokalaemia) which may contribute to the general weakness of the patient. This is especially likely if there is an anaplastic tumour that is producing large amounts of adrenocorticotrophin-like peptides and hence greatly increasing the synthesis of cortisol, the mineralocorticoid effects of which then become significant. Patients with inoperable malignant disease causing Cushing's syndrome can be treated with metyrapone, a drug which interferes with the biosynthesis of steroid hormones. Of course the effects of increased production of cortisol by the adrenal are also produced in patients treated with hormones with powerful glucocorticoid effects, such as cortisone and prednisone. If iatrogenic Cushing's syndrome develops as a result of this, then the therapy may have to be reduced: in this case care is necessary, since the production of adrenocorticotrophin will have been suppressed and the ability of the adrenal cortex to respond to stress will be impaired.

## Function of the zona glomerulosa

Aldosterone is produced exclusively in the zona glomerulosa (Fig. 3.6) and is the most potent hormone with mineralocorticoid activity produced by the adrenal gland.

EFFECTS OF ALDOSTERONE

The main sites of action of aldosterone are in the distal tubule and the collecting ducts of the kidney where it increases sodium reabsorption (so promoting retention of sodium) and increases the excretion of potassium and hydrogen ions. Sodium reabsorption is linked to the secretion of potassium and hydrogen ions, by a cation exchange mechanism. Aldosterone raises blood pressure, partly by increasing plasma volume and partly by increasing the sensitivity of the arteriolar muscle to vasoconstrictor agents. The response of an individual to administered aldosterone is only observed after a lag period of about 1 hour during which there is synthesis of a specific aldosterone-induced protein which promotes sodium transport. If administration of aldosterone is continued, the ability to excrete excess sodium is regained after 1−3 weeks, depending on sodium intake; this 'escape phenomenon' is almost certainly the result of re-adaptation of the feedback control system which is responsible for the regulation of the rate of reabsorption of filtered sodium in the proximal tubule.

SECRETION OF ALDOSTERONE

Despite the rate of aldosterone secretion being about 100 times lower than that of cortisol, it is responsible for about 80% of

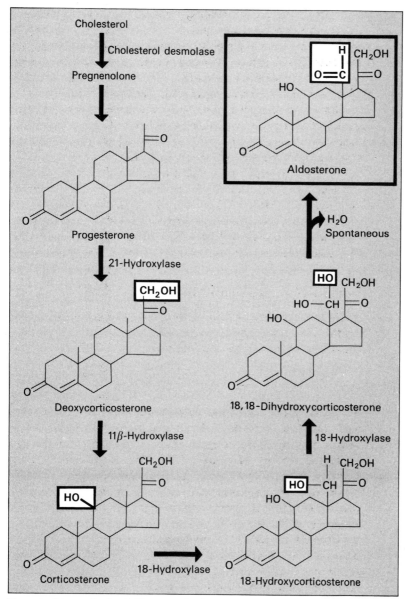

**Fig. 3.6** The synthesis of aldosterone in the zona glomerulosa.

the mineralocorticoid activity of the adrenal glandular secretion (Fig. 3.5). Aldosterone is more rapidly cleared from the circulation than cortisol, the half-life of disappearance is 20–30 minutes, as opposed to 100 minutes for cortisol. This rapid clearance of aldosterone is in part explicable by the fact that it is only bound to a limited extent by carrier proteins in the circulation. The circulating concentration of aldosterone is normally about 300 pmol/l, a thousand times lower than that of cortisol (300 nmol/l).

In animals maintained on low sodium diet, the secretion of aldosterone increases. The zona glomerulosa can double in thickness in 3 weeks. Initially, lipid is lost from the glomerulosa cells but this is gradually restored as the cells hypertrophy with an increase in the amount of smooth endoplasmic reticulum, Golgi complex and the number of mitochondria. Conversely, in animals maintained on high sodium diet the secretion rate falls and there is a decrease in the thickness of the glomerulosa by about 50%; cytoplasmic lipid content is reduced, while lysosomal bodies (autophagic vacuoles) are usually increased.

### THE RENIN–ANGIOTENSIN SYSTEM

This is the most important regulator of the secretion of aldosterone. It had been shown in the late 1890s that extracts of renal tissue could produce hypertension in experimental animals but it was not until 1936 that Goldblatt demonstrated that constriction of one renal artery (producing renal ischaemia) caused a slow rise in arterial pressure. This effect is due to the action of a substance called renin (Fig. 3.7) which is secreted by special cells in the juxtaglomerular region of the nephrons in the kidney (Fig. 3.8). These juxtaglomerular cells are found surrounding the afferent arteriole just before it enters the Malpighian corpuscle and breaks up into the glomerular capillaries. They are epithelioid in nature and replace the smooth muscle cells of the afferent arteriole at this point. They synthesize the proteolytic enzyme, renin, which is stored intracellularly in granules. Adjacent to the juxtaglomerular cells, are those of the macula densa which is a specialized part of the distal tubule. The juxtaglomerular cells and the macula densa form the juxtaglomerular apparatus. Release of renin is activated by a fall in plasma fluid volume; it is discharged from the cells by exocytosis and then diffuses into the lumen of the arterioles and thus into the circulation, where it has a half-life of about 20 minutes.

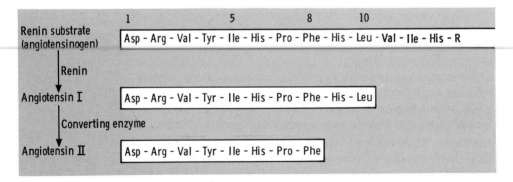

**Fig. 3.7** The human renin–angiotensin system; note that R in the substrate represents the rest of the $\alpha_2$ globulin.

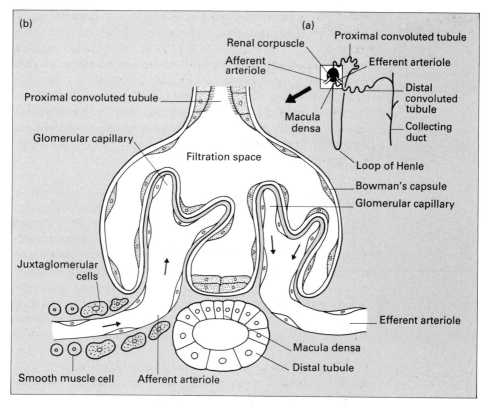

**Fig. 3.8** (**a**) *Top right*. The structure of a nephron. Note the renal corpuscle and its blood supply of an afferent and efferent arteriole. From the renal corpuscle arises the proximal convoluted tubule which straightens out to form the descending limb of the loop of Henle. The ascending limb forms the distal convoluted tubule before emptying into a collecting duct. Where the distal tubule lies between the afferent and efferent arterioles it forms the macula densa.

(**b**) The structure of a renal corpuscle, its blood supply and the juxtaglomerular apparatus. Note the afferent and efferent arterioles. Between them lie the glomerular capillaries which are surrounded by Bowman's capsule. The filtration space empties into the beginning of the proximal tubule. The juxtaglomerular apparatus consists firstly of the juxtaglomerular cells containing renin granules; these cells replace the smooth muscle cells of the afferent arteriole. In addition, the closely packed cells of the distal tubule form the second component of the juxtaglomerular apparatus, the macula densa.

Renin is a proteolytic enzyme which splits a leucine–valine bond (Fig. 3.8); its usual substrate is a circulating $\alpha_2$-globulin (angiotensinogen or renin substrate) which is made in the liver. Under the influence of renin, a decapeptide is split off from the angiotensinogen. The decapeptide is angiotensin I which is largely biologically inactive but is converted in several tissues into angiotensin II, an octapeptide and the most potent pressor substance known; it raises both systolic and diastolic blood pressures and so pulse pressure does not alter. The lung is the primary site of conversion of angiotensin I to angiotensin II, where its endothelial cells contain the appropriate endopeptidase.

Normally in man, the renin substrate of hepatic origin is present in adequate concentrations and the rate-limiting step for production of angiotensin II is the concentration of renin. For this reason plasma renin is usually taken to reflect any changes in plasma angiotensin II concentration, since the latter is more difficult to measure and its short half-life in the circulation is of the order of 1 minute.

Angiotensin II stimulates aldosterone secretion by an effect on the zona glomerulosa cells. It also has an action on peripheral arterioles and so can help maintain blood pressure both directly and indirectly. During sodium depletion, angiotensin II has a particularly potent effect on the renal circulation as it reduces the rate of glomerular filtration and in consequence reduces renal excretion of sodium. When injected in minute quantities directly into the hypothalamus of animals, it increases thirst, causing polydipsia. Since angiotensin II does not cross the blood–brain barrier, this effect may not be physiologically significant; however, renin has been found in brain tissue and so there may be local production of angiotensin II. Renin, or at least a closely related substance, is also present in the uterus and in salivary glands, but renin disappears from the circulation almost completely after nephrectomy so that the kidney must be the main source of circulating renin.

*Regulation of the production of renin*
Three factors control the secretion of renin by the kidney (Fig. 3.9). One of these is neural; the juxtaglomerular apparatus of the kidney is richly supplied by sympathetic neurones and destruction of this nerve supply leads to a blunting of the renin response to sodium depletion. The second important factor is the flux of sodium across the macula densa of the distal tubule. When the flux is high (as, for example, when sodium is plentiful) the secretion of renin is suppressed and it is clear that normally the renin–angiotensin system is not important in maintaining blood pressure in the sodium replete state. However, when the animal is sodium depleted, renin secretion increases and the effects of sodium on aldosterone production from the adrenal are largely mediated via the renin–angiotensin system, and this is essential for maintenance of blood pressure during sodium depletion. The third factor regulating renin production is the mean transmural pressure (as opposed to the pulse pressure); when the transmural pressure is high, renin secretion is suppressed, and when low the secretion of renin is stimulated. Another regulatory factor is the concentration of angiotensin II itself; it has been shown that infusion of angiotensin II into the renal circulation will sharply reduce the secretion of renin, forming a short-loop feedback system.

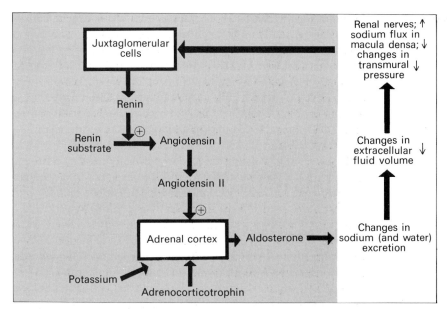

**Fig. 3.9** The factors which interact to control the secretion of aldosterone and renin and regulate extracellular fluid volume and total body sodium and water. For example, a fall in extracellular fluid volume produces increased activity in renal nerves, reduced sodium flux in the macula densa and a fall in transmural pressure (as shown by the thin arrows). These activate the juxtaglomerular apparatus which, through increased renin production, leads to more angiotensin and so stimulation of aldosterone secretion which helps restore extracellular fluid volume.

Plasma potassium has only a weak effect on the production of renin and what effect it does have is actually antagonistic to the direct effect which changes in potassium have on the secretion of aldosterone by the glomerulosa cells. For example, a low concentration of potassium in the plasma sharply reduces aldosterone secretion but at the same time it has a small but definite stimulatory effect on renin production. Because potassium can have a direct action on the adrenal as well as an effect on production of renin, there can be a dissociation between the production of aldosterone and the amount of renin present in some situations.

*Interplay of factors regulating the secretion of aldosterone*
Angiotensin II, potassium and adrenocorticotrophin can directly stimulate the rate of secretion of aldosterone (Fig. 3.9), as can melanocyte stimulating hormone, while somatostatin and atrial natriuretic peptide (see below) can inhibit aldosterone secretion. The effects of potassium can be seen when plasma volume is constant—then small changes of potassium within the physiological range affect aldosterone secretion. The dependence of the aldosterone secretion rate on plasma volume is mediated by the renin–angiotensin system which can override any opposing changes in the plasma concentration of potassium and adrenocorticotrophin. For example, the secretion of aldosterone

rises during the morning (because of the fall in plasma volume on assuming an upright posture) even though the secretion of adrenocorticotrophin falls during the day. Injection of adrenocorticotrophin can stimulate aldosterone production but this effect lasts only 24–48 hours even if adrenocorticotrophic hormone is administered repeatedly. This is because the aldosterone-producing cells no longer respond to adrenocorticotrophin. This is not due to salt retention affecting the glomerulosa cells since it can occur on a low sodium diet. Lack of adrenocorticotrophin as a result of hypophysectomy or disease does not significantly reduce aldosterone production and overproduction of aldosterone is not a consequence of prolonged excessive secretion of adrenocorticotrophin.

ATRIAL NATRIURETIC PEPTIDE

A number of physiological experiments have indicated the existence of natriuretic substances (i.e. substances that increase the excretion of sodium). In 1981 de Bold and his colleagues showed that extracts of the atrium of the heart could increase the excretion of sodium and of water. The atrial muscle cells (cardiocytes) synthesize a peptide which is stored in secretory granules. This peptide has been isolated from both the left and the right atria. The secretory granules contain a prohormone with 126 amino acids, while the secreted form of the hormone has only 28 amino acids, with an intrachain disulphide bond. The gene encoding the peptide has been cloned and expressed in eukaryotic systems and a synthetic peptide has been made. Secreted by the heart into the bloodstream, the peptide is rapidly removed from the circulation. Specific receptors for the peptide have been found in the glomeruli and in the medullary collecting ducts of the kidney, in the zona glomerulosa of the adrenal cortex and in peripheral arterioles. It also accumulates, for reasons which are not clear, in the paraventricular nuclei of the hypothalamus.

A graded release of atrial natriuretic peptide occurs in response to increased stretching of the isolated rat heart. In intact animals, a graded increase in blood volume also stimulates a progressive release of the hormone. Increase of sodium intake and of water can both stimulate the discharge of the secretory granules containing the peptide from heart muscle. The response to atrial natriuretic peptide is best studied in conscious animals, since anaesthesia itself affects renal handling of salt and water. Atrial natriuretic peptide causes a fall in plasma renin and in the concentration of circulating aldosterone, and increases renal blood flow. It promotes the excretion of water, possibly by inhibiting the action of antidiuretic hormone. The increase in sodium excretion is due largely to a rise in the rate of glomerular filtration, and also to inhibition of sodium reabsorption in the medullary collecting duct. Atrial natriuretic peptide relaxes vascular smooth muscle and inhibits vasoconstriction produced by angiotensin II. Although it is clear that atrial natriuretic peptide in animals is a potent hormone, its precise role in man still remains to be established.

## EFFECTS OF EXCESSIVE ALDOSTERONE SECRETION

The discovery of aldosterone led to the recognition of clinically important disorders of aldosterone production. These may arise either because of a primary abnormality of the adrenal zona glomerulosa or, secondarily, because of extrarenal disease leading to a sustained increase in the concentration of circulating renin. Conn recognized a syndrome characterized by systemic hypertension associated with potassium depletion, with low plasma and urine potassium, and alkalosis. This is primary hyperaldosteronism. The patient often complains of muscle weakness and might have cramps and even spasm, particularly of the hands (so-called carpopedal spasm). It might be expected, because of the sodium retaining effect of aldosterone, that there may be oedema. However, this is usually not the case because there is an 'escape' mechanism from sodium retention which operates after 1−3 weeks, depending on the initial stores of sodium.

Hyperaldosteronism, without hypertension, can occur when there is resistance to the cardiovascular effects of angiotensin; this is Bartter's syndrome, which is characterized by hypokalaemia causing muscle weakness. The resistance to the hypertensive effect of angiotensin is probably due to the presence of excess prostaglandins which are vasodilators, unlike angiotensin which is a vasoconstrictor. In this syndrome the overproduction of renin by the juxtaglomerular apparatus is probably due to over-stimulation by prostaglandins which increase renin release: this can be treated by administration of inhibitors of prostaglandin synthetase, such as indomethacin.

Secondary hyperaldosteronism can be caused by hypoprotein-aemia which can arise from liver or renal disease. Because of the reduced oncotic pressure, there is redistribution of the extra-cellular fluid so that more is present interstitially and hence plasma volume is reduced. This stimulates production of renin and the latter increases secretion of aldosterone; retention of sodium then occurs and oedema develops. Narrowing of the renal arteries can also cause secondary aldosteronism, with hypertension.

In the differentiation of the causes of hyperaldosteronism, the concentration of aldosterone in relation to renin is important. In primary aldosteronism the concentration of renin will be low, while in secondary hyperaldosteronism, the concentration of renin (and therefore angiotensin II) is high.

The production of sex steroids (androgens in the male and oestrogens and progestogens in the female) is mainly from the gonads and is therefore considered in Chapter 4. However, the adrenal cortex can contribute by production of androstenedione (Fig. 3.10). The two main androgens, testosterone and di-hydrotestosterone, are formed in peripheral tissues from andro-stenedione. Also some oestrogen can be released from the adrenals or formed peripherally from dehydro*epi*androsterone sulphate (DHEAS), a weak androgen secreted by the adrenals. The role of sex steroids produced as a result of adrenal cortical activity is not entirely clear: their synthesis is important to growth of body hair in females and may become more important in disease. Before the onset of puberty of a normal child the secretion of dehydro*epi*androsterone sulphate rises sharply. This coincides with the final maturation of the zona reticularis and is called the adrenarche. In man and other primates the circulating con-centration of the dehydro*epi*androsterone is high (about 10 times

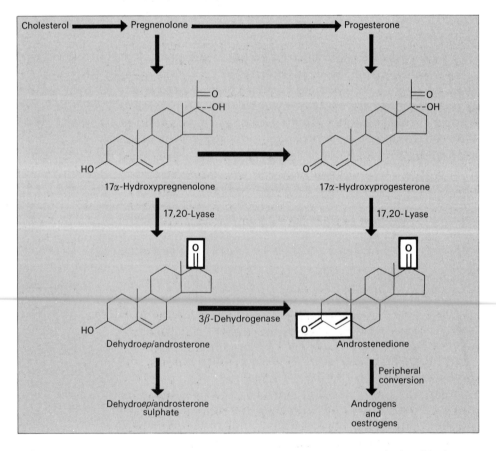

**Fig. 3.10**   The production of precursors of sex hormones in the adrenal cortex.

that of cortisol) but this is not so in other species and so the role of this steroid remains unclear.

## THE EFFECTS OF DEFICIENT FUNCTION OF THE ADRENAL CORTEX

In Addison's disease, there is adrenocortical failure, which causes deficiency both of cortisol and of aldosterone. The patient complains of weakness and lethargy and may present with severe loss of weight. On examination they will be found to be hypotensive and excessive pigmentation will be present. This is particularly noticeable in the skin folds but may also be found in the mouth. The increased pigmentation is the result of increased production of adrenocorticotrophin due to lack of suppression of the hypothalamic–pituitary axis (see Chapter 2). The serum potassium is raised while the serum sodium is low, and blood urea is generally raised. Addison's disease must be treated immediately. Acutely, it is necessary to give intravenous saline, while the long-term management requires administration of hormones with glucocorticoid and mineralocorticoid actions. Cortisone is generally given for its glucocorticoid properties: the dose in adults is about 25 mg/day given in divided doses, often 15 mg in the morning and 10 mg in the evening. This will suppress the overproduction of adrenocorticotrophin. For a mineralo-corticoid effect it is not feasible to administer aldosterone because it has a very short half-life, but a potent synthetic mineralocorticoid, 9$\alpha$-fluorohydrocortisone, can be given. It is important, of course, to note the difference between the management of adrenal insufficiency because of removal or destruction of the adrenal glands as opposed to the adrenal insufficiency that arises from pituitary failure; in the latter case aldosterone production is unaffected by the deficiency of adrenocorticotrophin and the only steroid therapy needed is cortisone (or hydrocortisone i.e. cortisol).

## THE EFFECTS OF DEFICIENCY OF THE ENZYMES INVOLVED IN THE BIOSYNTHESIS OF STEROID HORMONES

Specific enzyme deficiencies in the pathways of biosynthesis of steroid hormone have been recognized and study of them has advanced our understanding of these metabolic pathways, just as knowledge of the biosynthetic steps has helped to explain the clinical manifestations (Fig. 3.11). These enzyme deficiencies can occur in both the adrenal cortex and the gonads, if the particular enzyme involved is common to both steroidogenic tissues; then an adrenal disorder can be complicated by alteration in sexual maturation. A feature of many of these conditions is reduced capacity for synthesis of cortisol. Most commonly this

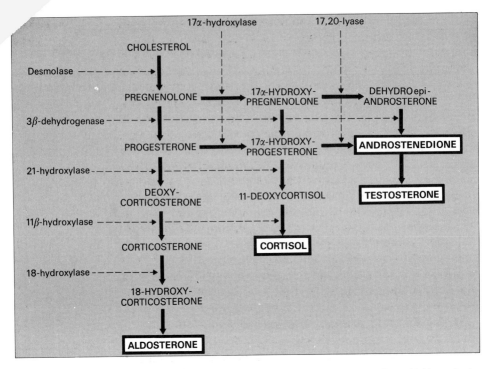

**Fig. 3.11** A schematic representation of the pathways of steroid biosynthesis.

The effects of deficiency of any of the enzymes involved can be deduced by consideration of these pathways. For example, deficiency of desmolase means that no steroids can be made and therefore there is a lack of aldosterone, cortisol and androgens. The results of this include sodium loss and, in the male infant, sexual ambiguity. If the condition is treated by administration of hormones with mineralocorticoid and glucocorticoid effects, then later another problem becomes apparent; that is a failure to enter puberty. Similarly, deficiency of 3β-dehydrogenase again causes a failure of production of aldosterone, cortisol, androstenedione and testosterone. The lack of testosterone causes sexual ambiguity in male infants, while in female infants there may be sexual ambiguity because dehydroepiandosterone is made and causes masculinization. There is failure of onset of puberty in both sexes.

By contrast, deficiency of 17α-hydroxylase causes increased production of hormones with mineralocorticoid activity as a result of overproduction of adrenocorticotrophin; a consequence of this is hypertension. Differentiation of female infants is normal but that of males is ambiguous. Later in life, because of lack of production of oestrogens, females do not enter puberty, nor do males. Deficiency of 21-hydroxylase is the commonest cause of congenital adrenal hyperplasia. Salt loss can be a serious feature of this deficiency as is sexual ambiguity in the female at birth.

Deficiency of 11β-hydroxylase has the same effect as that of deficiency of 21-hydroxylase, except that deoxycorticosterone can be made so that hypertension may be a problem.

All of these deficiences cause congenital adrenal hyperplasia because of compensatory overproduction of adrenocorticotrophin. Lack of 18-hydroxylase does not cause congenital adrenal hyperplasia because cortisol production is normal; however there is failure of aldosterone secretion and sodium loss. Lack of 17,20-lyase causes problems with sexual differentiation, without leading to adrenal hyperplasia and no sex steroids can be made, so there are problems with puberty in both sexes.

is due to a deficiency of 21-hydroxylase which, with an incidence in Europe and the USA of between 1 in 5000 and 1 in 15000, accounts for 90–95% of cases. To compensate, there is overproduction of adrenocorticotrophin which produces an important feature of this group of conditions—enlargement of the adrenal glands that gives them the generic name of 'congenital adrenal hyperplasia'. The increased secretion of adrenocorticotrophin stimulates growth of the adrenal gland and, in fact, may ensure that cortisol production is adequate. Therefore, the major feature of congenital adrenal hyperplasia is that the circulating concentration of cortisol is normal while that of adrenocorticotrophin is inappropriately high. The other features of congenital adrenal hyperplasia depend on which enzyme is deficient; there may be deficiency of aldosterone production which results in a sodium-losing state which leads to hypotension. There can also be a defect in the synthesis of testosterone; *in utero* this leads to a failure of masculinization of the fetus and the baby is therefore born with ambiguous genitalia. Later on, in females, a defect in the synthesis of oestrogen may lead to failure of onset of puberty with inability to menstruate, that is, primary amenorrhoea.

Apart from the effects of deficiency of production of aldosterone, cortisol or testosterone, the features of congenital adrenal hyperplasia may include the consequences of overproduction of some of the other hormones as a result of the increased drive from adrenocorticotrophin. For example, if there is overproduction of deoxycorticosterone then hypertension will be a feature. Similarly, if there is overproduction of dehydro*epi*androsterone, androstenedione or testosterone, masculinization of a female will occur because they are androgenic.

Identification of the enzyme deficiency depends on measuring circulating steroids and identifying those which are deficient and those which are produced in excess. For example, there is an accumulation of progesterone and 17$\alpha$-hydroxyprogesterone if there is a deficiency of the 21-hydroxylase in both the zona glomerulosa and the zona fasciculata/reticularis.

Treatment of these disorders requires provision of replacement of those hormones that are not being made in sufficient amounts and suppression of the overproduction of adrenocorticotrophin; the latter is achieved by treatment with cortisol in physiological amounts. Clearly an understanding of the pathophysiology is important if these conditions are to be treated logically, and effectively.

## FUNCTION OF THE ADRENAL MEDULLA

The principal hormones of the adrenal medulla are catecholamines and in the adult 80% of the catecholamine content consists of adrenaline; the remaining 20% is noradrenaline, which was identified by von Euler as a neurotransmitter. The adrenal medulla thus differs from the sympathetic nervous system which only releases noradrenaline. As has already been stated, while the adrenal medulla is not vital for survival, it does contribute to the response to stress.

Much of the volume of the cytoplasm of the cells in the medulla is occupied by granules which are the storage sites of the catecholamines (Fig. 3.12). They also contain proteins, some of which are soluble; at least 12 such soluble proteins have been identified including dopamine $\beta$-hydroxylase which can be either soluble or bound to the granule membrane. The remainder of the soluble proteins are called chromogranins and are found within the matrix of the granule. The storage granules

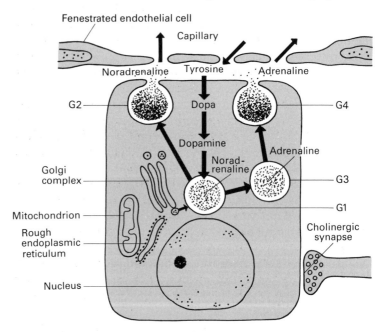

**Fig. 3.12** The synthesis, storage and release of catecholamines in an adrenal medullary chromaffin cell. The protein components of the storage granules (G), including the chromogranins, are sythesized on the rough endoplasmic reticulum and packaged in the Golgi complex to form the granule. Tyrosine enters the cell, is enzymically converted to dopa and then dopamine in the cytoplasm. Dopamine enters a granule (G1) and is converted by the enzyme dopamine $\beta$-hydroxylase to noradrenaline. The noradrenaline can then be released exocytotically (G2) when it then diffuses into the local fenestrated capillary. Alternatively, noradrenaline can be further converted by phenylethanolamine transferase to adrenaline in a different storage granule (G3), where it can also be released exocytotically (G4). Each cell has a cholinergic synapse, where acetylcholine is released which initiates the train of events leading to exocytosis. The nucleus and a mitochondrion are also shown.

Although the cell in this diagram is shown secreting both of the catecholamines, chromaffin cells usually only secrete either noradrenaline or adrenaline.

also contain phenylethanolamine *N*-methyl transferase, which is important in the methylation of noradrenaline, i.e. its conversion to adrenaline. In the granules, ATP forms a loose, high molecular weight complex with the catecholamines. The membranes of the chromaffin granules are characterized by their high levels of lysolecithin. Each chromaffin cell is innervated by a cholinergic, preganglionic sympathetic neurone which releases acetylcholine. These synapses are the terminations of fibres carried in the splanchnic nerves, whose cell bodies lie mainly between $T_3$ and $L_3$. Acetylcholine stimulates the release of catecholamines from the chromaffin cells by depolarizing them; an accompanying influx of $Ca^{2+}$ occurs, which leads to the membrane of the granules fusing with the plasma membrane. Exocytosis of the granule contents then occurs. The contents are released into the extracellular space where they diffuse into the local blood supply. This process is known as 'stimulus secretion coupling'. The granule membrane then seals off, detaches itself from the cell membrane and is ready for recycling again. It is also possible that catecholamines may leak out of the granules and leave the cell by diffusion through the plasma membrane.

The chromaffin cells of the adrenal medulla also synthesize and store a number of opioid peptides, particularly met-enkephalin and leu-enkephalin. The sequence of these two opioid peptides are Tyr-Gly-Gly-Phe-Met and Tyr-Gly-Gly-Phe-Leu respectively: thus they differ only in the carboxy-terminal residues and it is from these that they derive their names. They are formed by proteolytic cleavage of pro-enkephalin A which consists of 267 amino acids: within that sequence are six copies of met-enkephalin and one of leu-enkephalin. The structure of enkephalin A (Fig. 3.13) was deduced from analysis of the sequences of bases in a complementary DNA prepared from adrenal medulla. An additional sequence of a signal peptide with 24 amino acids was also identified in the DNA thus giving the structure of pre-pro-enkephalin A.

There are two important groups of larger opioid peptides, those that begin with a met-enkephalin sequence followed by additional amino acid residues on the carboxy-terminal side and those that begin with the sequence of leu-enkephalin. The former group (those containing the met-enkephalin penta-peptide) includes $\alpha$-, $\gamma$- and $\beta$-endorphins with 16, 17 and 31 amino acids respectively. They are found in $\beta$-lipotrophin which is formed from pro-opiomelanocortin along with adrenocorticotrophic hormone in the pituitary. These met-enkephalins are respectively derived from residues $61-76$, $61-77$ and $61-91$ of $\beta$-lipotrophin. Pre-pro-opiomelanocortin has 284 amino acids, including the 20 residues in its signal peptide (see Chapter 2). The leu-enkephalin-containing opioid peptides include the dynorphins with 8, 17 or 29 amino acids, $\alpha$-neo-endorphin

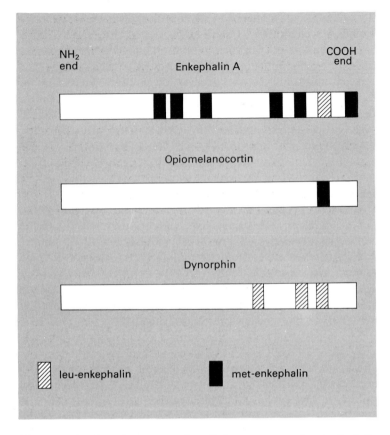

**Fig. 3.13** A schematic representation of the occurrence of met-enkephalin and of leu-enkephalin sequences in three larger peptides (see also Fig. 2.5 which shows the family of peptides derived from one of these).

with 9 and $\beta$-neo-endorphin with 10 residues. These are present in nerve fibres and may also be found in the adrenal medulla: they are neurotransmitters which can bind to opioid receptors without removal of the carboxy-terminal extension. They are all contained within and are derived from a single precursor protein called prodynorphin (or pro-enkephalin B). Thus there are three distinct parent proteins, namely enkephalin A, opiomelanocortin and dynorphin, each with a distinct family of peptides that can be formed from them (Fig. 3.13).

In the adrenal medulla met-enkephalin and leu-enkephalin are packaged with chromagranin A and adrenaline, noradrenaline and other peptides with which they are co-secreted. The roles of the adrenal enkephalins remain to be established. Leu-enkephalin reacts particularly with $\delta$ receptors (associated with inhibition of activation of adenalate cyclase) while met-enkephalin binds to the $\mu$-receptors that are associated with the classical effects of morphine such as analgesia. The secretion of enkephalins from the adrenal medulla may account for the ability of runners to overcome pain and the production of a euphoric state over long distances, through the production of endogenous analgesics.

SECRETION OF CATECHOLAMINES

The synthesis of noradrenaline and then of adrenaline from tyrosine occurs in four steps (Fig. 3.14). The first step, the conversion of tyrosine to 3,4-dihydroxyphenylalanine (dopa) by tyrosine hydroxylase, is the rate-limiting step. Regulation of this enzyme is controlled by negative feedback in the adrenal. Noradrenaline and dopamine reduce the activity of tyrosine hydroxylase

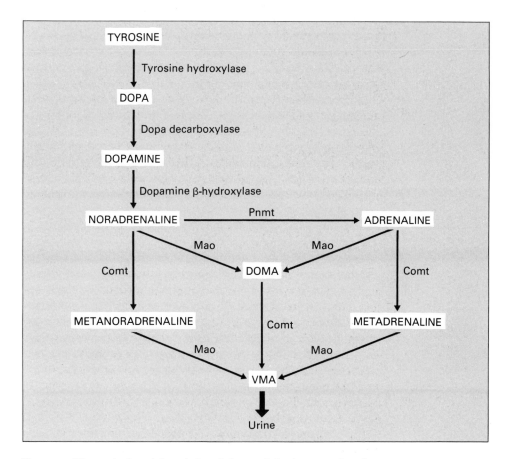

**Fig. 3.14** The synthesis and degradation of the catecholamines, noradrenaline and adrenaline.

Dopa = 3,4-dihydroxyphenylalanine; dopamine = 3,4-dihydroxyphenyl-ethylamine; Pnmt = phenylethanolamine-$N$-methyl transferase; Mao = mono-amine oxidase; Comt = catechol-$O$-methyl-transferase; doma = 3,4-dihydroxymandelic acid; VMA = vanillylmandelic acid (3-methoxy-4-hydroxymandelic acid).

by combining with its co-factor, tetrahydropteridine. The conversion of noradrenaline to adrenaline, by phenylethanolamine-$N$-methyl transferase requires the presence of a high concentration of glucocorticoids, which is provided by the portal vein system already described, within the adrenal gland (Fig. 3.2).

In addition to the action of acetylcholine on chromaffin cells, histamine, 5-hydroxytryptamine and acetylcholine-like substances (such as nicotine and carbachol) can also cause release of hormones. Any substance which increases the activity of the vasomotor centre in the medulla oblongata in the brain stem will also indirectly provoke release of catecholamines. The output of these hormones can be changed in a number of different ways. Thus, $\alpha$-methyltyrosine reduces hormone synthesis by inhibiting the rate-limiting step dependent on tyrosine hydroxylase. In contrast, treatment with reserpine depletes the vesicles of their hormone content; administration of ganglion-blocking drugs, such as hexamethonium, will impede access of acetylcholine to the nicotinic receptors on the adrenal medullary cells and so decrease catecholamine secretions.

There is some evidence to suggest that the proportions of adrenaline and noradrenaline released will differ according to the emotional circumstances; fear may provoke a preferential increase in plasma adrenaline concentration, while anger favours an increase in noradrenaline concentration, but the relative contributions of the sympathetic nervous system and the adrenal medulla to the rise of noradrenaline, however, are difficult to separate.

*The fate of adrenaline and noradrenaline*

Uptake in cells is also important in terminating the actions of the two hormones. Noradrenaline in particular can be taken up into postganglionic sympathetic nerve terminals (uptake 1) where it can then be metabolized by monoamine oxidase. Most of the noradrenaline taken up in this way from the circulation will enter the storage vesicles where it becomes available for re-use as a neurotransmitter. Adrenaline, and to a lesser extent noradrenaline, can also be removed by non-neuronal uptake (uptake 2) and since no storage occurs in such tissues, for example in platelets, the hormones will be almost wholly metabolized if taken up in this way.

Metabolism plays a minor role in terminating the action of circulating adrenaline and noradrenaline (Fig. 3.14). The enzymes involved in this are catechol-$O$-methyl transferase and monoamine oxidase and among the many end-products the main one is vanillylmandelic acid (VMA). These two enzymes are distributed widely throughout the body, particularly in the liver. Catechol-$O$-methyl transferase is found in non-neuronal tissue in association with its co-factor, $S$-adenosyl methionine, whereas monoamine oxidase occurs in mitochondria in both neuronal and non-neuronal tissues. The two hormones are found in urine; 5% is unchanged but 95% represents metabolites of adrenaline and noradrenaline. Removal of the adrenal medulla leads to loss of all urinary adrenaline.

EFFECTS AND MODE OF ACTION OF CATECHOLAMINES

Adrenaline increases systolic blood pressure but reduces diastolic blood pressure so that there is little change in mean pressure. Tachycardia occurs and gut motility is reduced with secondary closure of the sphincters. Adrenaline is a bronchodilator and can also cause piloerection. Topical application of high concentrations of adrenaline onto the conjunctivae causes dilation of the pupil (mydriasis). The systemic effects of noradrenaline are rather different; it raises both systolic and diastolic pressure and so increases the mean blood pressure, it causes bradycardia which is reflex and can be blocked by prior administration of atropine, it has much less effect in reducing gut motility than adrenaline, and it does not produce bronchodilatation. However, like adrenaline, noradrenaline causes piloerection and dilation of the pupils.

The metabolic effects of adrenaline are also important. It promotes hepatic glycogenolysis, which leads to the production of glucose-6-phosphate. This in turn leads to hyperglycaemia and lactic-acidaemia, due to further metabolism in the liver and muscle respectively (see Chapter 7). Adrenaline also increases the plasma concentration of free fatty acids. Noradrenaline is much less potent than adrenaline in producing hepatic glycogenolysis but is more potent in causing mobilization of free fatty acids.

The difference between the effects of adrenaline and noradrenaline are partially explained by the existence of two populations of receptors on the surface of effector cells, referred to as $\alpha$- and $\beta$-adrenoreceptors. The receptors have been defined on the basis of their blockade by certain other synthetic pharmacological agents. This blockade (antagonism) therefore provides a convenient method of classification of these receptors, although the physiological significance of $\alpha$- and $\beta$-type activities has not yet been resolved. Interaction with $\alpha$-adrenoreceptors produces effects which are predominantly excitatory while interaction with $\beta$-adrenoreceptors produces effects which are predominantly inhibitory. The $\beta$-adrenoreceptors can be further subdivided into $\beta_1$ and $\beta_2$-receptors by employing pharmacologically produced analogues. Noradrenaline interacts only with $\alpha$- and $\beta_1$-receptors, it cannot cause bronchodilatation and it is less potent on the gut. In blood vessels noradrenaline only has vasoconstrictor actions but in those blood vessels which have $\alpha$- and

$\beta_2$-receptors, adrenaline can cause dilatation in low concentrations. In studying the effects of injected noradrenaline, consideration of the reflex changes is important since noradrenaline reflexly reduces sympathetic activity while also increasing vagal activity.

Metabolically, as opposed to neurologically, the $\beta$-adrenoreceptor is closely associated with the adenylate cyclase system. In both cardiac and bronchial muscle, containing $\beta_1$- and $\beta_2$-adreno-receptors respectively, administration of adrenaline increases the production of cyclic AMP. However, the $\alpha$-adrenoreceptor is not linked to adenylate cyclase and the mechanism involved is not yet established.

THE EFFECTS OF OVERPRODUCTION OF CATECHOLAMINES

A phaeochromocytoma is a tumour of chromaffin tissue which can occur in 1:10000 of the population; in about 10% of the cases the tumours are multiple. Generally they are benign but a proportion (about 10%) are malignant. Usually the phaeo-chromocytoma arises in the adrenal medulla but occasionally it can arise in the paraganglia, anywhere from the base of the skull to the pelvic floor.

These tumours oversecrete adrenaline and noradrenaline in various proportions; they may do so continuously, or the secretion may be intermittent. The clinical manifestations depend on the relative amounts of noradrenaline and adrenaline. Since all phaeochromocytomata produce an absolute excess of noradrenaline, the predominant feature is nearly always systemic hypertension. This is sustained in most patients but can be paroxysmal in a minority (25%). Sudden release of catecholamines can cause attacks with severe symptoms, bursts of headache, sweating and apprehension; these symptoms may be precipitated by cold, by fasting, by exercise or by pressure on the tumour. Overt diabetes mellitus develops in about 10% of patients with a phaeochro-mocytoma and many patients may show an impaired glucose tolerance. Whether or not carbohydrate metabolism is affected will depend on the quantity of adrenaline secreted. If a child develops a phaeochromocytoma, carbohydrate metabolism is not affected, presumably because their adrenal glands produce predominantly noradrenaline. The increase in the metabolic rate and the apprehension that is produced, sometimes mimics thyrotoxicosis. In patients who have continuous secretion of noradrenaline alone, hypertension will be sustained and there will be no disturbance of carbohydrate metabolism, so differen-tiation from other causes of rise of blood pressure can be difficult.

Support for the diagnosis can be obtained by measurement of catecholamines and their principal metabolites, vanillylmandelic acid or metadrenaline and metanoradrenaline in urine. It can also be useful to measure the concentrations of circulating adrenaline and noradrenaline. Since adrenaline is only secreted by the adrenal medulla (unlike noradrenaline which is widely released from sympathetic tissue) measurement of circulating adrenaline can be very valuable. It is, however, necessary to exclude the effects of anxiety—this can be done by giving pentolinium, i.e. a ganglion-blocking agent. Although the majority of tumours arise in the adrenal glands, it is important to try to localize the tumour before attempting surgical removal. For this purpose analysis of adrenaline and noradrenaline in samples of blood obtained from different sites in the inferior and superior vena cava can sometimes be useful.

Treatment is by surgical removal of the tumour. Before the operation it is necessary to block the action of the catecholamines. For this purpose phenoxybenzamine, which is an $\alpha_1$-blocking agent, and propranolol, which has $\beta_1$- and $\beta_2$-blocking actions, are important. Phenoxybenzamine alkylates the receptors irreversibly, and recovery then requires synthesis of new receptors, so its effects can last 3 or 4 days. When a patient is adequately treated with these drugs, removal of the tumour is less hazardous. Although a phaeochromocytoma accounts for less than 1% of all cases of hypertension, it is one of the few causes of hypertension that can be cured; thus it is important to identify oversecretion of catecholamines as a cause for elevation of the blood pressure.

## SUMMARY

The adrenal cortex is a complicated structure with three clearly distinct cell types each performing a different function. The outer layer of zona glomerulosa cells synthesizes aldosterone and releases this steroid hormone in response to stimulation by angiotension II or increases in potassium concentration. Aldosterone has potent mineralocorticoid activity and is involved, along with other hormonal and neural systems, in regulating sodium balance and blood pressure. The adrenal cortex also contains two other cell types in the zona fasciculata and reticularis regions which respond to adrenocorticotrophin and yield cortisol (in man), plus a variety of other steroid hormones possessing mainly glucocorticoid activities. This region is probably also responsible for producing certain androgens and oestrogens secreted by the adrenal gland. The central region of the gland is the medulla, where the hormones adrenaline and noradrenaline are stored in granules. These require cholinergic, preganglionic sympathetic stimulation for release of their contents into the circulation. Adrenaline stimulates glycogenolysis and an increase in circulating free fatty acids, while noradrenaline is more potent in the latter action. Both hormones are vasoactive, although only noradrenaline increases blood pressure.

BALFOUR W. E. (1985) Blood volume regulation: on the right lines at last. *Nature* **314**, 226–7.

BESSER G. M. and REES L. H. (Eds) (1985) The pituitary–adrenocortical axis. In *Clinics in Endocrinology and Metabolism*, Vol. 14, No. 4. W. B. Saunder Co. London, Philadelphia, Toronto.

GELLAI M. *et al.* (1986) The effect of atrial natriuretic factor on blood pressure, heart rate and renal functions in conscious, spontaneously hyperactive rats. *Circulation Research*, **59**, 50–62.

IMURA H. *et al.* (1985) Endogenous opiods and related peptides: from molecular biology to clinical medicine. Sir Henry Dale Lecture. *Journal of Endocrinology* **177**, 147–57.

MAKIN H. L. J. (1984) *Biochemistry of Steroid Hormones*. Blackwell Scientific Publications, Oxford.

COOPER J. R., BLOOM F. E. & ROTH R. H. (1986) *The Biochemical Basis of Neuropharmacology*, 5th edn. Oxford University Press, Oxford.

# 4 Reproductive endocrinology

Reproductive endocrinology is concerned with the role of the sex hormones and the associated hypothalamic and pituitary hormones in the reproductive life. These are all important at various stages of life, starting with the formation of gametes, the development of the embryo and the fetus, and the differentiation of the phenotypic sexual characteristics. The changes at puberty are dependent on the sex hormones. These hormones have a special role in the female during pregnancy and at parturition; they are also required for lactation. Later, the changes at the menopause are attributable to an altered endocrine status.

Historically the scientific study of gamete formation can be regarded as having stemmed from 1647 when Leeuwenhoek and Ham first observed human sperm under the microscope, thus identifying the material basis of the male's contribution to conception. Twenty-six years earlier, Harvey had argued from his observations on hybrids that the female also contributed to conception and in his *De Generatione* generalized that 'an egg is the common origin of all animals'. Even so, the discovery of the development of the mammalian ovum in the ovarian Graafian follicle had to wait until 1822 when von Bauer published his description of its formation.

The thought that, besides the gametes, the gonads also produced substances which had more general effects on the body arose from Berthold's experiments in 1849. He showed that transplantation of a cock's testes into a capon induced normal development of a cock's comb in the castrated animal. Much later, in 1911, Pezard induced comb growth in capons by injections of testicular extracts. However, the active principle, testosterone, was not crystallized until 1935 when bulls' testes were used as the source. The thought that the ovary also produced substances which affected other bodily activities was suggested by Beard, after Sobotta in 1896 had described the origin of the corpus luteum in the ovary. Beard postulated a relationship between the activity of the corpus luteum and pregnancy, a concept confirmed by Ancel and Bouin in 1910. The ovarian oestrogens were isolated and crystallized between 1919 and 1930. This was followed by the purification of progesterone from the corpus luteum by Corner and Allen between 1918 and 1930; they showed that it could prevent the abortion that usually followed removal of the ovaries, that is ovariectomy or oophorectomy, in early pregnancy. In 1932 Moore and Price made the important suggestion that release of gonadotrophins from the pituitary was subject to feedback control by the gonadal sex hormones. Appreciation of the contribution of the Y chromosome in the determination of genetic sex had to await some 100 years after the recognition of the existence of chromosomes in 1820 and the role of testosterone in determining phenotypic sex differentiation was only more recently elucidated by Jost in the 1950s. Thus the scene was gradually set for our understanding of reproductive endocrinology.

In this chapter the male will be considered first, then the female and finally the endocrinological control of the development of the reproductive system will be described.

## THE MALE REPRODUCTIVE SYSTEM

The male gonad has two important functions: firstly, the production of the gametes (spermatogenesis) and secondly, the synthesis of the male sex hormones (androgens). The androgens are involved not only in the process of spermatogenesis but also in the initiation and maintenance of male characteristics and the secondary sexual glands. Indeed, a compound is defined as having androgenic activity on the basis of its ability to masculinize the genitalia and maintain the activity of the accessory sexual organs.

### Morphology

Spermatozoa are produced in the seminiferous tubules of the testes. Each testis is attached to an epididymis into which the tubules lead and in which maturation of sperm occurs. From the epididymis, the vas deferens leads to the urethra. In the testes there is a clear-cut separation between the seminiferous tubules (which make up the bulk of the tissue and produce sperm) and the lipid-laden, interstitial cells of Leydig (which lie between the tubules and are the steroid-synthesizing cells). In the seminiferous tubules there are two types of cell, the germ cells and the Sertoli cells (Fig. 4.1). Tight junctions between adjacent Sertoli cells produce two compartments in which the extracellular milieu is very different; there is a basal compartment and an adluminal compartment. In the basal compartment are found the spermatogonia and in the adluminal, the spermatocytes, spermatids and sperm.

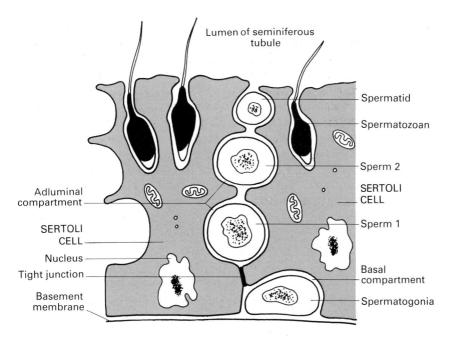

Lumen of seminiferous tubule

Spermatid

Spermatozoan

Sperm 2

SERTOLI CELL

Adluminal compartment

Sperm 1

SERTOLI CELL

Nucleus

Tight junction

Basal compartment

Basement membrane

Spermatogonia

**Fig. 4.1** The structure of the wall of a seminiferous tubule. Sertoli cells span the thickness of the tubule from the surrounding basement membrane to its lumen. Two Sertoli cells are shown (shaded) in the figure. Tight junctions between adjacent Sertoli cells separate the spermatogonia in a basal compartment from the other stages in spermatogenesis in an adluminal compartment. The Sertoli cells closely surround the primary (sperm 1) and secondary (sperm 2) spermatocytes, the spermatids and sperm.

## SPERMATOGENESIS

The primordial germ cells are laid down in the testes in the fetal period. Once they are committed to becoming spermatogonia, no further development to form spermatozoa takes place until puberty. In adolescent and adult life, spermatogonia continually augment their numbers by mitotic division. They appear to be of two types; type A which are reserve spermatogonia and which divide to give more of type A, or, after several divisions, type B which are destined to move from the basal compartment of the seminiferous tubule into the adluminal compartment where they divide and form primary spermatocytes. Primary spermatocytes then undergo the first meiotic division to form secondary spermatocytes which have half the chromosomal number of the original spermatogonium. The second meiotic division produces spermatids; when first formed the spermatid is a small rounded cell, which will gradually transform into a spermatozoon. Their intimate association with the Sertoli cells is essential for these processes. Indeed Sertoli cells are sometimes called 'nurse cells' and they secrete a steroidal, meiotic stimulating factor. The

123

spermatozoa are extruded by the Sertoli cells into the lumen of the tubule. Although apparently fully differentiated, the spermatozoa are not capable of independent motility or fertilization at this stage and further maturation is required; this occurs during passage through the epididymis. The mature spermatozoa are fully mobile when they leave the epididymis and become mixed with the secretions of the seminal vesicle and prostate at the time of ejaculation. In many mammals, however, the freshly ejaculated spermatozoa are still incapable of fertilization until they have undergone a further process called 'capacitation' in the female reproductive tract; this precedes the reactions brought about by the acrosome and it is the latter changes which enable spermatozoa to penetrate the ovum. The acrosome is a large, specialized lysosome in the head of the sperm, and contains a number of acid hydrolases. During fertilization, the hydrolases are released and extracellular materials in the path of the sperm are digested, thus allowing it access to the ovum. Semen appears to contain a factor that inhibits capacitation; this is important because capacitated sperm deteriorate very rapidly.

## Androgens

### SYNTHESIS AND SECRETION

A number of androgenic hormones are secreted by the testes including androstenedione, dehydro*epi*androsterone and testosterone. The most important (both in terms of the quantity secreted and its biological potency) is testosterone. Its synthesis takes place in the interstitial Leydig cells and proceeds via cholesterol and pregnenolone (Fig. 4.2) in the same way as the adrenal androgens are formed (see Figs 1.9 and Fig. 3.10). In the normal male the testis is the major site of androgen synthesis with only a very small contribution (<5%) from the adrenal. The action of testosterone at its target sites (except muscle) requires, however, its further metabolism by the enzyme $5\alpha$-reductase to $5\alpha$-dihydrotestosterone (see Fig. 4.2).

### ACTIONS OF ANDROGENS

Puberty is a period of rapid somatic growth and development, accompanied by increasing secretion of gonadal hormones and the consequent development of secondary sexual characteristics. The onset of puberty in the male can first be detected phenotypically by an increase in testicular volume which is brought about by an increase in germ cell layers and the appearance of a lumen in each seminiferous tubule. The Leydig cells also increase in number and size and are stimulated to produce and secrete testosterone. Following this increase in blood testosterone

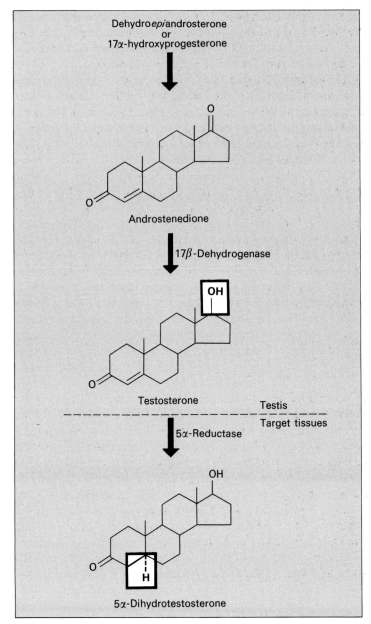

**Fig. 4.2** The biosynthesis of androgens. The formation of testosterone occurs in Leydig cells. The earlier steps are shown in Fig. 1.9. Dehydro*epi*androsterone is only a weak androgen which can masculinize but does not affect secondary sex organs. Testosterone is secreted and is converted in target tissues to dihydrotestosterone.

concentration, a deepening of the voice and beard growth occurs and spermatogenesis commences. Growth of the secondary sexual glands in response to increased testosterone secretion also occurs at this time.

Conversely, the removal of the testes in the adult leads to involution and atrophy of the epididymis, seminal vesicles, prostate and penis. Secondary sexual characteristics such as facial hair growth are either lost or diminished.

Before puberty, removal of the testes prevents pubertal changes. There is no hair growth on the face, trunk or axilla; laryngeal growth is arrested and the voice does not break; abnormal deposition of fat occurs on the hips and buttocks; the skeletal muscles are less well developed and the skin has a pale appearance and the penis remains small.

CONTROL OF TESTICULAR FUNCTION

Testicular function is regulated by the two pituitary gonadotrophins, follicle stimulating hormone and luteinizing hormone, both of which are glycoproteins. The initiation and maintenance of spermatogenesis normally requires the action of both follicle stimulating hormone and luteinizing hormone. Luteinizing hormone stimulates the synthesis of testosterone by the Leydig cells. Testosterone maintains spermatogenesis though it cannot initiate it. Thus if adult rats are hypophysectomized, immediate administration of luteinizing hormone will maintain spermatogenesis. If, however, administration of luteinizing hormone is delayed or if the experiment is done in immature rats, spermatogenesis does not occur, since follicle stimulating hormone is needed to initiate spermatogenesis.

The action of follicle stimulating hormone and testosterone (and hence of luteinizing hormone) on the process of spermatogenesis is not thought to be directly on the germ cells, but indirectly via their action on Sertoli cells, which are triggered to produce compounds necessary for sperm maturation. One such substance which has been identified in rat testicular fluid is androgen-binding protein. This is secreted by Sertoli cells into the lumen of the seminiferous tubule and its production is stimulated by follicle stimulating hormone and testosterone. In animals it binds, and hence provides a reserve of androgens in the testicular fluid, but its role in humans is still not certain.

The secretion of the two gonadotrophins controlling testicular function is regulated by a single gonadotrophin releasing hormone (GnRH), a decapeptide produced in the hypothalamus. The secretions of the hypothalamic–pituitary unit are regulated by a negative feedback mechanism (see Chapter 2) involving steroid hormones, gonadotrophins and a gonadal peptide hormone called 'Inhibin' from the Sertoli cells of the testis (see below).

Luteinizing hormone controls the rate of testosterone synthesis in Leydig cells by regulating the enzymic step involved in the conversion of cholesterol to pregnenolone; this requires cholesterol desmolase (see Chapter 1). The action of luteinizing hormone on Leydig cells is mediated by a receptor on the cell surface which is linked to an adenylate cyclase system. The gonads, in their turn, exert an influence on the hypothalamic–pituitary system by a negative feedback control whereby elevated concentrations of circulating testosterone inhibit the release of luteinizing hormone. Other steroids can also affect this feedback control, including oestradiol and 5α-dihydrotestosterone. At one time it was thought that oestradiol was the important controlling compound, following its formation from the aromatization of testosterone in the brain. However, this cannot be the only mechanism operating, since 5α-dihydrotestosterone also suppresses luteinizing hormone secretion yet it cannot be converted to oestradiol. The secretion of luteinizing hormone is pulsatile and seems to be much more sensitive to negative feedback by steroids than that of follicle stimulating hormone.

## Inhibin

A peptide is secreted from the gonads that can inhibit the secretion of follicle stimulating hormone, and it is called inhibin. It was originally detected in aqueous extracts of testis and subsequently it was isolated from ovarian follicular fluid. The isolation of inhibin was monitored by measuring follicle stimulating hormone production in cultured pituitary cells. Inhibin has a molecular weight of 32 000 and it is made up of two peptide chains, $\alpha$ and $\beta$ of molecular weights 18 000 and 14 000 respectively, linked by disulphide bonds. There are two forms of the $\beta$-chain, referred to as $\beta_A$ and $\beta_B$, so two forms of inhibin exist which have a common $\alpha$-chain. The two types of inhibin contain the chains $\alpha\beta_A$ and $\alpha\beta_B$. From a knowledge of the amino acid sequence, chemically-synthesized complementary DNA probes have been prepared. By using these probes it has been shown that the synthesis of the $\alpha$- and $\beta$-chains occurs separately, with the genes for the relevant chains being present on different chromosomes. The situation is thus similar to the synthesis of pituitary glycoprotein hormones, namely thyrotrophin and the gonadotrophins. It has been estimated that in the ovary the messenger RNA for the $\alpha$-chain is present in a 10-fold excess over the $\beta_A$- and a 20-fold excess over the $\beta_B$- chains.

Dimers of $\beta$-chains have also been found in follicular fluid. They have different properties from inhibin and, although it is uncertain how or under what conditions the dimers are secreted, they are actually capable of increasing the secretion of follicle stimulating hormone. Two dimers have been identified: one consists of $2\beta_A$-subunits which is called 'follicle stimulating hormone releasing protein', and the other consists of $\beta_A\beta_B$-subunits which is called 'Activin'. However, little is known of the control of either $\alpha\beta$ or $\beta\beta$ dimerization.

The $\beta$-dimers have structural similarities to transforming growth factor-$\beta$ (TGF-$\beta$), which is a dimer of two subunits of molecular weights 12 500 linked by disulphide bonds. Transforming growth factor-$\beta$ acts as a local hormone in a variety of tissues, and it can even increase the secretion of follicle stimulating hormone. It has been suggested that transforming growth factor-$\beta$, inhibin and activin may arise from a common gene family.

The concentration of inhibin in the testis falls after hypophysectomy and it increases when follicle stimulating hormone is injected. Inhibin occurs in the circulation and inhibits pituitary production of follicle stimulating hormone. These facts demonstrate that there is an endocrine loop controlling the production of the gonadal hormone, inhibin, which may act as a local hormone in the gonad, as well as having important actions on the pituitary.

### Male infertility

A defect of spermatogenesis, with reduced numbers of sperm or even total absence of sperm from the semen, is the cause of infertility in 10% of couples who find they cannot conceive. The failure of spermatogenesis may be due to lack of luteinizing hormone and follicle stimulating hormone. Prolactin is important in the control of gonadotrophin release and so high concentrations of prolactin may cause testicular involution and impotence. Infertility, however, more commonly arises from primary failure of the testis itself, e.g. due to cryptorchidism (undescended testes) or damage to the testes by mumps. In some cases where there has been testicular damage or the vas deferens has been resected, infertility may be due to the formation of anti-sperm antibody. Even if the sperm count is normal, there may be abnormal forms or reduced motility of the sperm; also the sperm may have a low capacity for fertilization, although at present it is difficult to demonstrate this. Chromosomal abnormalities can also cause infertility as in Klinefelter's syndrome. Investigation of infertility thus necessitates consideration of the endocrine, immunological and genetic mechanisms involved in reproduction, as well as psychological factors, of course.

## THE FEMALE REPRODUCTIVE SYSTEM

The function of the female reproductive system differs in many respects from that of the male; mature germ cells are only produced intermittently and usually only one germ cell reaches full maturity at a time; this occurs at intervals of approximately 28 days. Moreover, production of mature germ cells, once it has started at puberty, only continues for a limited time rather than continuing for the rest of the individual's life. Thus only

about 400 germ cells reach full maturity to be released at
ovulation. This cyclical production of mature oocytes in the
ovary is associated with cyclical changes in the production of
hormones from the ovary, and accompanying cyclical changes in
the uterus and the vagina.

## Morphology

### OOGENESIS

Oogenesis begins in the fetal ovary when the primordial germ
cells proliferate to become oogonia. At the 11th to 12th week
of gestation the oogonia enter the prophase of the first meiotic
division and then become arrested without completing the
division. At this stage they are called primary oocytes and, with
the surrounding granulosa cells from the sex cords, form the
primordial follicles (Fig. 4.3). The primordial follicles reach
a peak number of about $7 \times 10^6$ between the 20th and 28th
week of gestation but from then on their number declines.
At birth there are only about $2 \times 10^6$ and by puberty only
300 000, each surrounded by a single layer of flattened follicular
cells embedded in a cellular stroma. The centre or medulla of
the ovary consists largely of blood vessels. The ovaries are sited
close to the open ends of the Fallopian tubes, which pass to the
body of the uterus, whose cervix opens into the vagina.

### FORMATION OF THE GRAAFIAN FOLLICLE

At the beginning of a menstrual cycle, a group or cohort of
10–20 early follicles enlarge through the proliferation of the
flattened follicular cells, to form secondary follicles (Fig. 4.3).
These consist of several layers of membrana granulosa cells,
surrounding the oocyte. In any one menstrual cycle usually only
one of the follicles matures fully. Stromal cells become arranged
around the follicle to form the well-vascularized theca. Growth
of the follicle proceeds and a large cavity, the antrum, develops
within the tertiary follicle filled by the follicular fluid. The
oocyte is supported in the antrum by a stalk of granulosa cells,
the cumulus oophorus. Up to this time, the granulosa cells are
ionically coupled to one another and to the ovum by gap junctions.
Then in mid-cycle they become uncoupled and the Graafian
follicle ruptures liberating the oocyte (ovulation) which enters
the fimbriated opening of the Fallopian tube. If the ovum is
fertilized, development starts and usually reaches the blastocyst
stage before it enters the uterus to become implanted in the
uterine endometrium. If the ovum is not fertilized it dies.

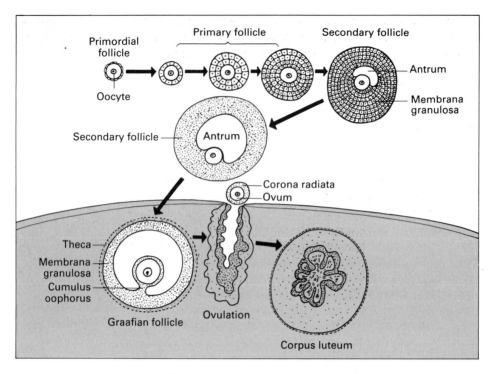

**Fig. 4.3** The growth, maturation and ovulation of a Graafian follicle followed by the formation of a corpus luteum. The earlier stages are shown above and the later stages are shown below in the shaded part representing the ovarian stroma. A primordial follicle consists of an oocyte surrounded by a layer of flattened cells. Growth of the primary follicle consists of multiplication and enlargement of the flattened cells to form a multilayered membrana granulosa. The appearance of a liquid-filled antrum indicates the formation of a secondary follicle. The antrum enlarges and the oocyte remains attached to the membrana granulosa by a stalk of cells, the cumulus oophorus. Stromal cells become organized around the maturing Graafian follicle to form a steroidogenic layer of cells, the theca. When the follicle ruptures at ovulation, the ovum is expelled from the ovary surrounded by a layer of cells, the corona radiata. The granulosa cells of the collapsed follicle and the theca cells divide, enlarge and form a round, steroidogenic cellular mass, the corpus luteum.

FORMATION OF THE CORPUS LUTEUM

The cells of the ruptured Graafian follicle proliferate, enlarge and fill the collapsed antrum of the follicle. This new structure becomes a solid, round mass of steroidogenic cells, called the corpus luteum which is initially red in colour but then becomes yellowish. If fertilization and blastocyst implantation do not occur, the corpus luteum, having been active for most of the latter half of the menstrual cycle, begins to involute. The luteal cells then cease their synthetic activity and disappear, and the whole structure, replaced with scar tissue, becomes the corpus albicans. However, if implantation occurs, the corpus luteum increases in size and remains active during the early weeks of pregnancy until its function of steroidogenesis is taken over by the placenta; thus the corpus luteum maintains the uterine endometrium in early pregnancy.

## Ovarian hormones

CONTROL OF OVARIAN HORMONE PRODUCTION

Hormone production in the ovary is cyclical and several different cells are involved at different points in the menstrual cycle. Two main steroid hormones are produced; oestradiol which is an oestrogen, and progesterone which possesses progestational activity (see Table 4.1). The biosynthesis of oestradiol (Fig. 4.4) is

**Table 4.1** The effects of female sex hormones.

| | Oestrogens | Progesterone |
|---|---|---|
| 1 | *At puberty*<br>Oestrogens stimulate the growth of the uterus and of the breasts and determine the female figure by controlling the deposition of fat. They contribute to closure of the epiphyses. They have important effects on personality and sexual responsiveness | |
| 2 | *During the menstrual cycle*<br>Oestrogens cause endometrial proliferation and secretion of clear mucus from the cervix together with maturation of the vaginal epithelium. They have positive and negative feedback effects on the hypothalamus and pituitary and cause maturation of the vaginal epithelium | Causes a rise in body temperature, the production of a secretory endometrium and secretion of thick cervical mucus with leucocytes. It has a negative feedback on the hypothalamus and pituitary |
| 3 | *During pregnancy*<br>Oestrogens cause growth of the breast duct system and myometrial hypertrophy together with fluid retention and increase in uterine blood flow | Causes a reduction of contractions and reduced smooth muscle tone. There is a rise in body temperature and growth of the alveoli of the breasts |
| 4 | *Cellular effects*<br>Oestrogens cause production of receptors for progesterone and so the response to progesterone is dependent on oestrogenization | Progesterone stimulates the formation of 17-hydroxysteroid dehydrogenase which leads to inactivation of oestradiol in target tissue by converting it to oestrone |

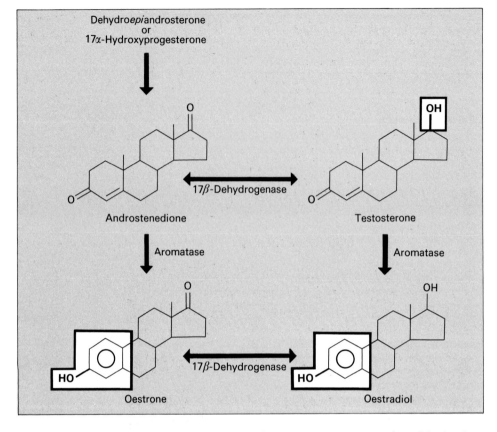

**Fig. 4.4** The biosynthesis of oestrogens: precursors are formed in the theca interna and aromatized in the granulosa cells (see Fig. 4.5).

remarkable in that its precursors (androstenedione and testosterone) are synthesized in the theca interna cells of the follicle and are then transported to the granulosa cells where they are aromatized to yield oestrone and oestradiol (see Fig. 4.3). Steroidogenesis is stimulated by luteinizing hormone, which activates the rate-limiting cholesterol desmolase by stimulating production of cyclic AMP (Fig. 4.5).

In the early follicular phase of the menstrual cycle, follicle stimulating hormone initiates the further development of a number of primary follicles and so increases the number of granulosa cells while the number of theca cells increases under the influence of luteinizing hormone. This combination gives rise to an increased production of oestradiol between the 8th and 10th days of the cycle. Just before ovulation, the granulosa cells of the follicle also develop receptors for luteinizing hormone and these begin to synthesize progesterone.

When the empty follicle becomes a corpus luteum, the theca interna cells are trapped between granulosa cells, and both types

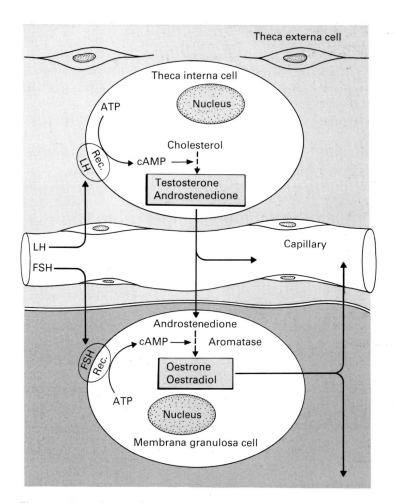

**Fig. 4.5** The structure of part of the wall of a Graafian follicle. Membrana granulosa cells are separated from the surrounding theca by a distinct basement membrane. The theca interna consists of androgen-synthesizing cells and capillaries; external to these are fibroblast-like cells of the theca externa. Luteinizing hormone (LH) stimulates receptors (Rec.) on the theca interna cells via cAMP to synthesize testosterone and androstenedione. This passes either into the local capillaries or crosses the basement membrane into the adjacent membrana granulosa cells. These are stimulated by follicle stimulating hormone (FSH) to produce oestrogens by the aromatization of the testosterone and androstenedione. The oestrogens then enter the circulation or pass into the antrum of the follicle and act on the oocyte.

of cells remain active producing oestrogen and progesterone. The combination of the production of oestradiol and progesterone then has a negative feedback effect, to suppress the production of luteinizing hormone and follicle stimulating hormone (Fig. 4.6), though luteinizing hormone is needed to support the corpus luteum.

EFFECTS OF OVARIAN HORMONES ON THE UTERUS
AND VAGINA

The changing ovarian steroid output (Fig. 4.7) throughout the
menstrual cycle is responsible for the changes that are observed
in the endometrium of the uterus and the rest of the female
genital tract. At the start of a new cycle, after menstruation is com-

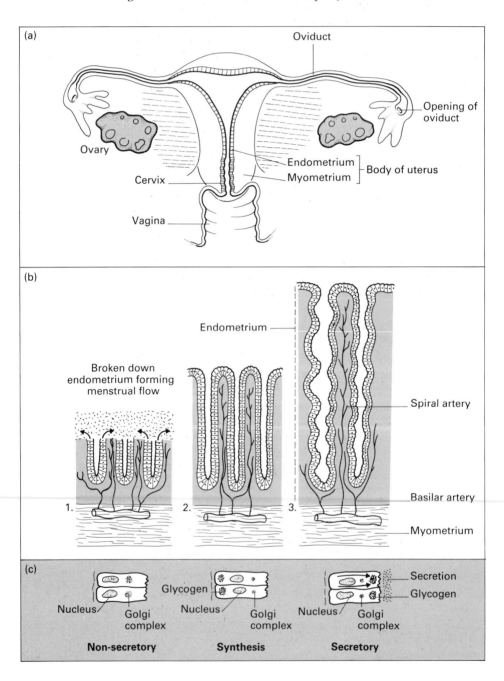

pleted, the increased secretion of oestradiol stimulates the repair and proliferation of the endometrium and the synthesis of receptors for progesterone and oestradiol in its cells. The rise in progesterone that follows ovulation leads to changes in the secretion of the endometrium which are essential if implantation of a fertilized ovum is to occur. In the second half of the cycle the endometrium doubles in thickness and the simple tubular glands become tortuous and saccular. The maintenance of the secretory phase is dependent on the continued stimulus of oestrogen and the additional stimulus of progesterone from the corpus luteum so that when luteolysis occurs the endometrium breaks down, sloughs off and menstrual bleeding occurs.

Cyclical hormonal changes also alter the consistency and pH of the cervical mucus. The changes in the mucus are sufficient to render the entry of sperm into the uterus less likely during the luteal phase when, because of high concentrations of progesterone, the mucus is viscous and of low pH, neither of which is conducive to survival of the sperm. In contrast, the mucus of the oestrogen-induced follicular phase is abundant, clear, watery and of higher pH and consequently is more suitable for sperm transport and motility.

The actions of progesterone on the female reproductive tract, outlined above, have been exploited in the 'progesterone only' contraceptive pill, which is probably achieved through its effect on cervical mucus and endometrium.

(Facing page)
**Fig. 4.6** Changes in the uterine endometrium during the menstrual cycle. (see also Fig. 4.7).
(a) Section showing the body and cervix of the uterus, the vagina. The body of the uterus consists of an inner endometrial layer containing the uterine mucosa and a surrounding thick myometrium consisting largely of smooth muscle.
(b and c) Changes in the uterine gland during the menstrual cycle.
1 Breakdown of the endometrium (days 1−3) occurs, in which the outer functional two-thirds is shed, the debris of the glands and endometrial stroma forms the menstrual flow. The basal third of the endometrium persists and its cells divide and grow over the exposed stromal tissue to repair the endometrium. The uterine gland cells show a basal location to the nucleus and the adjacent Golgi complex.
2 During the oestrogenic, proliferative phase (days 3−14), the uterine glands grow in length as the endometrium thickens. Glycogen appears in the base of the glandular cells, pushing the nucleus towards the centre of the cell.
3 During the progestational, secretory phase (days 14−28), the uterine glands double in length and become tortuous and sacculated. Glycogen in the glandular cells migrates to the apex of the cell and, with other materials, is released to form the endometrial secretion which reaches a maximum by day 20. Stromal oedema also increases to a maximum by day 21, approximately the time of normal blastocyst implantation. During the last 2−3 days of this phase vascular changes occur in the spiral blood vessels leading to their vasoconstriction. Blood vessel rupture and extravasation then occur and lakes of blood form in the stromal tissue. Endometrial breakdown follows.

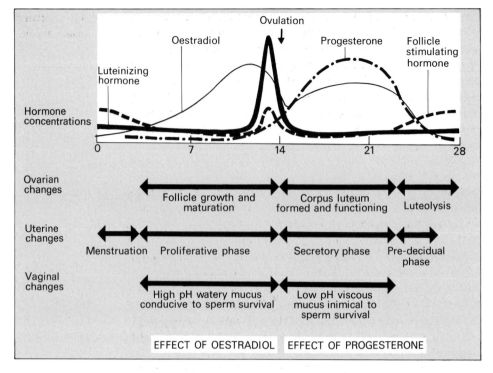

**Fig. 4.7** A schematic representation of the changes in the menstrual cycle shown as beginning with the start of menstruation on day 0 and lasting 28 days.

REGULATION OF THE MENSTRUAL CYCLE

Regulation of the menstrual cycle occurs as a result of a number of interactions between the hormones of the hypothalamic–pituitary–gonadal axis (Fig. 4.7). The important regulatory features which have to be accounted for are: firstly, why when a cohort of follicles begin to ripen, does only one usually ovulate; secondly, what is responsible for the initiation of ovulation; and thirdly, what causes the regression of the corpus luteum and so terminates the cycle?

*Control of follicle development*

Through the stimulus of follicle stimulating hormone a group of primary follicles begin to develop into secondary follicles, which produce oestradiol. Under the influence of increased concentrations of oestradiol the follicles then start to synthesize more receptors for follicle stimulating hormone in the granulosa cells. Secretion of oestradiol and also of inhibin by the follicles then begins to suppress the production of follicle stimulating hormone: the concentrations of oestradiol and of inhibin (see p. 127) in the circulation are closely correlated. Inhibin is found in the follicular fluid and probably comes from the granulosa cells; its circulating concentration may be a good measure of granulosa cell function.

The falling concentration of follicle stimulating hormone at this stage presents the cohort of ripening follicles with a competitive situation in which only one or two, with the highest concentration of receptors for follicle stimulating hormone, are able to sustain their development while the rest atrophy and regress. The availability of follicle stimulating hormone is thus crucial at this stage of the cycle. The role of $\beta\beta$-dimers, such as activin, in stimulating secretion of follicle stimulating hormone remains to be established (see p. 127).

### Initiation of ovulation

The occurrence of ovulation in the middle of the cycle is associated with a surge in the secretion of luteinizing hormone and, to a lesser extent, of follicle stimulating hormone by the pituitary. The surge of luteinizing hormone lasts for about 36 hours, which is also the time taken for the oocyte to mature. There is a local factor in the ovary that normally suppresses oocyte maturation and this can be overcome by raised concentrations of luteinizing hormone. The mid-cycle rise in circulating gonadotrophins leads to increased synthesis of plasminogen activator in the follicle, and this aids follicle rupture and release of the ovum (ovulation).

The cause of this surge in gonadotrophin secretion has been investigated in the Rhesus monkey and appears to be due principally to the action of oestradiol on the pituitary. Throughout the cycle, gonadotrophin output is stimulated by the continued, pulsatile output of gonadotrophin releasing hormone, at about 90-minute intervals, by the hypothalamus. In the early follicular phase of the cycle the output of gonadotrophin is restricted by the negative feedback on the pituitary of inhibin and oestradiol from the ovary. As the follicle ripens, oestradiol output increases. At about the 12th day of the cycle, if a certain threshold concentration of oestradiol is exceeded, and if this elevated concentration is maintained for at least 36 hours, there is a switch from negative to positive feedback. Oestrogen-mediated positive feedback gives rise to the surge in the release of gonadotrophins and so to ovulation.

### Luteolysis

After ovulation the collapsed follicle develops into the corpus luteum and continues to produce oestradiol and progesterone under the stimulus of the low concentration of luteinizing hormone which remains after the mid-cycle surge. However, the output of luteinizing hormone continues to fall as the negative feedback of oestradiol on the pituitary is resumed.

The continued function of the corpus luteum depends on the stimulatory effect of luteinizing hormone and so, by about the 25th day, the falling output of this hormone results in failure of steroidogenesis. Menstruation follows as there is no longer oestradiol and progesterone available to maintain the endometrium. This absence of oestradiol and progesterone removes the inhibition on the pituitary, which, under the stimulus of gonadotrophin releasing hormone, resumes secretion of follicle stimulating hormone and luteinizing hormone and so the next cycle commences.

If implantation of a blastocyst occurs at about the 20th day of the cycle, the resulting trophoblast begins to secrete human chorionic gonadotrophin, a glycoprotein hormone that has luteinizing hormone-like activity. This hormone maintains the corpus luteum to continue the production of oestradiol and progesterone and so prevents menstruation.

## Puberty

In the United Kingdom about 95% of girls reach the menarche (i.e. start to menstruate) by the age of 15. Breast development (thelarche) starts a few years earlier, under the influence of ovarian oestrogens which stimulate the proliferation of the duct system of the breast and the accumulation of fat in the breast. At the same time the characteristic female distribution of hair develops under the influence of androgens secreted from the adrenals (hence the term adrenarche). The pulsatile release of luteinizing hormone is first demonstrable at puberty. To begin with it only occurs at night, but as puberty progresses it occurs in the day as well. It has been suggested that luteinizing hormone is released in a pulsatile manner to enable the receptors to remain active; if there is continuous stimulation from luteinizing hormone the receptors become unresponsive. In this state the receptors are sometimes referred to as being 'down regulated' (see Chapter 1). The fact that luteinizing hormone is released in pulses can cause confusion clinically, when the concentration of luteinizing hormone is measured to investigate disorders of the reproductive system. To avoid this error it is necessary to assay serial samples.

## Pregnancy

### Conception and implantation

Normal conception requires that a spermatozoon should fertilize an ovum in the Fallopian tube. To achieve this, large numbers of sperm (approximately 25–50 million) have to be ejaculated into the vagina, whence they make their way through the cervix and body of the uterus to the Fallopian tube to encounter the ovum. Although only one sperm is necessary for final fertilization, the penetration of the ovum seems to require a sustained attack by many sperm, which release hydrolytic enzymes from their acrosomes to loosen the corona radiata cells around the ovum to allow the sperm access. Once fertilized the ovum is transported down the Fallopian tube by peristaltic contractions and the action of its ciliated epithelial cells. During this descent, it undergoes a series of cell divisions to reach the blastocyst stage of development, with about 16 cells. The secretion of a glycogen-rich mucus is necessary for nutrition of the blastocyst at this stage, and the uterine endometrium must be in a suitable secretory and receptive state for implantation to occur.

The life of sperm in the female genital tract is probably less than 72 hours; there is a similarly short period during which the ovum is in the Fallopian tube, and the cervical mucus is favourable to survival of sperm. Thus there is a relatively short period (perhaps a couple of days on either side of ovulation) when coitus is likely to result in conception. This necessary coincidence of events provides the underlying rationale for the rhythm method of birth control and is also of use in counselling couples who are attempting to achieve conception.

### The fetoplacental endocrine unit

When the blastocyst is successfully implanted in the endometrium it continues to develop. The trophoblast begins to secrete human chorionic gonadotrophin into the maternal bloodstream; it is the detection of this glycoprotein hormone in maternal blood or urine that is the basis of most tests for early detection of pregnancy. Human chorionic gonadotrophin sustains the oestradiol and progesterone secretion by the corpus luteum and thus supports the fetoplacental unit. The increase in concentration of these steroids produced under the stimulus of human chorionic gonadotrophin suppresses the pituitary production of follicle stimulating hormone, and so prevents further ovulation. At about the ninth week of pregnancy the fetoplacental unit acquires cholesterol desmolase activity and so is able to synthesize both pregnenolone and progesterone (Fig. 4.8). Pregnenolone crosses to the fetus and the developing fetal adrenal converts it to dehydro*epi*androsterone sulphate; this goes back and in the placenta aromatization occurs with the formation of oestriol. Oestriol production begins from the 12th week and with the onset of steroid production by the placenta, the corpus luteum of pregnancy regresses gradually. The fetoplacental unit provides a continuously rising output of progesterone and oestriol throughout pregnancy. This provided the rationale for measurement of maternal serum and urinary oestriol, and urinary pregnanediol (which is a metabolite of progesterone), as indices of fetal well-being and placental function respectively, though neither is a totally satisfactory index. Better information is obtained by ultrasound scans during pregnancy.

### Changes in the breasts during pregnancy

Growth and development of the alveoli of the breasts occurs during pregnancy under the influence of several hormones. In early pregnancy, the most important of these are the oestrogens which

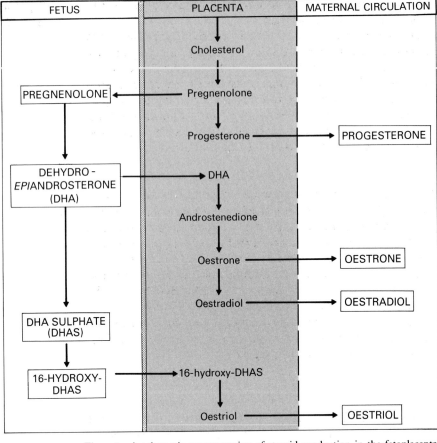

| FETUS | PLACENTA | MATERNAL CIRCULATION |
|---|---|---|

Cholesterol

PREGNENOLONE ← Pregnenolone

Progesterone → PROGESTERONE

DEHYDRO-*EPI*ANDROSTERONE (DHA) → DHA

Androstenedione

Oestrone → OESTRONE

Oestradiol → OESTRADIOL

DHA SULPHATE (DHAS)

16-HYDROXY-DHAS → 16-hydroxy-DHAS

Oestriol → OESTRIOL

**Fig. 4.8** A schematic representation of steroid production in the fetoplacental unit. The placenta also produces protein hormones, particularly chorionic gonadotrophin and placental lactogen.

stimulate growth of the ducts. Later on glucocorticoids from the adrenal, prolactin from the pituitary and placental lactogen (a prolactin-like hormone from the placenta) are important to inducing the enzymes necessary for the production of milk (lactogenesis). However, the high progesterone concentrations prevent synthesis of milk proteins and lactation from starting until after delivery, even though the concentration of prolactin is high throughout pregnancy. The number of lactotrophs in the pituitary increases in pregnancy and prolactin is the only pituitary hormone to be present in high concentrations in the circulation during pregnancy. The role of the high prolactin concentration in pregnancy is not clear. It may, in part, be important to the stimulation of the 1-hydroxylase in the kidney to increase the hydroxylation of 25-hydroxycholecalciferol (see Chapter 6). Thus the concentration of 1,25-dihydroxycholecalciferol increases to facilitate calcium absorption, and maintain calcium balance during pregnancy and lactation. Prolactin may also be involved in the maintenance of osmolality of fetal fluids and its concentration is high in amniotic fluid.

The onset of lactation after delivery is made possible by the fall in the circulating concentration of oestrogen and progesterone at parturition and is dependent upon the continued production of prolactin. The ejection of milk in response to suckling requires the action of oxytocin, secreted by the posterior pituitary in response to the suckling reflex. If lactation is maintained the normal cycling of pituitary gonadotrophin release is delayed and fertility is reduced while breast feeding is continued.

### Parturition

The gestation period for the human fetus is normally about 9 months. The nature of the signal for paturition is still not entirely clear, and may vary in different species. Glucocorticoids from the large fetal adrenal are probably very important in this respect. The concentration of progesterone falls and there is an increase in circulating oxytocin (from the posterior pituitary) and of prostaglandins (from the uterus itself). Expulsion of the fetus is dependent on the production of prostaglandins, which stimulate the early uterine contractions, and on oxytocin, the release of which increases by positive feedback as the fetus moves down and distends the vagina.

## The menopause

The menopause is defined as the time of the last menstrual period, usually between 45 and 52 years of age. The ovaries gradually cease to function cyclically; this is referred to as the climacteric. Ovarian failure results from exhaustion of primordial follicles and causes low oestrogen and inhibin production and hence raised concentrations of luteinizing hormone and especially follicle stimulating hormone. Because of the fall in oestradiol production, the vaginal mucosa becomes atrophic and at the same time the mammary glands atrophy. Flushing attacks may occur, but the cause of this vasomotor instability is not known. After the menopause, for reasons which are not entirely clear, bone mass declines more rapidly than previously and osteoporosis may develop. This is presumably associated with the reduced production of oestradiol. After the menopause, oestrogen production depends entirely on peripheral aromatization of androstenedione, that has been produced in the adrenal, to oestrone.

Hormone replacement therapy in the menopausal period can therefore be used. If oestrogen alone is given it produces endometrial hyperplasia and in consequence the risk of a neoplasm developing may be increased. Consequently, progesterone should be given as well; this reduces the oestrogen receptors in the target-cell cytoplasm and increases the activity of oestradiol $17\beta$-dehydrogenase which inactivates the oestradiol by converting it to oestrone which has a lower affinity for oestrogen receptors. This form of therapy is given intermittently and produces withdrawal bleeding.

### Disturbances of the menstrual cycle

*Primary amenorrhoea*
If menstruation has not started by the age of 16, the condition of primary amenorrhoea may be said to exist. This may be of no significance since periods may develop normally later. However, there are a number of other possible causes; for example, the ovaries may be absent or damaged, or rudimentary. If breast development has occurred, there must have been some production of oestrogens and therefore there must have been functional ovaries present; however, if breast development has not occurred then there may be a lack of active ovaries. Primary amenorrhoea can also be caused by depletion of oocytes and follicles because of chromosomal abnormalities, or by abnormalities of the hypothalamus or pituitary. A defect of gonadotrophin production may be part of a generalized disturbance of the hypothalamus or pituitary or there may be isolated deficiency of gonadotrophins.

*Secondary amenorrhoea*
Most commonly menstruation occurs regularly at intervals of 28–31 days. Pregnancy, of course, is the commonest cause of amenorrhoea but, apart from this, about 2% of women get bouts of amenorrhoea during their reproductive life. The term secondary amenorrhoea is used when an interval of 6 months or more occurs without a period in a girl or woman who has previously had normal periods. There are many causes for secondary amenorrhoea including, for example, ovarian failure (i.e. a premature menopause), excessive androgen production, pituitary disease (including, particularly, prolonged overproduction of prolactin), disturbances in gonadotrophin production arising from a defect of negative feedback or a failure of initiation of cyclical release of the gonadotrophins. Measurement of the concentrations of luteinizing hormone and follicle stimulating hormone is useful, since if there is no feedback from ovarian secretions the concentrations of gonadotrophins will be high. Psychiatric disturbance and abnormalities in the nutritional pattern can also cause amenorrhoea: these two occur together in the condition known as anorexia nervosa in which amenorrhoea is an important feature.

*Failure of ovulation*
At the beginning and end of reproductive life, i.e. after the menarche and before menopause, it is common for women to have menstrual cycles without ovulation occurring. In some

women failure to ovulate also occurs during the reproductive period of life. In a few women ovulation rarely occurs because of a lack of positive feedback by oestrogens. Lack of adequate, pulsatile secretion of gonadotrophin releasing hormone also causes failure of ovulation. Failure to ovulate may be associated with a short cycle but is more often associated with irregular or long cycles. In a normal menstrual cycle, the endometrium is stimulated first by oestrogen and then by progesterone and the breakdown of the endometrium occurs with a fall in the concentration of circulating progesterone and oestrogen. If there is no ovulation, the only stimulus to proliferation of the endometrium is the secretion of oestrogen, and menstrual bleeding is due to oestrogen withdrawal after non-ovulatory follicles have atrophied.

*Detection of ovulation.* There are a number of indirect ways of inferring that ovulation has occurred; these depend on the assumption that a corpus luteum has been formed. For example, in the second half of a normal ovulatory cycle, there is a rise in the basal body temperature of about $0.5°C$; if the temperature is taken daily before getting out of bed, or eating or drinking, a rise in the basal temperature indicates that ovulation has occurred. Similarly, examination of the vaginal epithelium may give an indication, since under the influence of both oestrogen and progesterone, the vaginal epithelium matures; if the vaginal smears are examined weekly, then evidence of ovulation can be obtained. Likewise, if the endometrial mucosa is examined, the finding of a secretory endometrium in the second half of a cycle indicates that progesterone stimulation has occurred and that ovulation has preceded it. More direct evidence that a corpus luteum has formed may be obtained by measurement of progesterone in plasma obtained in the second half of the cycle; it is easier, however, to measure the excretion of a metabolite of progesterone, namely pregnanediol glucuronide in urine. Easier still and more direct, is to look at the ovaries using ultrasound to see follicles.

*Artificial induction of ovulation.* It is possible, if necessary, to stimulate ovulation. Before doing so it is essential to know that the ovary contains ova (i.e. that the patient is not suffering from ovarian failure). If the pituitary is capable of secreting gonadotrophins and the ovary is capable of producing more than basal levels of oestrogen, it is feasible to treat the patient with the drug clomiphene which is an 'anti-oestrogen' and hence stimulates the release of gonadotrophins. The response to treatment with clomiphene can be followed directly by ultrasound or indirectly by measurement of body temperature or plasma progesterone, to see if ovulation has been induced. Before ovulation the diameter of the follicle is $8-10$ mm, and it can be seen to increase up to $20-22$ mm in diameter.

It is also possible to induce ovulation by administration of gonadotrophins, of which two preparations are available: 'human menopausal gonadotrophins', which are extracted from the urine of postmenopausal women and are a mixture of luteinizing hormone and follicle stimulating hormone; and 'human chorionic gonadotrophin', which is isolated from the urine of pregnant women and has predominantly the effects of luteinizing hormone. To induce ovulation, human menopausal gonadotrophins are first given (this stimulates many follicles to develop but caution is needed, since it may produce overstimulation and cyst formation). Treatment with human menopausal gonadotrophin is then followed by administration of human chorionic gonadotrophin, used to replace the normal mid-cycle surge in luteinizing hormone production and trigger ovulation. The dose of human menopausal gonadotrophin required to produce a satisfactory response varies from patient to patient and the response must be monitored. The urinary total oestrogen, oestradiol or oestrone excretion should be measured during treatment with human menopausal gonadotrophin, and the dose adjusted appropriately. If the response is too small, the dose should be increased, but if the response is too great, then human chorionic gonadotrophin should be withheld because there is then a risk of overstimulation. Once a satisfactory response to human menopausal gonadotrophin has been achieved, then human chorionic gonadotrophin can be given. Ultrasound scans, or measurement of the plasma progesterone or urinary pregnanediol glucuronide excretion can be followed to establish whether ovulation has occurred. In judging the effectiveness of this type of therapy, it should be remembered that in normal women who have regular intercourse, only 60% will become pregnant within 6 months and 85% within a year. It cannot be expected, therefore, that artificially induced ovulation will be successful immediately in all cases, and so repeated courses of treatment may be needed.

Administration of luteinizing hormone releasing hormone is obviously the treatment of choice in patients whose infertility arises from a hypothalamic defect causing secondary deficiency of pituitary gondotrophins and consequently hypogonadism. The initial defect can be congenital, because there is a failure of hypothalamic development which can be associated with a reduced sense of smell. This syndrome, in which there is an association of hypogonadism and hyposmia, was first described by Kalman. Pulsatile infusion of luteinizing hormone releasing hormone to induce ovulation can overcome this 'hypothalamic–hypopituitary–hypogonadism'. The object is to induce ovulation from a single follicle, as occurs normally. Pulsatile infusion of synthetic luteinizing hormone releasing hormone at a constant frequency of a fixed amount of hormone is given to stimulate the pituitary. The ovary can then respond to the change in pituitary gonadotrophin secretions.

It is possible to fertilize an oocyte *in vitro*, allow it to divide, and then implant it in the uterus, after which pregnancy can follow a normal course. This method is useful when a woman has normal ovulatory cycles but is infertile because her fallopian tubes are blocked. The likelihood of success is dependent on the number of fertilized ova that are implanted: with one or two, the success rate for pregnancy concluding in normal delivery is 10−12%, while with implantation of three or four fertilised ova it is 15−20%. The rate of successful fertilization of ova *in vitro* is about 80% so, to get three or four oocytes fertilized, it is necessary to have five or six available for fertilization. Thus, the aim in inducing ovulation for *in vitro* fertilization is different from that of *in vivo* fertilization.

In normal conception, one ovum is produced at a time and it leads to one baby: when ovulation is induced for *in vivo* fertilization, again one ovum is all that is needed, although there is a risk of inducing maturation of multiple follicles during hormone therapy. For *in vitro* fertilization the aim is to induce maturation of multiple follicles, to be able to harvest six ova, if possible, in order to get one that matures to a full-term delivery of a single healthy baby. Thus, multiple ovulation has to be induced by high-dose gonadotrophin therapy. The response is followed by ultrasound scans of the ovaries and measurements of oestradiol. With (say) six follicles maturing, there is a proportional increase in the amount of oestradiol in the circulation, and this may produce a premature rise in luteinizing hormone and cause premature ovulation. This can be prevented, however, by giving injections of an analogue of luteinizing hormone releasing hormone to inhibit pituitary gonadotrophin release. The ova can be collected in a variety of ways, such as laparoscopy, which is done through the anterior abdominal wall. However, this needs a general anaesthetic, while ultrasound-guided needle aspiration can be done through the bladder in a conscious patient. A third approach is culdoscopy via the back of the vagina. Once the oocytes have been obtained they are mixed with a washed suspension of the husband's sperm and incubated until cleavage is seen under the microscope. The embryos can then be introduced into the uterus through the vagina.

## Endocrine regulation of fertility

The 'rhythm' control or 'safe period' method of contraception is based on the fact that the ovum once released is only viable for a short time, probably less than 24 hours, and that the sperm do not survive in a state in which they are able to achieve fertilization for more than 2 or 3 days. By avoiding intercourse for 4 or 5 days either side of the expected date of ovulation, there is a reduced prospect of pregnancy. The major difficulty in this method of control is in forecasting the exact time of ovulation, particularly in a woman with irregular menstrual cycles.

The most commonly used oral contraceptive pill contains a progestogen (a progesterone-like compound) and an oestrogen. Commonly, a fixed daily dose of oestrogen and progestogen is taken for approximately 21 days followed by a placebo or treatment-free period for 7 days. These preparations act by suppressing the hypothalamic−pituitary axis, depressing the gonadotrophin output and so preventing the maturation of follicles. In addition, the condition of the endometrium remains unsuitable for implantation and the cervical mucus is not conducive to passage of sperm, so that even if ovulation occurs, fertilization is less likely to follow. The failure rate of these mixed preparations is 0.08/100 woman-years. These preparations may produce adverse reactions such as depression, loss of libido, weight gain, mild hypertension and, less commonly, thrombosis. They should not be taken by women who have had thromboses or emboli, or have severe liver disease or malignant tumours that are thought to be sensitive to oestrogens. It should also be noted that if taken in combination with other drugs, either the contraceptive effect may be reduced, or the action of the other drug may be modified.

Another form of oral contraceptive has only a progestogen in low dose to be taken daily. This is less effective, the failure rate being 1.1/100 woman-years. In many women this 'mini' pill, however, causes irregular and frequent bleeding. Its mode of action is less certain. Ovulation is not inhibited in all cases and the major contraceptive action is thought to be a consequence of the unsuitable conditions of the endometrium and cervical mucus.

SEX DETERMINATION AND SEXUAL DIFFERENTIATION

The genetic sex of an individual is initially determined at the time of fertilization when an X or Y chromosome-bearing spermatozoon fuses with a normal X chromosome-bearing ovum, which produces a female (XX) or male (XY) zygote, respectively. Thus the genetic sex of the male human subject is normally determined by the presence of a Y chromosome. However, the mechanism involved in the translation of the zygote's genetic sex into the sexual dimorphism of the adult male or female phenotype is dependent on a complex interplay of genetic, hormonal, psychological and social factors, of which only the first two will be discussed here.

CHROMOSOMAL DETERMINANTS

The X and Y chromosomes are called the sex chromosomes and the remaining 44, the autosomes. In man the Y chromosome normally carries the genetic determinants essential for the development of masculine traits, while the female traits are carried on the autosomes or the X chromosomes or both. Study of chromosomal disorders has shown that no matter how many X chromosomes (e.g. the XXY male) are present, if a Y chromosome is also present, then testes will develop and phenotypically (i.e. anatomically) the individual will be a male. This suggests that the Y chromosome bears the genetic determinants for differentiation of the testis.

Until recently, there was little information available as to how the Y chromosome brought about testicular morphogenesis. In 1955 the H-Y histocompatibility antigen was discovered in the skin of male mice, which causes rejection of male skin grafts in female mice. In 1975 Wachtel discovered the invariant expression of the H-Y antigen in cells from the XY mammalian male but not the XX female. Moreover, the cells of XYY men have about twice the amount of H-Y antigen as normal XY males. Although the H-Y antigen is normally associated with a Y chromosome, this is not invariably the case.

The antigen is a component of the cell membrane and is found on the surface of all cells of mammalian males except immature germ cells and red blood cells. It is expressed early in development since it is found on cells of the early blastocyst and it is thought either directly or indirectly to induce differentiation of the testis from the primitive gonad, which has an inherent tendency to form an ovary in the absence of the H-Y antigen. This antigen is probably important for spermatogenesis while another locus on the Y chromosome is important for testicular morphogenesis.

In the human, in contrast to the mouse for example, two X chromosomes are necessary for the bipotential gonad to develop as a normal ovary. It is also clear that the autosomes carry genes essential for both normal male and normal female development. So far, at least 19 genes have been implicated in the control of sexual differentiation.

HORMONAL DETERMINANTS

The human gonads start to develop at about the 5th week of gestation. They appear initially as the two urogenital ridges, thickened areas of coelomic epithelial cells covering the mesonephros and associated underlying mesenchymal cells. The germinal ridges are then progressively invaded by primordial germ cells which have migrated from the endoderm of the yolk sac. By amoeboid movement the primordial germ cells leave the endoderm, migrate dorsally in the mesentery and enter the germinal epithelium (Fig. 4.9). The thickened germinal epithelium containing the dividing germ cells, now called gonocytes, proliferates and sends cords of cells (the primary sex cords) into the underlying stroma. The establishment of these primitive gonads and the urogenital tract is indistinguishable in the two sexes, up to about 6 weeks of development. Then, presumably through the influence of the H-Y antigen, the sex cords of the male become separated from the germinal epithelium and eventually develop into the seminiferous tubules. Leydig cells also begin to differentiate at this stage. In the female the sex cords break up into clusters of cells each containing a gonocyte to form the primordial follicles (Fig. 4.9). Indifferent gonocytes become spermatogonia in the testes and oocytes in the ovaries.

At the end of the indifferent phase of differentiation, the urogenital tract consists of two components. Firstly, there is a dual duct system, the mesonephric (or Wolffian) duct and the paramesonephric (or Müllerian) duct. These form the anlagen of the internal accessory reproductive organs. The second component is made up of the urogenital sinus and tubercle which differentiate to form the external genitalia and in the male the terminal urethra. The Müllerian duct develops later than the Wolffian duct and its caudal portion is derived from the Wolffian duct itself. The cranial portion (mesonephric tubules) of the Wolffian duct connects to the gonad (i.e. the testis) but the cranial end of the Müllerian duct never does so. During differentiation of a male fetus the Wolffian duct develops to form the rete testis, epididymis, vas deferens and seminal vesicles while the urogenital sinus gives rise to the prostate. In the differentiation of the female, the Fallopian tubes, the uterus and the upper half of the vagina develop from the Müllerian duct.

During differentiation of the respective sexes, the duct which is not needed regresses. Regression of the Müllerian duct and virilization of the Wolffian duct in the male is an active process dependent upon the secretions of the fetal testis. In the absence of testicular secretion, the female form develops even in the absence of the ovaries. The fetal testis secretes a Müllerian duct regression factor called anti-Müllerian hormone. This is a glycoprotein, which is initially synthesized by the fetal Sertoli cells early in fetal life. In adults it is secreted in small amounts; in women it is secreted into the follicular fluid by mature granulosa cells. It has a molecular weight of 145 000 with 13.5% of carbohydrate; it is a homodimer, i.e. made up of two identical chains. Messenger RNA has been isolated from fetal bovine testis and it codes for the two 560 amino acid peptide chains each with a molecular weight of 62 000. The messenger RNA has been used to prepare complementary DNA (see Chapter 1), and the genes for both human and bovine anti-Müllerian hormone have been cloned. The Müllerian duct is only sensitive to this hormone's action for a short period between the 7th and the 8th week of intra-uterine life. The action of the Müllerian regression hormone is ipsilateral. Failure of its synthesis

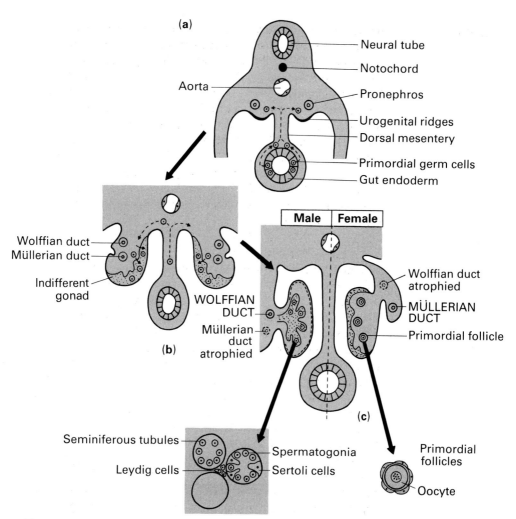

**Fig. 4.9** The early stages in the differentiation of the genital system.

(a) Shows a cross-section of a 5 week human embryo showing the primordial germ cells migrating from the gut endoderm up the dorsal mesentery to the thickening urogenital ridges. The neural tube, notochord, pronephros and aorta are also shown.

(b) A later stage (6 weeks) shows the invasion of the primordial germ cells into the urogenital ridges to form the indifferent gonads and the appearance of the Wolffian and Müllerian ducts.

(c) The male, seminiferous tubules differentiate and show spermatogonia and Sertoli cells. The steroidogenic Leydig cells appear between the tubules and the Müllerian duct regresses. In the female, primordial follicles consisting of an oocyte and flattened surrounding cells appear and the Wolffian duct regresses.

or action results in the persistence of female structures into postnatal life.

The fetal testis also secretes testosterone which is responsible for virilization of the Wolffian duct. Conversion of testosterone to 5α-dihydrotestosterone is necessary for virilization of the fetal external genitalia and the development of the prostate. This conversion is produced by $5\alpha$-reductase in these fetal derivatives of the urogenital sinus. During fetal development, sex hormone-dependent changes occur in the urogenital epithelial tissue of both sexes even though the cells do not have sex hormone receptors. These developmental changes only occur if the developing epithelium is in close proximity to the sex hormone receptor-containing mesenchymal tissue. Factors secreted by the mesenchymal tissue in response to sex hormone act on the nearby epithelium. The epithelium later develops sex hormone receptors and then it can respond directly to endocrine factors.

Thus, five factors are important in the development of the male reproductive system. The first is the Y chromosome product responsible for testicular differentiation while the second is the H-Y antigen which is responsible for spermatogenesis. The third is Müllerian duct regression hormone needed to produce regression of the ovarian duct. The fourth is testosterone which virilizes the Wolffian duct, and the fifth is $5\alpha$-dihydrotestosterone required for differentiation of the external genitalia. Under the influence of these five, the gross anatomy of the phenotypic male is established by the end of the third month.

In the latter two trimesters of pregnancy the testes descend from their position by the kidneys to the adult position in the scrotum. This process requires gonadotrophin from the developing pituitary as well as testosterone. The descent is usually completed by birth but is sometimes delayed: if descent does not occur, synthesis of testosterone in later life can occur, but spermatogenesis will fail since this requires the lower temperature of the scrotum. However, this can be corrected effectively by surgery, provided this is done before the age of 6 years.

In the differentiation of the female, the Fallopian tubes, the uterus and the upper half of the vagina develop from the Müllerian duct. The development of the female lags behind that of the male. Regression of the Wolffian duct and development of the female structure only commences towards the end of the first trimester and the development of the gross anatomy of the female is not completed until the third trimester.

Then the reproductive systems are established in fetal life but their further development, and development of the germ cells, occurs later in life while full maturation occurs only after puberty.

### Abnormalities of sexual differentiation

With the extended and complex nature of the processes involved in the expression of the true phenotype, it is not surprising that disorders of sexual differentiation occur. Since normal development is a sequential process, failures in fetal life can be recognized in postnatal life by characteristic abnormalities. Some of these are detailed below.

## FAILURE OF ANTI-MÜLLERIAN HORMONE

If testosterone were the only hormone to be produced by the fetal testis, males would also have a vestigial uterus, upper two-thirds of vagina and Fallopian tubes. A rare familial condition in which this occurs has been identified. In normal males these Müllerian-derived structures are normally suppressed by the elaboration of anti-Müllerian hormone but when this effect fails these structures persist.

### PSEUDOHERMAPHRODITISM

In pseudohermaphroditism the genetic and gonadal sex are at variance with the phenotypic sex.

#### *Male pseudohermaphroditism*

A male pseudohermaphrodite is an individual whose karyotype is XY and whose gonads are exclusively testes but whose phenotypic characteristics are to varying degrees female. This condition may arise as a result of a number of abnormalities some of which are described below.

*Failure to respond to testosterone.* In this condition, testosterone fails to act on its target-cells owing to 'end-organ' resistance or their insensitivity to the actions of testosterone. Anti-Müllerian hormone still has its local action and an individual is born with female external genitalia, a short vagina (the upper two-thirds having been obliterated). However, they have no uterus

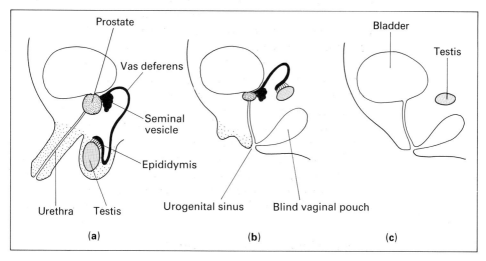

**Fig. 4.10** (a) The normal male genital tract and the changes which occur in (b) 5α-reductase deficiency and (c) testicular feminization. In the enzyme deficient animal, structures arising from the genital tubercle (shaded areas) are absent (e.g. penis) and a blind vaginal pouch is present. In the testicular feminization syndrome only the testis is found. The epididymis, vas deferens, seminal vesicle, prostate and penis are all absent. (Modified from Imperato-McGinley *et al.* (1974) *Science* **186**, 1213.)

or Fallopian tubes. These individuals are reared as females (Fig. 4.10).

The underlying biochemical failures in two types of end-organ insensitivity have been recognized.

1 Testicular feminization. In one form, the individual's target-cells do not contain the androgen-binding cytoplasmic receptor protein. At puberty these patients will develop breasts but they will have no pubic or other body hair and usually present with primary amenorrhoea. They have a male karyotype (46XY) and develop testes that may be found in an inguinal hernia; spermatogenesis is impaired. Because of tissue resistance the testosterone produced by the testes is inactive and this explains why body hair does not develop. However, the testosterone can still be aromatized to oestradiol so these patients will develop normal breasts at puberty. This condition is referred to as the androgen insensitivity syndrome, or 'testicular feminization syndrome'.

2 Failure to metabolize testosterone. There is another form in which there is lack of the enzyme 5α-reductase which converts testosterone to 5α-dihydrotestosterone. There will be no development of the external genitalia and so these individuals have penile-scrotal hypospadias and ambiguous female external genitalia. They have labial testes and all the testosterone-dependent internal structures but a reduced prostate. At puberty, hair development and production of sebum are impaired because of reduced formation of dihydrotestosterone, breast development does not occur because there is no excess production of oestrogens, but there is a rise in testosterone production at puberty with increased muscular development and an increase in the size of the phallus. Testicular descent and spermatogenesis can occur but there is infertility because of hypospadias. Because of the ambiguity of the genitalia at birth, these children are reared as females. However, at puberty they change gender and become masculinized and behave as males, with heterosexual orientation as males: their infertility can then be corrected by surgical treatment for hypospadias.

*Defects of steroid biosynthesis.* Deficiencies of the enzymes in the pathway of biosynthesis of testosterone (Fig. 4.2) have been recognized clinically; a consequence can be that testosterone and hence dihydrotestosterone are not synthesized in normal amounts. Since their effects are not all-or-none, but are related to the circulating concentrations, ambiguity of the genitalia occurs.

*Female pseudohermaphroditism*

A female pseudohermaphrodite has an XX karyotype, and ovaries are present but there are varying degrees of phenotypic masculinization. There is no abnormality of the ovary or its functional capacity and no abnormality of internal genital development, so reproductive function is often possible after appropriate treatment. Female pseudohermaphroditism usually arises as a result of enzyme abnormalities involved in adrenal steroid biosynthesis. In some of the varieties of congenital adrenal hyperplasia there is excess production of androgens (see Chapter 3). This results in the masculinization of the genitalia of the female fetus.



*True hermaphroditism*

Only when both female and male gonadal elements can be definitely demonstrated in the same individual can true hermaphroditism be said to exist. The chromosomal pattern may be XX, XY or a mosaic. There may be a testis on one side of the body and an ovary on the other; more commonly, there is an 'ovotestis' present on one or both sides. The phenotype depends on the number of Leydig cells; the amount of testosterone which such gonads produce at puberty is inadequate for a male or excessive for a female. Thus at puberty a 'male' patient may develop gynaecomastia or a 'female' develop excessive body hair.

### EFFECT OF ABNORMAL EXPOSURE TO HORMONES *IN UTERO*

Administration of androgens before the 12th week of pregnancy leads to fusion of the labia (scrotalization) of a female fetus. Oestrogen administration can also have serious effects. In the late 1950s diethylstilbestrol (a synthetic compound that has oestrogenic activity even though it does not have a steroid nucleus) was used in an attempt to improve the prognosis of pregnancy in diabetic patients because the morbidity and mortality of infants of diabetic mothers is considerable. This treatment had no effect on the outcome of pregnancy but it became apparent that some of the daughters of mothers who had been treated in this way developed a carcinoma of the vagina when they were about 20 years old. Similar changes could be reproduced in rats treated with diethylstilbestrol early in pregnancy; neoplastic change subsequently developed at the time of puberty. In other words there were two endocrine events in the development of this tumour, the first *in utero* and the second at the time of puberty, and if puberty was prevented in the rats, neoplasms did not develop.

## SUMMARY

The maintenance of the male reproductive system and secondary sexual characteristics depends on androgens secreted from the testes. The male continuously produces a very large number of gametes (spermatazoa), whereas the female produces only one (or two) each month. The control of gametogenesis in the male depends on testicular stimulation by follicle stimulating hormone and luteinizing hormone, whose secretion is inhibited by a negative feedback of the testicular hormones, androgens and inhibin. In the female, the production of ova depends on a cycle of hormonal changes involving follicle stimulating hormone (FSH) and luteinizing hormone (LH) with negative feedback by ovarian hormones, oestrogens, progesterone and inhibin. Ovulation is initiated by a surge of LH at mid-cycle resulting from a switch from negative to positive feedback by oestrogens on the pituitary. The cycle of hormonal changes brings about follicular development, luteolysis and menstruation and in so doing maintains the female genital tract in a condition which allows fertilization and implantation to occur at the appropriate time. Oestrogens also maintain the secondary sexual characteristics.

In pregnancy, the fetoplacental unit acts as an endocrine organ, secreting human chorionic gonadotrophin, human placental lactogen, oestrogens, progesterone, and adrenocortical steroids into the maternal circulation and so maintains pregnancy and eventually initiates parturition.

Sexual differentiation and development over an extended period, from conception to puberty, depends on a complex interplay of genetic and hormonal factors. In the absence of a functioning testis the female phenotype prevails despite a 46XY chromosome karyotype.

Disorders of the reproductive system are very varied ranging from the commonest endocrine cause of infertility, i.e. over-secretion of prolactin, to rare genetic disorders such as end-organ insensitivity.

## FURTHER READING

Austin C. R. & Short R. V. (1985) *Reproduction in Mammals*. Book 4. Reproductive Stress, 2nd edn. Cambridge University Press, Cambridge.
Yen S. S. C. & Jaffe R. B. (1986) *Reproduction Endocrinology*, 2nd edn. W. B. Saunders, Philadelphia & London.

# 5 The thyroid gland

In man the thyroid gland is a discrete organ situated just caudal to the larynx and adherent to the front of the trachea. The characteristic feature of the gland is its ability to concentrate iodide from the bloodstream and synthesize the iodine-containing thyroid hormones, thyroxine and triiodothyronine. The thyroid gland is dependent upon a constant supply of dietary iodide, and when this element is scarce the gland enlarges in response to demands for the gland to trap more iodine and hence make more thyroid hormone; this visible swelling in the neck is called a goitre. Because of the relatively common occurrence of goitres in iodine-deficient regions of the world, references to the condition date back to the second millennium BC in Chinese literature. However, Thomas Wharton in 1656 gave the first unequivocal modern description of the normal thyroid and he gave the gland its name, which is derived from the Greek word meaning 'shield-like'; the name approximately describes the flat, oval shape of each of the two lobes of the normal thyroid gland.

It was not until the latter part of the 19th century that the various symptoms related to disorders of the thyroid were recognized. The association of sporadic cretinism (impaired neurological development) in infants with atrophy of the thyroid was described by Fagge in England in 1871. Soon after this, Ord reported atrophy of the thyroid at autopsy in two cases of the newly described Gull's disease, which he renamed myxoedema, referring to the apparent oedema or subcutaneous mucus deposits that caused fluid retention visible in these patients. In 1883 thyroidectomy of goitrous patients was noted to cause an initial improvement of their condition but they later developed symptoms resembling myxoedema. Experimental thyroidectomy on animals was initially complicated by the simultaneous and inadvertent removal of the parathyroid glands; the dual effects of their removal were resolved by Gley in 1891. In the last decade of that century, the beneficial effects of thyroid grafting into myxoedematous patients was quickly replaced by the equally effective oral administration of lightly cooked animal thyroids.

In 1820 Coindet was the first to describe the effects of treatment of patients with goitre using potassium iodide or tincture of iodine. The idea stemmed from the observation of Courtois

(1813) that seaweed contained iodine and the knowledge that burnt sponge had for centuries been a recognized remedy for goitre. The suggestion of Kocher in 1895 that the thyroid itself might contain iodine was confirmed a year later by Baumann but it was not until Christmas Day, 1914, that Kendall in the USA first purified an iodine-containing substance from extracts of thyroid tissue: 30 years later Pitt-Rivers and Harrington determined the structure of thyroxine and suggested how it was synthesized. Since the middle of the 20th century, the availability of radioisotopes of iodine and the technique of chromatography have revolutionized the study of the thyroid. Radioactive iodine has been used extensively in the study of disorders of the thyroid, in thyroid ablation, and in the labelling of thyroid hormones used for metabolic studies or in the technique of radioimmunoassay.

Apart from thyroxine, the thyroid gland also secretes another hormone, triiodothyronine which has one fewer iodine atom per molecule. In contrast to most other hormones in the body, the concentrations of circulating thyroid hormones are maintained relatively constant, and only very small alterations occur throughout the life of a normal human. The presence of thyroid hormone is absolutely essential for normal growth and development. In the adult virtually every tissue in the body has a requirement for the thyroid hormones to a greater or lesser degree. Administration of thyroid hormones leads to an increase in basal metabolic rate (BMR) in an adult. Thyroid hormones restore normal growth patterns in thyroid-deficient immature animals in addition to these calorigenic effects.

## MORPHOLOGY

### Development

In the human embryo, the early stages of development of the thyroid gland and parathyroid glands are closely associated and will, therefore, be considered together. Thyroid development commences at day 24 as a midline thickening and then as an out-pouching of the endodermal floor of the pharyngeal cavity. This primordium of the thyroid eventually forms a sac-like diverticulum between the first and second pharyngeal pouches (Fig. 5.1a). At about one month of development, when the fetus is nearly 4 mm in length, the diverticulum comprises a solid mass of cells and weighs about $1-2$ mg. By the 6th to 7th week it is clearly bilobed, and as the embryo elongates and the tongue grows forward the thyroid descends in the neck but remains attached to its point of origin by a narrow canal, the thyroglossal duct. During the 5th and 6th weeks of development, the distal ends of the IIIrd and IVth paired pharyngeal

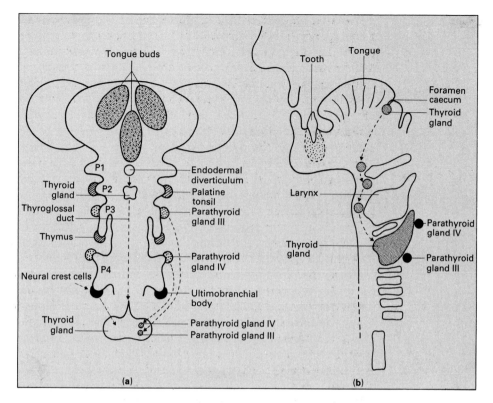

**Fig. 5.1** (a) A horizontal section of a human fetal pharynx, looking down on its floor, and showing the origin of the thyroid and parathyroid glands. The thyroid originates as an endodermal diverticulum in the floor of the pharynx at the level of the first pharyngeal pouch (P1). It moves caudally ( ↓ ), becoming bilobed, but remaining for some time attached to its origin by the thyroglossal duct. As the thyroid moves caudally, paired cell masses detach themselves from the third (P3) and fourth (P4) pharyngeal pouches respectively, become positioned on the thyroid's posterior surface and form the parathyroid glands III and IV. Neural crest cells, which have invaded the fourth pharyngeal pouch (P4) to form the ultimobranchial bodies, migrate into the caudally moving thyroid and form its C-cell component. The origins of the thymus, palatine tonsils and tongue buds are also shown.

(b) The thyroid gland and its caudal migration ( ↓ ) to just below the larynx. Its point of origin in the tongue persists as the foramen caecum. Common sites of thyroglossal cysts (⊚) are also shown and the position of paired parathyroid glands III and IV are indicated (●). A developing tooth is also indicated. (After K. L. Moore, *The Developing Human*; W. B. Saunders, Philadelphia.)

pouches differentiate into the primordia of the four parathyroid glands (Fig. 5.1a). Caudal movement of the developing thyroid brings it down to the level of parathyroids IV, which do not appreciably alter their position relative to the thyroid. However, parathyroids III bud off from the pharyngeal body during this time, pass the parathyroids IV in their caudal descent, and come to rest on the posterior surface of the thyroid gland. Parathyroids IV thus become the *superior* and parathyroids III become the *inferior* parathyroid glands in humans, lying on the posterior surface of the thyroid gland.

The lower (ventral) portion of the IVth pharyngeal pouches, the ultimobranchial bodies, come into contact with the thyroid anlagen, and eventually a fusion of the two organs occurs with a mixing of the two cell types. These latter cells become the C-cells of the thyroid gland, making up about 10% of the adult cell-mass of the gland, and they secrete the hormone calcitonin (see Chapter 6). The thymus is derived from cells which arise from the ventral portion of the IIIrd pharyngeal pouch and which migrate caudally with the thyroid and parathyroids. If the parathyroids or ultimobranchial bodies do not become attached to or incorporated into the thyroid, they form ectopic glands.

Normally, the thyroglossal duct ruptures and the cells atrophy or are resorbed by the second month, leaving only a small dimple (the foramen caecum) at the junction of the middle and posterior third of the tongue: persistent thyroglossal duct tissue may give rise to cysts (Fig. 5.1b). Cells in the lower portion of the duct differentiate into thyroid tissue, forming the pyramidal lobe of the gland as an upward, finger-like extension. The thyroid develops laterally into two distinct lobes connected by a narrow isthmus of thyroid tissue at the midline. The lobes come to rest on either side of, and slightly behind, the trachea, with the isthmus running across its front, just below the larynx in humans and most mammals; this, therefore, provides a convenient landmark for locating the thyroid gland.

The thyroid gland of higher vertebrates appears to have evolved from an open, ventral pharyngeal groove found in such lowly chordates as *Amphioxus* and the larval lamprey. In these animals it is an exocrine structure secreting mucus, but in higher vertebrates it has the unique capacity to concentrate iodide and secrete the thyroid hormones.

By the 7th week of development, when connection of the human thyroid to the pharynx is lost, the cells of the thyroid are grouped into clusters. At about 11 weeks, a central lumen appears in each cluster, completely surrounded by a single layer of cells. Although the thyroid is functionally capable of trapping iodide and releasing hormone at this stage, it does not actually respond to pituitary secretion of thyrotrophin until this occurs at around the 22nd week. In the rat and rabbit, however, the pituitary-linked response does not occur until approximately 5 days after birth.

ABNORMALITIES

Developmental abnormalities of the thyroid are fairly common in human subjects. In approximately 15% of the population, the thyroglossal duct fails to atrophy, or it is partially resorbed, and so may still be present in the adult, yielding a midline pyramidal lobe of active thyroid tissue. In the same way, development abnormalities of the isthmus may occur which are not noted until the gland is investigated later in life. If the thyroid fails to descend to the correct level, or else descends too far, then the thyroid gland may be found in sublingual or intrathoracic positions. Absence of the left lobe is also observed in some individuals, owing to development of only a single thyroid lobe. Usually these developmental abnormalities do not affect thyroid function, and it is only during investigation of thyroid dysfunction that these abnormalities may be found. Occasionally, a congenital complete absence of the thyroid occurs; this requires immediate detection and treatment with thyroid hormone within 1 week of birth, otherwise severe and largely irreversible neurological damage occurs to the neonate, resulting in the state of 'sporadic cretinism'.

The adult human gland is a pad of pink tissue, weighing between 10 to about 20g. Thyroid glands are usually smaller in regions of the world where supplies of dietary iodine are abundant. It is nearly always asymmetric, with the right lobe often twice the size of the left lobe. The thyroid is usually larger in women than men, and it enlarges during adolescence, and in pregnancy, during lactation and in the latter part of the menstrual cycle; seasonal changes have also been reported between summer and winter, during which period a decrease in thyroid mass frequently occurs.

The gland is enclosed by two connective tissue capsules. The outer capsule of the gland is not well defined and attaches the thyroid to the trachea. On the posterior surface of the thyroid, the two pairs of parathyroids are situated between the two capsules. From the inner capsule trabeculae of collagen fibres pervade the gland and carry nerves and a rich vasculature to the cells (Fig. 5.2). In humans, the sympathetic and parasympathetic supply to the gland appear to regulate the rich vascular system. Secretomotor fibres to follicular cells have not been convincingly demonstrated. The arterial blood supply arises from the external carotids and subclavians and enters the gland via the superior and inferior thyroid arteries respectively. The thyroid has a blood flow which has been estimated to range from 4 to 6 ml/min/g of tissue, which is nearly twice that of the kidney. In conditions of severe hyperplasia very much greater flow-rates may occur, as is evidenced by an audible bruit when a stethoscope is placed on or near an overactive gland.

## Histology

The functional unit of the gland is the thyroid follicle or acinus (Fig. 5.2). This consists of cuboidal epithelial (follicular) cells

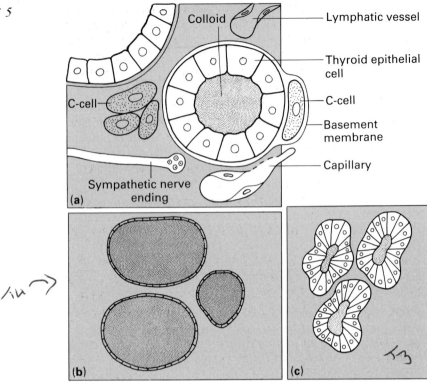

**Fig. 5.2** The histological components of the mammalian thyroid gland.

(a) Euthyroid follicles are shown, consisting of hollow spheres of cuboidal, epithelial cells, the lumens of which are filled with colloid. Surrounding each follicle is a basement membrane enclosing C-cells in a parafollicular position. In the interfollicular stroma are found fenestrated capillaries, lymphatic vessels and sympathetic nerve endings.

(b) Underactive follicles are shown with flattened thyroid epithelial cells and increased colloid.

(c) Overactive follicles are shown with tall, columnar epithelial cells and reduced colloid.

arranged as roughly spheroidal sacs, the lumen of which contains colloid. The latter is almost entirely composed of the iodinated glycoprotein called thyroglobulin which yields an intensely pink periodic acid-Schiff (PAS) positive stain. The normal human follicle varies in diameter from 20 to 900 μm, and many thousands of these are present in the gland; several follicles are usually grouped together in arbitrary units separated by blood vessels and connective tissue. Each follicle is surrounded by a basement membrane, and lying between this membrane and the follicular cells are the parafollicular, calcitonin-secreting, C-cells.

A loose framework of reticular fibres holds the follicles together, and an abundance of short, fenestrated capillaries surround them (Fig. 5.2). An extensive network of lymphatic vessels is also present, and small amounts of thyroglobulin have been found to be absorbed by this lymph system. However, this is not thought to be quantitatively significant in thyroglobulin removal and is probably unrelated to thyroid hormone release from the gland, although it may be relevant in thyroid autoimmune states (see below). As mentioned above, postganglionic sympathetic nerve fibres from the middle and superior cervical ganglia supply blood vessels and hence control the blood flow through the gland. By this means, they alter the delivery-rate of thyrotrophin, iodide and other metabolites such as amino acids etc., to the cells of the gland. Preganglionic parasympathetic fibres from the vagus also enter the gland: adrenergic nerve terminals may be associated principally with mast cells in the thyroid, but it is impossible to rule out a direct, although probably minor, effect of the biogenic amines on thyroid follicular cells.

In the situation where the gland is essentially normal, but underactive (such as occurs in an iodine-deficient hypothyroid state), the follicles are distended with colloid and the acinar cells are thin and flattened with little cytoplasm visible under the light microscope, and the nuclei are the characteristic feature at the edges of the follicles. On the other hand, in the overactive or hyperactive gland, the acinar cells are tall and columnar and periodic acid-Schiff staining of droplets of colloid may be seen within some cells under the light microscope. Different follicles appear to be activated to different extents, as is evidenced by differing densities of staining of the luminal colloid and colloid droplets in surrounding cells. Under the electron microscope, large pseudopodia and an extensive network of microvilli may be observed at the apical or colloid end of the active cells.

## CIRCULATING THYROID HORMONES

### Chemical structure

The structures of the iodothyronine hormones produced by the thyroid, and some other important metabolites, are shown in Fig. 5.3: thyroxine (or $3,3',5,5'$-tetraiodothyronine) is frequently abbreviated to $T_4$, and triiodothyronine is abbreviated to $T_3$, with the numbers representing the number of iodine atoms attached to each thyronine residue. A biologically inactive iodothyronine called 'reverse-$T_3$', that is $3,3',5'$-triiodothyronine, is also found in significant concentrations in human serum.

### Thyroid hormones in the circulation

In serum, both of the active iodothyronine hormones (thyroxine and $3,5,3'$-triiodothyronine) are strongly bound to serum proteins; about 0.015% of the total circulating thyroxine and

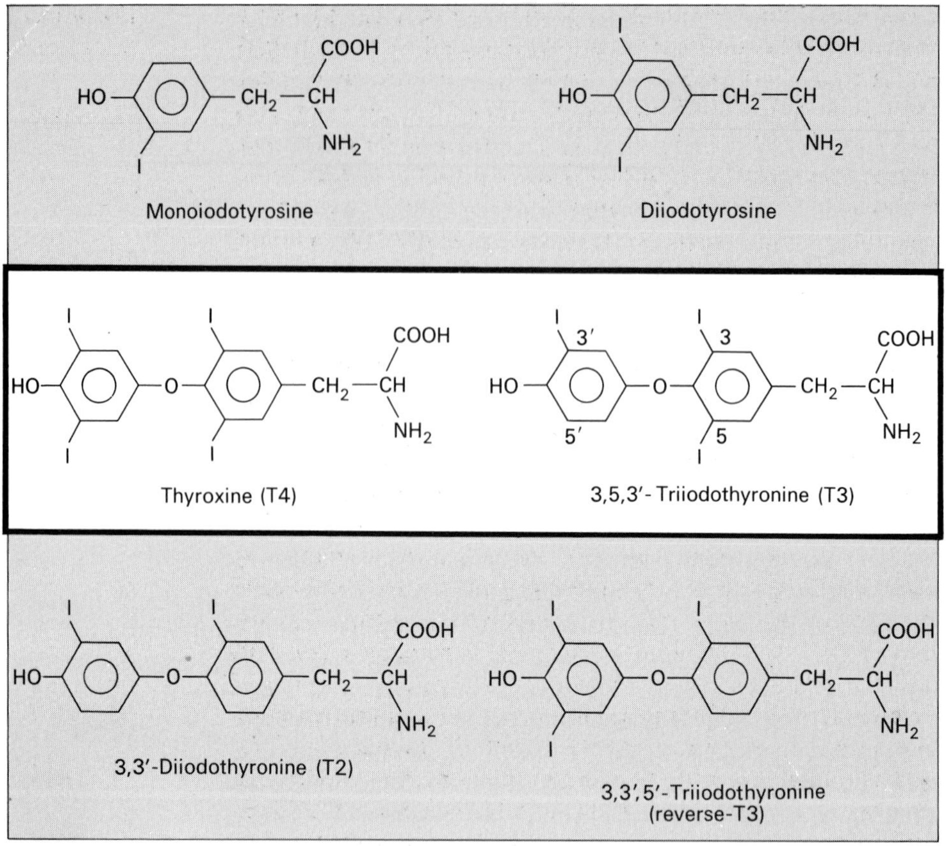

**Fig. 5.3** Structures of intrathyroidal iodoamino acids. Mono- and diiodo-tyrosines are precursors of the thyroid hormones (see text). Thyroxine (T4) and triiodothyronine (T3) are the two biologically active forms of the thyroid hormones. Triiodothyronine is secreted by the gland and can also be formed peripherally from thyroxine by specific enzymic deiodination. 'Reverse' T3 and T2 are inactive metabolites formed by deiodination of the thyroid hormones by peripheral tissues of the body. The numbering of critical positions is shown on the structure of T3.

0.33% of the total serum triiodothyronine are present in the free form. Triiodothyronine is bound slightly less strongly to each of the three principal serum binding-proteins than is thyroxine, and the strength of binding (affinity) of both iodo-thyronines decreases in the following order: thyroxine-binding globulin (TBG) > thyroxine-binding pre-albumin (TBPA) > serum albumin. Albumin is a relatively non-specific binder of thyroid hormone present in the circulation.

The two *iodothyronine* binding proteins (misleadingly referred to as 'thyroxine'-binding) are the principal thyroid hormone binding proteins in serum. They may be demonstrated in serum by adding radioiodine-labelled iodothyronine and separating the serum proteins by electrophoresis in an appropriate buffer system, when three radioactive peaks are observed. Thyroxine-binding globulin migrates between the $\alpha_1$- and $\alpha_2$-globulins; thyroxine-binding pre-albumin, as its name suggests, migrates faster than the labelled albumin peak in the anodal direction at pH 8.6. The relative affinities of binding-proteins for the iodothyronines may be demonstrated by diluting the labelled hormone with different concentrations of non-radioactive hormone: redistribution of labelled hormone, which is initially attached principally to TBG and TBPA, occurs with a larger proportion of the total radioactivity binding to albumin.

*Measurement*

Thyroid status is now usually assessed by radioimmunoassay of the concentration of thyroid hormones and thyrotrophin in serum, and these methods have virtually completely replaced other methods of assessing thyroid function. Some of the older techniques such as determination of radioiodine uptake by the thyroid gland, measurement of the circulating 'protein-bound iodine' (PBI) in the serum and indirect methods such as measuring serum cholesterol levels are still employed in some countries of the world. The success of the radioimmunoassay technique has resulted in its widespread use, and the reproducibility of results has led to establishment of relatively well-defined 'normal ranges' for concentrations of thyroid hormones in the serum which are now very similar throughout the world. Measurement of the total thyroxine or triiodothyronine concentrations in serum is achieved by adding a blocking agent, which displaces the bound hormone from serum proteins. Usually, 8-anilino-1-naphthalene sulphonic acid (ANS) or salicylic acid are used to displace the thyroid hormones from their serum binding-proteins. The released iodothyronines are then free to equilibrate with added antiserum in an immunoassay system. The normal range for thyroxine is about 60 to 170 nmol/l, and that for triiodothyronine is about 0.8 to 2.7 nmol/l.

Free thyroid hormone concentrations may also be estimated in specially adapted immunoassays. In theory, the free iodothyronine concentration in the circulation should provide a more accurate assessment of thyroid status, since it will compensate for changes in binding protein concentrations which may occur under different conditions (see 'free thyroid hormones', below). Several different types of free thyroid hormone assays are available. Some of these assays provide only an approximation to the actual free thyroid hormone concentration in serum, because the assay system may be affected by the presence of interfering substances such as free fatty acids, greatly altered serum binding-protein concentrations, etc.

Sensitive and precise immunoassays for thyrotrophin are now available, with the replacement of radioimmunoassays by immunometric assays that use monoclonal antibodies. With the latter assays, the normal range for thyrotrophin has been defined between about 0.4 and 5 mIU/l. It is sometimes possible to make an initial assessment of patient thyroid status on the basis of thyrotrophin measurements alone. However, it is more usual to base the assessment on results from more than one of the foregoing immunoassay tests in conjunction with physical signs and symptoms. In certain circumstances (such as in the recognition of hypothyroidism in newborn infants) an assessment of thyroidal function may be based solely on biochemical evidence from thyrotrophin or thyroxine immunoassays, before physical signs or symptoms have become apparent.

## Kinetics

Studies on the kinetics of release and metabolism of iodothyronines in the body show that triiodothyronine has a shorter half-life (about 1−3 days) than has thyroxine (about 5−7 days). In addition, triiodothyronine has about twice the volume of distribution of thyroxine; in normal humans, thyroxine has a distribution volume of about 12 litres, which is a little larger than the volume of circulating blood, while triiodothyronine must be bound intracellularly to achieve a distribution volume in excess of 26 litres. Depending on the biological response monitored, estimates of the relative potency of the two hormones show that triiodothyronine is from 2 to 10 times more active than thyroxine, and the kinetic data, above, are consistent with the observation that triiodothyronine is biologically more active than thyroxine. However, the total serum concentration of triiodothyronine is only about 2% of that of thyroxine, i.e. about 2 nmol/l for T3 versus approximately 100 nmol/l for T4.

### FREE THYROID HORMONES

The differential binding to serum proteins results in free T3 concentrations being about 30% of those of free T4 (about 6 pmol/l for free T3, and about 18 pmol/l for free T4). In spite of the higher concentrations of thyroxine in serum, triiodothyronine is turned over in the body at a faster rate, and it is also biologically the more active hormone.

The majority of cells of the body do not appear to take up the binding-proteins from the serum and so these cells can only respond to the free thyroid hormones in serum. Under most normal circumstances, the serum binding-proteins remain at relatively constant concentrations, and measurements of the total thyroid hormone concentrations therefore mirror the levels of the free thyroid hormones present. However, in conditions where serum binding-protein concentrations are altered, the total thyroid hormone concentrations no longer reflect the free hormone concentrations in the serum. This arises because altered binding-protein concentrations in serum cause a change in the fraction of circulating free thyroid hormones, and the hypothalamo-pituitary—thyroid control mechanisms readjust to maintain the concentrations of iodothyronines that are free. Thus, when binding-protein concentrations fall, as can occur in starvation or in some disease states, e.g. liver disease or renal failure, less total iodothyronines are required to maintain adequate free concentrations at the euthyroid level. Conversely, when liver synthesis of binding-proteins is increased by steroid action on the liver during pregnancy or when oral contraceptives are taken, then more total thyroid hormone is required to maintain the concentrations of free idothyronines in the circulation.

Certain drugs can also compete with iodothyronines for binding to the serum proteins, and they therefore elevate the free thyroid hormone concentrations and cause the control mechanisms to lower the total iodothyronine concentrations in the serum. Typical of such drugs are the salicylates, the hydantoins used in the treatment of epilepsy, or anti-inflammatory drugs such as fenclofenac whose structure resembles that of the iodothyronine molecule. In order to monitor thyroidal status by biochemical measurements of the circulating concentrations of iodothyronine hormones in the presence of altered serum binding-protein concentrations, two courses of action are possible. Either a correction for the altered serum concentrations of thyroid hormone-binding proteins is required, or direct measurements of the free hormone concentrations must be performed.

Once the serum iodothyronine concentrations have settled to constant values within about 3 days after birth, little change occurs in the normal individual throughout the remainder of life, except perhaps for a very slight decline in thyroxine with age in some individuals. Thyroid status of such patients should be assessed by thyrotrophin measurements, rather than total thyroid hormone estimations.

## EFFECTS AND MECHANISM OF ACTION OF THYROID HORMONES

### General effects

A study of the mechanism of action of the thyroid hormones has proved to be extremely difficult. Constant exposure of cells of an adult animal to thyroid hormones implies that there is an essential requirement for iodothyronines in the maintenance of normal metabolic functions. Virtually the only definitive action of the thyroid hormones in intact animals is recognized to be an effect on increasing the basal metabolic rate (BMR). Although several short-term effects of the thyroid hormones have been observed at various subcellular sites, it is now recognized that the principal, and probably primary, site of action of the iodo-thyronine hormones is on the cell nucleus. Most of the actions of the thyroid hormones are mediated by triiodothyronine which is secreted by the thyroid, and produced by deiodination of thyronine in peripheral tissues.

## Cellular effects

### NUCLEAR SITE OF ACTION

The elegant studies of Tata and Widnell in the early 1960s were performed by injecting thyroidectomized rats with relatively low doses of triiodothyronine which were lower than the phar-macological doses used up until that time. An increase in nuclear RNA as a result of activation of DNA-dependent RNA poly-merase was found to precede all the other intracellular changes, as shown in Fig. 5.4. Increases were subsequently observed in ribosomal and messenger RNAs, which were followed by increased protein synthesis. This led to changes in amounts of various enzymes, shown as amino acid incorporation/mg of ribosomal RNA in Fig. 5.4, and ultimately of liver weight.

Triiodothyronine binds to specific nuclear receptors, but its

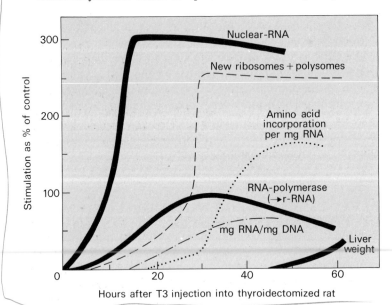

**Fig. 5.4** Effects of an injection of a relatively low dose of triiodothyronine into a thyroidectomized rat. The time course of synthesis of some intracellular nucleic acids and enzymes are shown as a percentage increase over the control with time after injection. An increase in nuclear RNA is the first significant event to be observed following the administration of thyroid hormone and it results in increased ribosomal RNA and polysome formation. This produces increased protein (mainly catabolic enzyme) synthesis within the cell, shown as amino acid incorporation/mg of ribosomal RNA. (Redrawn with permission from Tata (1967) *J. Clin. Path.* **20**, 323–6.)

exact site of action at a particular molecular site and the mechanism of stimulation of subcellular events is not known. The mechanism of entry of the iodothyronine hormone into the nucleus appears to be different from that of the steroid hormones. Because of the nuclear site of action, it is usually several hours after an injection of triiodothyronine (or a day or two after thyroxine administration), before a biological expression of the response to hormone action is observed *in vivo*.

## Mitochondrial actions

Thyroid hormones *do not* exert a physiological action by uncoupling oxidative phosphorylation as was once postulated, although these iodothyronine hormones may have some actions, either directly or indirectly, on certain mitochondrial or microsomal enzymes. The general metabolic increases which gave rise to an enhanced BMR are most likely to be due to an increase in the intacellular concentrations of enzymes involved in catabolic processes within the body; this is suggested because no convincing evidence has yet been presented for allosteric or conformational effects of the thyroid hormones at physiological concentrations on the affinity constant ($K_M$) or the reaction rate ($V_{max}$) of the many enzymes so far examined.

## Membrane transport of iodothyronines

Certain cells have been found to have a specific membrane-transport mechanism for the iodothyronines, which facilitate the uptake of free thyroid hormones from the serum into the cells. Although intracellular binding-proteins for the iodothyronines have been demonstrated in cell cytosol, no specific role for these proteins has yet been demonstrated. However, they do *not* appear to act in the same way as has been determined for the steroid hormone intracellular binding-proteins.

### DEIODINATION OF THYROXINE

A large proportion of thyroxine is mono-deiodinated by a specific enzyme to yield triiodothyronine within the cell, and it is estimated that between 30 and 80% of the daily requirement for triiodothyronine is derived from thyroxine by this extrathyroidal mechanism. It appears that another iodothyronine mono-deiodinase is also present in target-cells which, along with the enzyme converting T4 to T3, regulates the amount of biologically active T3 produced: the second enzyme deiodinates thyroxine at the inner ring, rather than the outer ring, to produce inactive reverse-T3 (see Fig. 5.3).

## Peripheral regulation of iodothyronines

It is suggested that regulation could be achieved when the cell has sufficient triiodothyronine for its metabolic requirements, by switching to the second enzyme which yields the biologically inactive product, reverse-T3, and this would explain the presence of the latter as a metabolite of thyroxine in the serum. In neonates and in certain elderly individuals, T3 and reverse-T3 exist in an inverse concentration relationship in serum, with one increasing as the other decreases; this inverse relationship has led to the suggestion that deiodination of T4 to one or other T3 derivative may represent a peripheral control mechanism to regulate thyroid hormone delivery to its intracellular receptors. These results suggest that thyroxine may be merely a pro-hormone, whose presence in the adult is required only to maintain a constant supply of triiodothyronine. However, it is not possible to verify this suggestion on the basis of current evidence, and it is also possible that thyroxine may have other specific and as yet unidentified actions on certain cells, e.g. during fetal development, on the thyrotroph cells of the pituitary, or perhaps on neural tissues.

MODULATION OF ACTIONS OF OTHER HORMONES

Thyroid hormones also influence the actions of many other hormones, but the effects are difficult to differentiate from a general action in increasing cellular metabolism. Probably the most dramatic and clinically important effect is the ability of triiodothyronine to exert a synergistic effect on the heart in conjunction with the actions of catecholamines to increase the heart rate: the effect of the two hormones combined produces an effect greater than the sum of the effects that either exerts alone at the same concentrations. Except for the latter single example, it is usually extremely difficult to discriminate the general effects of the thyroid hormones on virtually all metabolic processes from a direct modulation of the actions of other hormones. Most of the effects of other (non-thyroid) hormones are modified in conditions of under- or over-activity of the thyroid. However, with few exceptions, the changes can usually be attributed to the overall alterations in cellular metabolic processes in the target-cells which are influenced by prevailing levels of iodothyronine hormones. Thus, insulin responses to intravenous glucose-tolerance tests are slightly exaggerated in hyperthyroidism or significantly depressed in hypothyroidism, when compared with the test on the same individuals after corrective therapy. Note that comparison of intravenous glucose tolerance tests, rather than oral tests, is necessary since iodothyronine hormones can also alter the efficiency of carbohydrate absorption from the gastrointestinal tract.

**Synthesis of thyroid hormones**

Synthesis of thyroid hormones by the gland involves uptake of iodine from the blood and incorporation of iodine atoms into tyrosyl residues of thyroglobulin, the glycoprotein which is synthesized by follicular cells. The thyroid gland is remarkable and unique amongst the endocrine systems in that the storage form of the hormone is located in an extracellular depot, the colloid, which is contained within the follicles of the gland. The hormones are actually synthesized within the structure of the thyroglobulin molecule. The mechanisms of thyroid hormone synthesis, storage and release are considered in further detail below.

## IODIDE PUMP

The basal plasma membrane of the follicular cells contains a system for the active transport of iodide from the bloodstream into the cells against a steep iodide concentration-gradient. While this iodide pump appears to be linked to the activity of the $Na^+/K^+$-pump in the basal state, a second pump is distinguishable in stimulated glands, leading to the suggestion that there might be two separate, but physically closely associated systems in the basal cell membrane. The iodide pump shows all the characteristics of an energy-dependent and relatively specific transport system, as it requires ATP and follows Michaelis–Menten kinetics. The concentrating ability of the iodide pump may be judged from its capacity to produce intrathyroidal concentrations of iodide 20 to 100 times that of serum or the surrounding medium, even when the other reactions which utilize iodide within the follicular cell and hence deplete the intracellular concentration have been inhibited.

### Inhibitory anions
A variety of ions with approximately the same van der Waals radii as iodide are capable of completely inhibiting the iodide pump, with the following approximate potencies:

$$TcO_4^- > ClO_4^- > SeCN^- > SCN^- > I^- > NO_2^- > Br^-$$

Pertechnetate ($^{99m}TcO_4^-$) is mainly used as a short-lived radioactive ion which is taken up by the thyroidal iodide pump and then provides a method by which the gland may be imaged by monitoring radioactive emissions using scintiscanning or a gamma-camera. Perchlorate ($ClO_4^-$) is employed as a competitive inhibitor of the iodide pump, and large doses may be administered as a short-term measure to block iodide uptake by the gland. This is useful when studying the kinetics of thyroid hormone secretion, or as a prophylactic measure in inhibiting uptake of radioiodide by the thyroid if an individual has been contaminated by or has ingested radioactive iodine, in order to minimize the radiation hazard that arises from radioiodine accumulation within the gland. Perchlorate is additionally used in the so-called 'perchlorate-discharge test', in which the ability of the thyroid to synthesize iodothyronine hormones is assessed. The thyroid is

169

first allowed to accumulate tracer doses of one of the short-lived radioisotopes, $^{131}I^-$ or $^{123}I^-$, and following administration of perchlorate to block further radioiodine uptake, the rate of release of the radioisotope is followed over a period of time. The rate of radioiodine release is measured to assess whether the thyroid gland is normal, or whether there is reduced incorporation of iodine into thyroid protein as occurs in some inherited deficiency diseases. The administration of high doses of radioiodine is used in the treatment of thyroid overactivity: radioiodine emissions, for example from iodine-131, are used to ablate thyroid tissue.

Bromide $(Br^-)$ and nitrite $(NO_2^-)$ can competitively inhibit the iodide pump if their dietary intake is sufficiently high, as actually occurs in some regions of the world. Iodide $(^{127}I^-)$ itself does *not* inhibit the iodide pump, even at quite high circulating concentrations. Thiocynate $(SCN^-)$ and selenocyanate $(SeCN^-)$ are two anions which are not transported into the gland, but can inhibit the thyroidal iodide pump by a competitive mechanism.

THYROGLOBULIN SYNTHESIS

Follicular cells synthesize this large glycoprotein which is unique to the thyroid gland, and which is iodinated after it is synthesized. Thyroxine is subsequently made within this large precursor.

*Structure*
Thyroglobulin is a glycoprotein, containing approximately 10% carbohydrate, which is composed of two major types of polysaccharide units, one of which terminates in sialic acid: this sugar residue is responsible for the intense pink periodic acid-Schiff staining reaction observed in the colloid. Thyroglobulin is a large molecule with a molecular weight of 660 000 and contains a variable amount of iodine (about 1% iodine by weight) and it has a sedimentation coefficient of approximately 19S in the ultracentrifuge. The molecule is composed of two apparently identical subunits which can be dissociated under mild reducing conditions; this indicates that the subunits are either non-covalently associated, or weakly attached through one or two disulphide bridges. The subunits have sedimentation coefficients of 12S corresponding to molecular weights of 330 000. It is not yet certain whether the 12S subunits are composed of one or more peptide chains; they are heavily cross-linked by disulphide bridges, and analysis of the number of terminal amino acid residues present in thyroglobulin has proved to be unfruitful in resolving the problem of the number of peptide chains in each 12S subunit.

Protein synthesis in follicular cells follows the usual sequence.
Messenger RNA is synthesized in the follicular cell nucleus and
the peptide chains of thyroglobulin are translated from specific
messenger RNA on polysomes found in the rough endoplasmic
reticulum (Fig. 5.5). The exact number of peptide chains, and
therefore the number of species of messenger RNA required to
synthesize thyroglobulin, are still somewhat uncertain. However
a messenger RNA capable of yielding a peptide of about 300 000
molecular weight has been isolated and used to synthesize
thyroglobulin in a cell-free system *in vitro*.

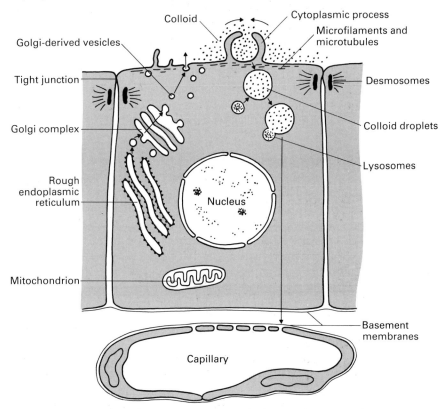

**Fig. 5.5** The intracellular organelles of a thyroid epithelial cell concerned in the
synthesis, storage and degradation of thyroglobulin. Thyroglobulin is
synthesized on the rough endoplasmic reticulum, packaged in the Golgi complex
and released from small, Golgi-derived vesicles into the follicular lumen (shown at
the top of the figure) to be stored as colloid. When stimulated by thyrotrophin,
colloid is engulfed by cytoplasmic processes and re-introduced into the cell as
colloid droplets. Lysosomes fuse with the colloid droplets and their acid hydrolases
degrade the thyroglobulin, leading eventually to release of the thyroid hormones
into local capillaries. Note also cytoplasmic microfilaments and microtubules
under the apical surface of the cell, the nucleus and mitochondrion. The capillaries
are fenestrated and surrounded by a basement membrane. Desmosomes (which
hold cells together) and tight junctions (which seal off the colloid) are also
shown.

Radioactively labelled amino acids and sugars may be followed in a time-sequence as they pass through the follicular cell using autoradiographic techniques, and the incorporation of the components which go to make up thyroglobulin between the rough endoplasmic reticulum and Golgi complex have been determined (Fig. 5.5). Radioactively labelled leucine is initially seen over the rough endoplasmic reticulum, and it then migrates via the smooth endoplasmic reticulum to the Golgi complex. Labelled mannose is located initially over the smooth endoplasmic reticulum, while other sugars such as galactose, fucose and sialic acid appear to be added in the Golgi apparatus. Newly synthesized thyroglobulin is found in small vesicles which are apparently packaged in the Golgi, and these vesicles move towards the apical cell membrane. Under the electron microscope, these apical vesicles appear as clear (i.e. not electron-dense) membrane-bounded inclusions within the cytoplasm. The apical vesicles then fuse with the apical cell membrane and release their contents into the lumen of the thyroid follicle by exocytosis: these vesicles are therefore referred to as exocytotic vesicles.

### Iodination of thyroglobulin

Radioactive iodine has been used to locate iodide within the follicular cell after it is transported across the basal membrane of the cell. Quickly, within 10 seconds of an injection of radioactive iodide, autoradiography shows high concentrations of iodine located over the apical cell membrane, with little radioisotope present elsewhere within the follicular cell. At longer time intervals, the band of radioiodine is seen to diffuse into the lumen of the colloid, and after some days the colloid becomes completely labelled with radioiodine. Analysis of the iodine content of the thyroglobulin extracted from thyroid tissue, or after removal of the protein from individual follicles by micromanipulation, has shown that it contains about 1% of its weight as covalently bound iodine in normal individuals.

The enzyme system carrying out the iodination of thyroglobulin is a peroxidase. This enzyme is synthesized and packaged in the Golgi complex into vesicles in an inactive form, probably along with thyroglobulin. At the apical cell membrane, the peroxidase enzyme is activated, either by changes which occur during membrane fusion or owing to the presence of iodide and co-factors required to activate the enzyme, such as an $H_2O_2$-generating system. A thyroid peroxidase has been purified from thyroid tissue and it requires a hydrogen peroxide-generating system, which may be linked to an NADP/glutathione redox cycle within the cell. The enzyme functions in a complex manner, in that it binds and oxidizes iodide to an active form which is then transferred to the acceptor tyrosyl residue of thyroglobulin which is itself bound at another site on the same enzyme:

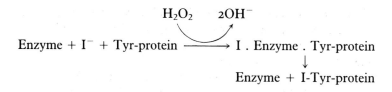

$$\text{Enzyme} + \text{I}^- + \text{Tyr-protein} \xrightarrow{\quad\quad} \text{I . Enzyme . Tyr-protein}$$

$$\downarrow$$

$$\text{Enzyme} + \text{I-Tyr-protein}$$

This enzyme system has a particularly high efficiency for catalysing the iodination of thyroglobulin *which has not previously been iodinated*; this efficiency decreases somewhat with thyroglobulin which already contains some bound iodine.

*Drugs inhibiting iodination.* The peroxidase enzyme, and hence the iodination reaction, is sensitive to inhibition by a number of antithyroid drugs such as thiourea, propylthiouracil (PTU) or methimazole (methyl mercaptoimidazole, MMI), all of which contain the N—C—SH grouping. These drugs, and particularly the mercaptoimidazoles, are employed to inhibit the iodination of thyroglobulin and hence stop or minimize production of the thyroid hormones by an overactive thyroid gland. Methimazole is favoured in the USA, while carbimazole is the drug of choice in the UK, but since the latter is hydrolysed to methimazole almost immediately it is administered there is no advantage of one form of the drug over the other. This is an effective method of suppressing the synthesis and secretion of thyroid hormones, and these drugs have less unwanted side-effects during long-term administration than does percholorate, which inhibits the iodide pump.

Naturally occurring substances have occasionally been found to cause goitres in a local population, and these substances are therefore called goitrogens. Naturally occurring goitrogens have been isolated from drinking supplies (water wells), the milk of cows fed on certain green fodder, and the *Brassicae* (cabbages, etc.) which contain particularly high concentrations of goitrogens. These naturally occurring goitrogens act by inhibiting the iodination of thyroglobulin, and hence the synthesis of thyroid hormones (see below). Release of negative feedback control at the pituitary results in increased thyrotrophin secretion and hence stimulation of the thyroid in an attempt to maintain circulating thyroid hormone levels: the prolonged stimulation results in thyroid hyperplasia and so a goitre forms.

*Importance of the structure of thyroglobin*

The iodination reaction described above occurs with the tyrosyl residues of thyroglobulin acting as acceptor molecules. Thyroglobulin contains about 125 tyrosyl residues, but only about one-third are available for iodination because they are situated at or near the surface of the glycoprotein; the other two-thirds are buried within the molecule. The iodination reaction not only causes iodination of tyrosyl residues, but it initiates formation of the thyroid hormones within the structure of thyroglobulin.

The structural similarity of thyroxine to two molecules of diiodotyrosine coupled together, originally led Pitt-Rivers and Harrington to suggest this as the probable mechanism of synthesis of the thyroid hormones. At one time a coupling enzyme was thought to be involved in the synthesis of thyroxine and triiodothyronine from mono- and diiodotyrosine. However, it is now accepted that the coupling reaction occurs within the thyroglobulin structure during the peroxidase-mediated iodination reaction: no coupling enzyme is therefore required (Fig. 5.6). During the oxidizing conditions of the iodination reaction, a molecular rearrangement occurs between two iodotyrosyl residues: the bond between the aromatic ring of a mono- or diiodotyrosyl residue and its alanyl side-chain is ruptured and the ring is transferred to the phenolic hydroxyl group of another peptide-linked residue of diiodotyrosine. This coupling reaction occurs within the structure of the thyroglobulin molecule as is shown diagrammatically in Fig. 5.6. The receiving diiodotyrosyl residue is linked to another part of either the same or perhaps another peptide chain as that of the transferred mono- or diiodotyrosyl residue, and either triiodothyronine or thyroxine is formed within the thyroglobulin structure. There is uncertainty as to whether the peptide chain is broken, or whether an alanyl or seryl residue may be left as a remnant of the original iodotyrosyl residue, after coupling to form the iodothyronyl residue elsewhere in thyroglobulin. Thyroglobulin which has been iodinated contains a multitude of small peptide fragments and these fragments are absent in iodine-deficient thyroglobulin. This observation suggests that the peptide chain is broken during the iodination and coupling reactions within thyroglobulin.

Iodination of thyroglobulin results in production of a maximum of four molecules of the two iodothyronine hormones linked within the structure of each protein molecule (see Fig. 5.7): the small number of iodothyronines and the large size of thyroglobulin (660 000 molecular weight) suggest that specific active sites for iodothyronine synthesis occur in the thyroglobulin molecule. The iodinated protein is stored in the lumen of the thyroid follicle and some further iodination of the protein may take place within the follicle, presumably because some of the peroxidase iodinating enzyme is released from membranes during the exocytotic process.

THE EFFECT OF DIETARY IODIDE ON HORMONE SYNTHESIS

The amount of iodine incorporated into thyroglobulin is directly related to the concentration of iodide reaching the thyroid gland from the circulation. Thus, when dietary iodide is limited or deficient, there will be little iodine incorporated into thyroglobulin.

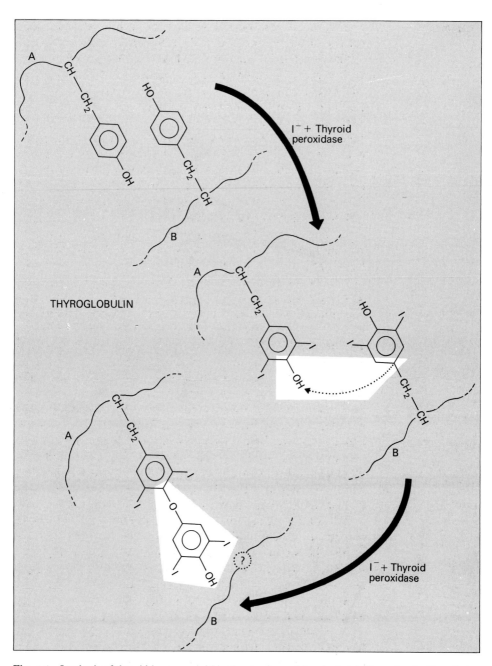

**Fig. 5.6** Synthesis of thyroid hormones within the structure of the thyroglobulin molecule. Two chains of thyroglobulin (labelled A and B to distinguish between them) each carrying a tyrosyl residue are shown at the top left. Iodination by the thyroid peroxidase introduces two atoms of iodine into each tyrosyl residue in the ortho-position relative to the hydroxyl group, in the central diagram. The dotted arrow indicates the molecular rearrangement which follows to yield the structure of thyroxine (T4) linked to the chain labelled A at the lower left of the figure. This rearrangement requires the presence of oxidizing conditions and may be spontaneously induced when particular key tyrosyl residues of thyroglobulin are iodinated. The fate of the B-chain of the protein and the alanyl side-chain of the tyrosyl residue is uncertain: either the chain breaks or a seryl side-chain may form. If the tyrosyl residue on the B-chain is only monoiodinated, then a 3,5,3'-triiodothyronyl residue (T3) is formed in the thyroglobulin molecule.

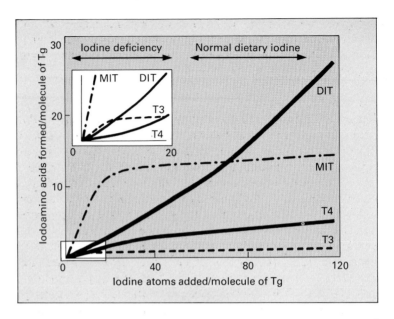

**Fig. 5.7** The proportion of iodo-amino acids formed within the structure of thyroglobulin (Tg) as a function of the number of iodine atoms incorporated. MIT = monoiodotyrosine; DIT = diiodotyrosine; T4 = thyroxine, T3 = 3,5,3′-triiodothyronine. Initially, T3 is synthesized in a relatively higher proportion than T4 at very low levels of iodine incorporated (as shown in the inset to the figure), when the precursor MIT/DIT ratio is high. At higher levels of iodine, T$_4$ is formed preferentially, up to a maximum of about four molecules of thyroxine/molecule of thyroglobulin.

This will yield mainly monoiodotyrosine and only a few di-iodotyrosine residues in thyroglobulin; this situation is described graphically in Fig. 5.7. An increase in the number of iodine atoms added yields progressively more diiodotyrosine. Under normal conditions of dietary iodide sufficiency, thyroglobulin will contain more diiodotyrosine than monoidotyrosine.

Under conditions of iodide sufficiency, where a lot of diiodo-tyrosine is present, thyroglobulin will contain from two to four molecules of thyroxine: there will be relatively little triiodo-thyronine because there is insufficient monoiodotyrosine to couple with diiodotyrosine. Iodide sufficiency, which would require a dietary iodine intake of greater than 50 μg per day, would correspond to about 80 atoms of iodine per molecule of thyroglobulin on the abscissa of Fig. 5.7. It has been estimated that thyroglobulin in the normal human thyroid stores about two month's supply of preformed thyroxine. This reserve is available to maintain the individual in the euthyroid state should adverse conditions of iodine deficiency be encountered.

In iodine-deficiency, thyroglobulin will contain relatively more monoiodotyrosine than diiodotyrosine, compared with iodine-sufficient regions. In consequence, there will be smaller amounts of thyroid hormones: in addition, because of the higher ratio of monoiodotyrosine to diiodotyrosine available to couple, iodine-deficient thyroglobulin contains more triiodotyronine than thyroxine (see inset to Fig. 5.7).

### Iodine deficiency and endemic goitre

Iodine deficiency is still a major problem in some areas of the world. In adults a reduced iodine intake (below $50\,\mu$g per day) causes compensatory changes, with the thyroid secreting triiodo-thyronine preferentially to thyroxine. Eventually, thyrotrophin secretion is increased to maintain the concentrations of circulating thyroid hormones. The increased thyrotrophin concentration induces thyroid enlargement. Although they have goitres, these adults produce sufficient thyroid hormone and so are euthyroid and are not hypothyroid, because the state of iodine deficiency is never total and sufficient thyroid hormone may be produced for the immediate needs of the individual. However, an important problem created by iodine deficiency is that during pregnancy the fetus is at risk from neurological damage. The syndrome of intellectual impairment, deafness and diplegia has been termed 'cretinism'; this condition is quite different from 'sporadic cretinism' which results from an athyrotic fetus (mentioned above in connection with neonatal hypothyroidism). Prophylaxis with iodine supplements has proved most effective in reducing the incidence of cretinism in many areas of the world, although the effect of iodide on reducing well-established goitres is small. Supplementation of essential or common dietary constituents such as salt or bread is not always possible, however, and resort is sometimes made in extremely isolated communities to depot injections of iodized oils which provide the thyroid with iodide supplies over periods of a few years.

Variations in dietary iodide intake may be associated with increased incidence of latent hyperthyroidism. Such conditions are encountered in some regions of western Europe, for example in areas of Germany where iodine supplements to food or water supplies are forbidden. A sudden increase in dietary iodide can precipitate expression of autoimmune disease of the thyroid, but the incidence is related to other unknown factors that appear to affect a given community.

### Iodine excess

Large doses of iodine, e.g. 5 mg/day, will initially inhibit the synthesis and release of thyroid hormones from the gland. This paradoxical effect arises from inhibition of two intrathyroidal reactions. Excess iodide inhibits the adenylate cyclase response to thyrotrophin, and it also inhibits iodine incorporation into thyroglobulin (which is sometimes called 'organification of iodide'). Thyroidal inhibition by excess iodine is known as the

Wolff—Chaikoff effect, and it may sometimes be seen as a transitory thyroid enlargement when certain preparations (such as cough mixtures which contain high concentrations of iodide) are administered. The rapid and acute inhibitory effects of excess iodide can be used in a thyrotoxic patient before thyroidectomy. This treatment is designed to restore the patient to a euthyroid state, and the excess iodide also has a pharmacological effect to decrease the vascularity and increase the firmness of the gland. It also prevents a condition known as 'thyroid storm', which is a severe and acute escalation of hyperthyroidism that may occur during or after surgery to the thyroid.

After a few days of high iodide intake, thyroidal iodide transport diminishes to near zero, the intracellular iodide concentration falls, and the block of iodine incorporation into thyroglobulin is relieved, i.e. the Wolff-Chaikoff effect is reversed. In this way, humans can generally adapt to prolonged excesses of iodide intake and they will eventually stabilize with normal circulating thyroid hormone concentrations. These observations demonstrate the ability of the thyroid to maintain the euthyroid state in spite of wide fluctuations in dietary iodide intake.

## REGULATION OF THE THYROID

The activity of the thyroid gland is controlled by thyrotrophin from the anterior pituitary gland: the secretion of this is in turn controlled by thyrotrophin releasing hormone from the hypothalamus (see Chapter 2). Thyrotrophin stimulates the secretion of thyroid hormones: these can themselves, by negative feedback, supress secretion of thyrotrophin.

### STIMULATION OF THE THYROID BY THYROTROPHIN

The anterior pituitary hormone, thyrotrophin or thyroid stimulating hormone (TSH), is bound to a specific receptor on the thyroid follicular cell surface and activates adenylate cyclase within the cell. Thyrotrophin action on the thyroid cell results in general stimulation of metabolism and it also has a trophic effect on the cell size and activity. Virtually all the actions of thyrotrophin appear to be mediated by cyclic AMP, presumably by means of a variety of protein kinases or similar enzymes. However, as with the other trophic hormones, it is somewhat surprising that the particular enzymes involved have not yet been identified. One of the few metabolic functions within the follicular cell which does not appear to be mediated by cyclic AMP is the turnover of phospholipid, and in particular of phosphatidyl inositol, which may be related to translocation of $Ca^{2+}$ or changes

induced in membrane conformation by the binding of thyrotrophin to its receptor.

The sequence of events following thyrotrophin action, which
is initiated by its binding to specific cell-surface receptors on the
thyroid follicular cell, *increases* the following:

1   Intracellular cyclic AMP concentration.
2   Transmembrane ion fluxes, with influx of $Na^+$ and *efflux*
of iodide; translocation of $Ca^{2+}$ and activation of calmodulin also
occur.
3   Activation of various protein kinases which lead to protein
or enzyme phosphorylation by phosphate transfer from ATP
(see Chapter 7).
4   Iodination of thyroglobulin and also thyroid hormone release.
5   Intracellular volume and number of colloid droplets, and the
numbers, form and activity of microvilli at the apical cell surface.
6   Cellular metabolism, including that of carbohydrate which
occurs principally via the pentose phosphate pathway; also
phospholipid turnover.
7   Protein synthesis, (including that of thyroglobulin) and also
RNA turnover.
8   Iodide *influx* to the cell, because the iodide pump requires
synthesis of a new protein for its activation.
9   DNA synthesis, although very limited mitosis and cell division occurs in the adult *in vivo*.

The thyroid contains very little glycogen, so it is not surprising
that the pentose phosphate pathway provides the major source of
metabolic energy for the various reactions stimulated within the
cell. An important response to thyrotrophin action appears to be
the effect on the iodide pump, first resulting in an efflux of
iodide, and only later resulting in an activation of the influx
mechanism. Increased membrane activities, protein iodination,
and release of the thyroid hormones are also observed in response
to thyrotrophin action; but apart from the increase in numbers
of colloid droplets and their fusion with lysosomes, thyrotrophin
does not appear to cause an enhancement of lysosomal enzyme
activities themselves.

The net result of thyrotrophin action on the gland is to increase
the synthesis of fresh thyroid hormone stores, as well as causing
an increase in release of the thyroid hormones within about an
hour. Most recently synthesized thyroglobulin is the first to be
removed from the follicle, because it is nearer to the microvilli at
the apical cell membrane than older thyroglobulin at the centre
of the follicle. Because newly iodinated thyroglobulin around the
edge of the follicle has a lower iodine content than the mature,
centrally positioned thyroglobulin, this new glycoprotein has a
relatively higher triiodothyronine to thyroxine ratio than that of

the older thyroglobulin stores (see Fig. 5.7). Hence a relatively subtle control mechanism exists within the gland, based on the turnover of thyroglobulin and its degree of iodination, which can produce not only more thyroid hormone, but also alter the amount of the more active triiodothyronine which is secreted by the gland.

### Thyroid hormone secretion

In order to release thyroid hormones from the thyroglobulin stores at the centre of the follicle, the glycoprotein must first be taken back into the thyroid cell where lysosomal enzymes can release the iodothyronines for secretion into the circulation.

COLLOID DROPLET FORMATION

The apical cell membrane of thyroid follicles is covered by microvilli and pseudopods (Fig. 5.5) which may be observed under the electron microscope. In stimulated thyroid glands, the number and length of the microvilli increase, and three-dimensional pictures obtained from a scanning electron microscope show structures rather like individual rose petals. These cellular extensions protrude into the colloid and encircle a droplet of thyroglobulin by fusion of the edges of the membrane, after which the top of the now cylindrical membrane fuses to form a vesicle which is thus positioned within the cell. The junction with the remainder of the apical membrane is broken to yield an intracellular 'colloid droplet'. This process is known as endocytosis, and it may also be accompanied by a similar process known as pinocytosis, in which smaller droplets of colloid are transferred into the cell. Only the larger colloid droplet vesicles may be seen under the light microscope after staining with periodic acid-Schiff reagents. They may be distinguished from other vesicles seen under the electron microscope because they have the same electron-density as the colloid (which is slightly more electron opaque, by virtue of the electron-absorbing mass of the large iodine atoms). Those vesicles that contain uniodinated thyroglobulin in exocytotic vesicles are less dense.

*Microfilaments and microtubules*
It is possible to observe filamentous structures of two general types within the follicular cells by using suitable variations of the normal fixation procedures for electron microscopy. A dense network of microfilaments is observed principally in the apical region of the cell, and microtubules are also present in the cell cytoplasm. Treatment of thyroid tissue or animals with colchicine, vinblastine or vincristine (drugs which inhibit polymerization of tubulin, the protein monomer which forms microtubules) also

inhibits the formation of colloid droplets within thyroid cells. Since colloid droplets are no longer formed, these drugs thus inhibit secretion of the thyroid hormones. It is interesting to note that lysosomes and other vesicular particles within the cell appear to clump together after treatment by these drugs, but this may not be due to a direct action of the drugs on these vesicles.

Microfilaments of 5–6 nm contain a major protein component which appears to be very similar to the actin component in muscle. The cytochalasin group of drugs, which are derived from mould secretions and which are cytotoxic, are also capable of inhibiting colloid droplet formation and hence thyroid hormone secretion, through a direct action upon thyroidal microfilaments. It is now thought that microfilaments are involved in some specific contractile activities which are related to the formation of colloid droplets and to the subsequent specific directional movement of subcellular vesicles, both towards and away from the apical membrane within thyroid follicular cells.

### Lysosomal fusion and release of thyroid hormones

Lysosomes are additional intracellular structures observed under the electron microscope; they appear as electron-dense vesicles of about 0.2 μm in diameter, and are usually located quite close to the nucleus of the follicular cell (Fig. 5.5). When thyroid cells are stimulated by thyrotrophin, the lysosomes migrate towards the colloid droplets and fusion of the membranes of these two types of vesicle then occurs. The hydrolytic enzymes of the lysosome degrade the thyroglobulin molecule, releasing iodo- and other amino acids and sugars. The latter are recycled within the gland, and mono- and diiodo-tyrosine are relatively specifically deiodinated by microsomal enzymes to release iodide which is also recycled within the cell and hence conserves the iodine supply of the gland. The iodothyronine hormones are released from the gland by some mechanism which remains to be elucidated: they pass across the cell membrane, then across the basement membrane of the follicle to gain access to the serum carrier-proteins through the fenestrated capillary bed (see Fig. 5.5) which surrounds the follicles.

## INAPPROPRIATE SECRETION OF THYROID HORMONES

### The effects of undersecretion

Lack of thyroid hormones occurs either because of disease of the thyroid itself or from lack of stimulation by the pituitary. The first of these situations represents primary hypothyroidism (or myxoedema) while the latter is secondary hypothyroidism. The effects of hypothyroidism are the result of a lowered metabolic rate. The subjects feel the cold and may want extra clothing or bedding. They gain weight and become very slow. These changes can develop insidiously and may be difficult to recognize—it may be thought that they are 'just slowing down' or 'getting old'. The skin becomes coarse and extremities feel cold. The pulse becomes slow. There may be a characteristic change in tendon reflexes—the muscles contract normally but relax slowly: the reason for this is not clear.

In children, thyroxine is necessary for normal growth and if the thyroid is underactive, then there is failure of growth. Lack of thyroid hormone is particularly serious in the newborn because this can cause irreversible brain damage (cretinism). The incidence of neonatal hypothyroidism in Western society is about 1 in 5000 births. It is most readily diagnosed by finding high circulating concentrations of thyrotrophin: this can now be measured in routine screening tests shortly after birth.

In hypothyroidism the concentrations of thyroxine and of triiodothyronine are low. In primary hypothyroidism the circulating concentration of thyrotrophin is high, in an attempt to stimulate the failing thyroid gland. In fact, in the early phase of the latter disease the concentration of circulating thyroid hormones is normal but is only maintained by increased pituitary activity. In secondary hypothyroidism the concentration of thyrotrophin is low. If this is due to pituitary disease, then administration of thyrotrophin releasing hormone will have little or no effect, but if it is due to hypothalamic disease, the releasing factor given intravenously can stimulate the pituitary.

Hypothyroidism can be treated very successfully by giving thyroxine by mouth; about 0.15 mg/day is usually sufficient in an adult.

*Effects of overproduction*

Hyperthyroidism (thyrotoxicosis) is the result of overactivity of the thyroid gland. Many of the effects of this are associated with the increase in basal metabolic rate and $\beta$-adrenergic overactivity. Thus there is often loss of weight even though appetite may increase enormously. The patient is anxious and irritable and may notice palpitations due to a tachycardia or atrial fibrillation. They may have diarrhoea. Muscle weakness and wasting may also be consequences.

The concentration of both thyroxine and triiodothyronine is usually raised although occasionally it is only the concentration of triiodothyronine that is raised. In interpreting the concentration of thyroid hormones there is of course the possibility that changes are due to alterations in the concentration of the circulating binding-proteins—the concentration of thyroxine-binding globulin is, for example, raised by oral contraceptives and this increases the total concentration of T4 but the free T4 concentration is normal. In thyrotoxicosis the concentration of thyrotrophin circulating is usually low since overproduction of thyrotrophin by a pituitary tumour is an extremely rare cause of thyroid overactivity. In fact the pituitary is suppressed by the high concentration of thyroid hormones and is unable to respond to thyrotrophin releasing hormone.

Thyrotoxicosis can be treated in various ways. Drugs can be used to suppress thyroid hormone synthesis: the drugs used include carbimazole and propyl thiouracil. While the drug treatment is being started it may be necessary to give a $\beta$-blocking agent (e.g. propranolol) until the overactivity is suppressed—this takes about 6 weeks. Treatment with the antithyroid drug usually has to continue for 6 to 18 months and the condition may relapse when treatment is stopped, or even months or years later. Radioactive iodine (e.g. $^{131}I$) can also be used to destroy the gland; such treatment must never be given during pregnancy as radioactive iodine would ablate the fetal thyroid. The over-active gland can also be removed surgically: about four-fifths is removed and often the remainder will provide normal function; not infrequently, however, the patient becomes hypothyroid post-operatively. Because of the close proximity of the parathyroid glands and the recurrent laryngeal nerves, hypoparathyroidism and vocal cord palsies are hazards of thyroid surgery.

THE GENESIS OF DISORDERED FUNCTION

*Thyroid disease originating from autoimmune disorders*

Disorders that affect the thyroid gland and which are most commonly seen in the Western world do not usually result from defects of the thyroid or pituitary system: curiously, they arise mainly from disorders of the immune system. In situations where the immune system no longer treats tissues of the host as normal constituents of the body, but attacks these tissues to cause disease states, then the condition is known as an 'autoimmune disorder'. Non-thyroidal autoimmune diseases which are now recognized include pernicious anaemia, idiopathic adrenal insufficiency, type I diabetes mellitus, myasthenia gravis, rheumatoid arthritis and systemic lupus erythematosus. Autoimmune reactions with thyroid tissue can lead either to hypothyroidism (myxoedema), or in the case of autoimmune thyroid stimulation, to hyper-thyroidism. The trigger that initiates an autoimmune response is not known, but the mechanism may involve class II HLA antigen DR3 elaborated by the follicular cell. These cells may present their cell components to T-lymphocytes; an activity usually under-taken by macrophages when they associate with an immunogen. These thyroidal autoimmune disorders are approximately five times more common in females than in males, and they frequently have a familial incidence.

The spectrum of autoimmune disease ranges from cell-mediated (rather than humoral) destruction of the thyroid, to stimulation of follicular cells by binding of antibodies. There are other facets of the latter autoimmune disorder which result in 'thyroid eye disease', goitre and dermopathy (changes in skin texture and pigmentation). Autoimmune disease frequently has a familial incidence, and this applies not only to thyroid disease but also to Addison's disease, pernicious anaemia, certain forms of juvenile diabetes and vitiligo (patchy loss of skin pigmentation) and possibly hypoparathyroidism.

*Hyperthyroidism, Graves' disease and thyrotoxicosis.* Autoimmune hyperthyroidism is unusual in the sense that antibodies (of the IgG class) bind to the thyroid follicular cell membrane either at or sufficiently close to the thyrotrophin receptor to cause stimulation of adenylate cyclase. This results in hypertrophy of the follicular cells (see Fig. 5.2c) and increased synthesis and secretion of thyroid hormones without significant destruction of acinar cells. These antibodies are called 'thyroid stimulating antibodies or immunoglobulins' (TSAb or TSI). These thyroid autoantibodies are unusual in that they stimulate this endocrine system. Adams and Purves in 1956 observed that a substance in the serum of some hyperthyroid patients would stimulate thyroid function when injected into themselves or in an *in vivo* bioassay using guinea-pigs. They named this substance long acting thyroid stimulator (LATS) because of the slow onset and extended time-course of its stimulatory activity when compared with stimulation by thyrotrophin.

Subsequently, the stimulation was shown to be caused by an antibody. This activity has now been measured in a variety of *in vitro* bioassay systems, such as those using incubated animal thyroid glands or cultured thyroid cells-stimulation of cyclic AMP accumulation or of iodide uptake is measured. Although the generalized nomenclature adopted for these stimulating auto-antibodies is thyroid stimulating antibodies or immunoglobulins, they are also frequently referred to by names derived from the particular bioassay used to detect them, e.g. human thyroid adenylate cyclase stimulators (HTACS). They, or a related group of autoantibodies, can also be detected by their ability to inhibit thyrotrophin binding to its receptor, and these are referred to as thyrotrophin receptor antibodies (TRAb). Monoclonal antibodies directed against the thyrotrophin receptor have been experimentally produced, both by using solubilized thyrotrophin receptors as the antigen and by fusion of lymphocytes from patients with Graves' disease. Some of these monoclonal antibodies block binding of thyrotrophin to its receptor but do not activate adenylate cyclase systems, whilst others mimic the stimulation of thyroid tissue observed with thyroid stimulating antibodies and thyrotrophin in a variety of bioassay systems.

In mothers with high levels of thyroid stimulating antibodies there is the risk of the fetus being affected by antibody crossing the placenta to produce fetal thyroid stimulation and hyperthyroidism; this is called 'neonatal thyrotoxicosis'. Individuals with latent and undiagnosed hyperthyroidism can often be precipitated into a 'thyrotoxic crisis' by sudden severe stress such as infection or surgery, or in some cases in iodine deficient regions by the sudden acute oral administration of normal levels of supplementary iodide. The thyrotoxic crisis results from an acute and potentially dangerous increase in circulating thyroid hormones.

*Hypothyroidism, Hashimoto's thyroiditis and myxoedema.* Hashimoto's thyroiditis is also an autoimmune disorder, but this condition is characterized by thyroid enlargement and lymphocytic infiltration. There may sometimes be a phase of oversecretion of thyroid hormones observed clinically, and quite often the disease progresses to destruction of the thyroid with consequent hypothyroidism. In addition to the pronounced cellular immune response, there are also high concentrations of humoral antibodies to thyroglobulin and to thyroid 'microsomes' (actually assessed against a heterogeneous subcellular fraction from thyroid tissue).

*Thyroid neoplasms*

The normal thyroid gland contains cells and follicles that are in different states of activity. Histological examination demonstrates that adjacent follicles, and even different cells within the same follicle, may be present in various states ranging from quiescent to active. This is described as follicular microheterogeneity. An exaggeration of follicular microheterogeneity can occur and this may lead to macroheterogeneity of the thyroid, where one or more nodules of stimulated thyroid follicular cells are formed: a non-toxic nodular or multinodular goitre results. A variety of toxic nodular goitres can also be found. Some are benign adenomas and others are multi-nodular adenomas.

Even though there are a variety of neoplasms affecting the thyroid, from the endocrine point of view we are concerned with only two problems: functioning benign thyroid adenomas and functioning thyroid carcinomas. Benign thyroid adenomas can produce sufficient thyroid hormone to result in thyrotoxicosis. This hormone production is autonomous, i.e. the cells are unresponsive to stimulation by either thyrotrophin or thyroid stimulating antibodies. The remainder of the thyroid is normal, and the abnormality can be corrected either by surgical removal of the adenoma or by its selective destruction with radioactive iodine.

Some malignant thyroid carcinomas retain some ability to take up iodine and synthesize thyroid hormone, but this is never sufficient to produce thyrotoxicosis. Carcinomas in the thyroid take up very little radioactive iodine during a diagnostic scan, and are therefore usually called 'cold' regions or nodules. The low level of cellular activity does, however, allow destructive treatment of tumour metastases, as they may take up radioactive iodine in the absence of competition from the thyroid, i.e. following thyroidectomy, provided they are stimulated by thyrotrophin.

## SUMMARY

The actions of the thyroid hormones are regulated by synthesis and secretion from the thyroid gland which is controlled acutely by thyrotrophin from the anterior pituitary and which in turn is under negative feedback control from the iodothyronine hormones (see Chapter 2). Dietary levels of iodide have a subtle regulatory action on the relative amounts of the two thyroid hormones synthesized in the thyroid gland. Thyroxine may function principally as a prohormone in the adult, since triiodothyronine is biologically more potent and the majority of thyroxine is converted to triiodothyronine by peripheral tissues: the latter conversion may be another site of regulation of thyroid hormone action. Triiodothyronine appears to act primarily at the nucleus and results in changes in enzyme concentrations within the cell, which produce an overall balance in favour of catabolism with a consequent increase in basal metabolic rate. In the normal state, the thyroid hormones appear to regulate the metabolic state of the individual. In hypothyroid states the metabolic rate of individuals slows down in adults; severe neurological damage can result from iodothyronine deficiencies in fetal and neonatal life, while hypothyroidism during childhood results in retardation of the individual's growth.

## FURTHER READING

BAYLISS R. I. S. (1982) *Thyroid Disease: The Facts.* Oxford University Press, Oxford.

INGBAR S. H. (1985) The Thyroid Gland, In *R H Williams' Textbook of Endocrinology*, 7th edn., Eds. J. D. Wilson and D. W. Foster, pp. 682–815. W. B. Saunders, Philadelphia & London.

INGBAR S. H. & BRAVERMAN L. E. (Eds.) (1986) *Werner's The Thyroid.* J. B. Lippincott, Philadelphia.

# 6 Calcium regulating hormones

Rickets, a disease of bone that causes deformity, was described vividly by Whistler and by Glisson in the 17th century in this country. Popular recognition that fish liver oil was a cure for rickets long preceded its recognition by the medical profession and the realization that it contained vitamin D. Rickets became more common in Britain with the Industrial Revolution and the movement of populations to the cities where exposure to sunlight was reduced and the first suggestion that rickets might be due to lack of sunlight came from a study of the distribution of the disease around the world by Palm in 1890. This preceded the development of the concept of vitamins which stemmed from the work of Gowland-Hopkins and of Funk at the beginning of this century. Subsequently, Mellanby succeeded in producing rickets experimentally in puppies and curing it with cod liver oil, although at first there was confusion between vitamin A and vitamin D, both of which are fat-soluble vitamins.

After the First World War, rickets became very common in central Europe. Then, in Vienna, it was shown that cod liver oil or exposure to sunlight could cure rickets. At about that time, Huldschinski found that rickets could be cured by irradiating babies with a mercury vapour lamp and later it was found that irradiation of some foods could cure experimental rickets. All these studies led to the realization that irradiation could yield vitamin D and that this was important for the calcification of bone. The natural form is cholecalciferol (or vitamin D3) which is produced from 7-dehydrocholesterol in the skin, while ergocalciferol (vitamin D2) is produced by irradiation of ergosterol in plants.

For some time, rickets in children and the corresponding disease in adults (called osteomalacia) were confused with another disease of the bone that was described in 1881 by Von Recklinghausen; this condition he called osteitis fibrosa cystica. He associated it with enlargement of the parathyroid glands, the existence of which had been first recognized only 35 years earlier. Owen, who was studying the thyroid of the rhinoceros, had first found the parathyroid glands attached to, but separate from the thyroid and later the histological features of these glands were described by Sandstrom in 1880. When studying the effects of removal of the thyroid, Gley in 1896 found that tetany (that is spasm of the muscles) occurred only if the parathyroid glands were removed as well. Subsequently, in 1900, Vassalli and Generali found that removal of the parathyroids (a term which they introduced themselves) caused tetany and, in 1909, MacCallum and Voegtlin showed that the tetany was due to a lowering of the serum calcium. In 1924 Collip and Clark produced the first extracts of the parathyroid glands that were capable of correcting the tetany by raising serum calcium.

A few years later, it was realized that enlargement of a parathyroid gland was the cause of osteitis fibrosa cystica, rather than a response to the bone disease, and the first parathyroid tumour was successfully removed from a patient with osteitis fibrosa cystica. Knowledge of the physiology of the parathyroid glands and the fact that parathyroid hormone could raise serum calcium and increase urinary excretion of calcium then led Albright to wonder whether parathyroid tumours would also be found in some patients who formed stones in their kidneys; a suggestion which was soon shown to be quite correct.

Thus two factors controlling calcium, namely vitamin D and parathyroid hormone, were recognized. A third factor was identified in 1960 by Copp who postulated that in addition to parathyroid hormone (which raises serum calcium) there must be a hypocalcaemic factor (i.e. one that lowered serum calcium). This factor was called calcitonin and is secreted by specialized cells in the thyroid gland.

## Calcium in the body

Calcium is an important intra- and extracellular ion which comprises a major component of the skeleton, and is needed for blood clotting and for the activity of many enzyme systems. Movement of calcium across cell membranes occurs all the time and change in flux is an important event, with physiological consequences. The importance of changes in calcium within the cell acting as a 'messenger' for hormones was described in Chapter 1. Release of calcium within the cell can be an important 'signal' activating the cell and leading, for example, to activation of secretion processes or to muscular contraction. Even quite small alterations in extracellular calcium concentration affects the excitability of cells in various ways, and hypocalcaemia (that is, a lower than normal concentration of calcium in the blood) can lead to epilepsy, or tetany.

The concentration of calcium in extracellular fluid is very carefully regulated. In human serum the calcium concentration is normally 2.2–2.55 mmol/l. This calcium exists in three forms. Approximately 0.7 mmol/l is bound to albumin and so is not readily diffusible, unlike the other two forms. About 0.25 mmol/l is complexed, for example, to citrate, and the remainder, the most important fraction, is free (i.e. ionized) calcium (about 1.3 mmol/l). The importance of circulating ionized calcium can be illustrated by considering the effects of overbreathing. Overbreathing can cause tetany because of a fall in the ionized calcium concentration in serum. This results from the disturbance of the following equilibria:

$$CO_2 + H_2O \rightleftharpoons H_2CO_3$$
$$H_2CO_3 \rightleftharpoons H^+ + HCO_3^-$$
$$Protein{-}H \rightleftharpoons Protein^- + H^+$$
$$Protein^- + Ca^2 \rightleftharpoons Protein{-}Ca$$

With a fall in the $P$CO$_2$ produced by overbreathing there is increased uptake of calcium ions on to negatively charged protein molecules in blood, and so the *ionized* calcium concentration is decreased, although the total circulating concentration is unaltered. Despite the importance of ionized calcium however, it is total serum calcium that is generally measured, since measurement of the free calcium ion concentration is difficult.

CALCIUM BALANCE

There is a continuous exchange of calcium between different sites in the body (sometimes called 'calcium pools'), and a balance between these various sites is usually maintained. There is a total of about 1 kg of calcium in the body, and of this about 99% is in bone, in the form of hydroxyapatite, $3Ca_3(PO_4)_2 . Ca(OH)_2$. Thus, outside bone there is only about 10 g of calcium available for other cellular processes in the body.

In the adult an equilibrium is reached between absorption and excretion (Fig. 6.1). Dietary intake provides about 25 mmol (that is 1 g) of calcium; intestinal secretions add another 7 mmol of calcium to the contents of the intestinal lumen and only part of the calcium in the lumen is absorbed into the bloodstream. Absorption is balanced by the renal loss of calcium (which ranges between 3−7 mmol in 24 hours). Excreted calcium in the urine is only a small proportion (about 2 or 3%) of the calcium that is filtered through the glomeruli, since the majority is absorbed by the renal tubules. In the growing child there is, of course, calcium retention and intestinal absorption of calcium exceeds renal excretion by about 10 mmol/day, to provide for the needs of skeleton. The child is therefore in positive calcium balance. In the adult calcium net absorption in the gut and renal excretion are approximately equal but there is still exchange between extracellular fluid and calcium in bone, amounting to about 10 mmol/day.

Regulation of calcium balance within the body is closely associated with that of phosphate, though regulation of the latter is rather less precise. The normal range of serum phosphate in adults lies between 0.6 and 1.3 mmol/l; it is higher in young children. A higher proportion of dietary phosphate is absorbed

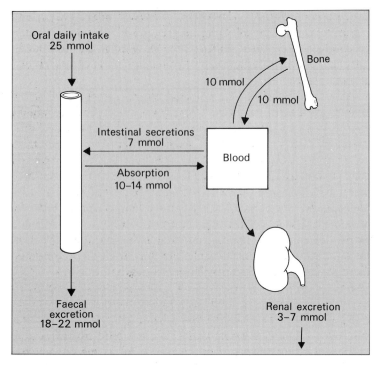

**Fig. 6.1** A schematic representation of calcium exchange in an adult who is in calcium balance, and in whom daily net absorption from the gut (total absorption less intestinal secretion) equals urinary loss. In a growing child, net absorption exceeds renal excretions, to allow for retention of calcium in the skeleton and so the child is in positive calcium balance.

than is the case for calcium, and so urinary excretion is much more variable (depending on the phosphate intake) and can vary from 15 to 50 mmol/24 hours, varying especially with meat intake. A gene on the short arm of the X chromosome is important in the renal regulation of phosphate excretion.

## CONTROL OF CALCIUM BALANCE

There are three ways in which mineral metabolism can be regulated; by alteration in bone turnover, by changes in absorption from the diet and by alteration of renal excretion. These homeostatic mechanisms are subject to control by three factors; parathyroid hormone (from the parathyroid gland), calcitonin (from the thyroid gland) and vitamin D.

### Bone

FUNCTION, COMPOSITION AND MORPHOLOGY

Bone has a number of functions, such as supporting the body and protecting vital organs (including brain and bone marrow).

It acts as a reservoir of calcium and phosphate and can contribute towards acid – base regulation (through phosphate and carbonate). In childhood and early adult life the skeleton is growing but in later life (especially after the menopause) there is an overall loss of bone mass.

Apart from calcium, the skeleton contains about 90% of the body's phosphate, 50% of its magnesium and 33% of its sodium. It is a hard, calcified connective tissue consisting of cells (osteo-progenitor cells, osteoblasts, osteocytes and osteoclasts) and a calcified extracellular matrix. The constituents of the matrix will vary in relative amounts according to the particular bone type and the age, sex and species from which it has come. In general, the inorganic or mineral component accounts for 65% of the bone's weight, while the organic constituents such as collagen fibres make up the rest. As there are relatively few cells per unit mass of bone, they make a negligible contribution to bone mass. Collagen accounts for 90–95% of the organic matrix of bone; the rest is made up of proteoglycans, glycoproteins, sialoproteins and a small amount of lipid. Osteocalcin accounts for 1–2% of the protein in bone: it is also called 'bone gla-protein' because it contains $\gamma$-carboxyglutamic acid. This can bind hydroxyapatite with high affinity (1 mg of osteocalcin binds 17 mg of hydroxy-apatite). Osteocalcin is also found in plasma and since this osteocalcin is derived from newly formed bone, it is used as an index of osteoblast activity. Osteonectin is a glycoprotein found in the bone matrix. It can bind collagen and hydroxyapatite, and *in vitro* it can facilitate calcification of type I collagen, so that it may be important *in vivo* as a mineral nucleator.

*Osteoblasts*
Osteoblasts are cells with the ultrastructural features of active protein-synthesizing cells (i.e. numerous polyribosomes, an extensive rough endoplasmic reticulum, and a large Golgi complex). Osteoblasts synthesize the organic constituents of bone (osteoid) and subsequently, are also involved in the mineralization (i.e. calcification) of the newly secreted osteoid. The precursors of osteoblasts are fibroblast-like cells. These proliferating osteo-progenitor cells appear on bone surfaces and differentiate into osteoblasts. In rats this process, which involves several mitotic divisions, takes about 5 days. The mineralization of osteoid occurs subsequently, after 10 days: the primary mineralization is rapid (60–70% is completed within 6 to 12 hours of initiation), but secondary mineralization takes 1 to 2 months for completion. Once osteoblasts have completed their function in matrix form-ation, they become surrounded by the new matrix and change into relatively inactive cells called osteocytes. They make contact with their neighbours by means of cytoplasmic processes which lie in tiny channels within the matrix called canaliculi. The canaliculi are in continuity with the extracellular spaces of the

Haversian canals, in which lie the blood supply of the bone. Thus, the canaliculi provide the means by which osteocytes get their nutrients, eliminate their unwanted products of metabolism and receive hormonal stimulation. Osteoblasts play an important role in the calcium homeostasis.

## Collagen

Collagen synthesis occurs on the rough endoplasmic reticulum of osteoblasts (Fig. 6.2) where a large molecule, procollagen, is assembled. This consists of three polypeptide chains organized in an alpha-helical conformation. Once translocated into the lumen of the rough endoplasmic reticulum several post-translational modifications to this larger molecule occur, including hydroxylation of the prolyl and lysyl residues, and glycosylation of the hydroxylysyl residues. Scission of the extension peptides to yield the final smaller molecule of collagen occurs extracellularly, after the procollagen has been extruded into the extracellular space, probably by exocytosis.

Collagen is rich in the amino acids glycine, proline and hydroxyproline and has the general formula $(Glycine. Proline. X)_{333}$ where $X$ is another amino acid. Extracellular collagen exists as a macromolecule with a molecular weight of about 300 000. It is a semi-rigid, rod-like molecule approximately 300 nm long and 1.5 nm in diameter. These rod-like collagen molecules polymerize in a highly specific manner extracellularly, with like-ends orientated in the same direction. Adjoining linear aggregates of collagen molecules are staggered with respect to one another, at positions which are approximately one-fourth to one-fifth of their length (Fig. 6.2), and are held firmly together by intermolecular cross-linkages. Linear arrays or bundles of collagen molecules form a microfibril and several microfibrils aggregate to form a collagen fibril. The 'hole zone' between the end of one tropocollagen molecule and the next becomes filled with calcium salts during the process of calcification, as do the spaces within the between microfibrils. Both collagen and its associated proteoglycans probably contribute to the initiation of hydroxyapatite crystallization by epitaxy, holding the components of the apatite in position so that the process of 'seeding' can start.

During bone formation, the calcified matrix and especially the collagen fibres, are laid down either:

1  As a series of concentric lamellae with a central blood vessel to form a Haversian system or osteone. This lamellar bone is found in the cortex of adult long bones and is called compact bone. Metabolically it is relatively inert.

2  Or as woven bone, where the collagen fibres are in the form of loosely woven bundles. Spongy (cancellous) and trabecular

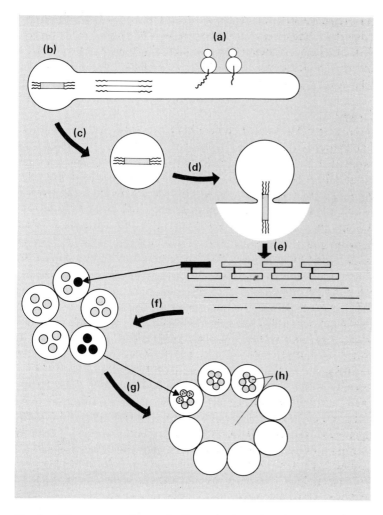

**Fig. 6.2** The sequence of events leading to the formation of collagen fibres in a fibroblast and the process of osteoid mineralization.

(**a**) Ribosomes attached to the endoplasmic reticulum translate messenger RNA for collagen, and polypeptide chains are translocated into the lumen of the endoplasmic reticulum.

(**b**) Three polypeptide chains align and then helically coil except for the extension peptides, to form procollagen.

(**c**) The procollagen molecule is processed into a secretory vesicle, probably through the Golgi complex.

(**d**) Procollagen is released from the osteoblast by exocytosis and the collagen molecule is formed after scission of the extension peptides.

(**e**) Linear and side-to-side alignment of collagen molecules by cross-bridges results in the formation of microfibrils. Hole zones are found between the ends of a linear array of collagen molecules.

(**f**) Cross-section of five linear aggregates of collagen forming a microfibril.

(**g**) Several microfibrils align to form a collagen fibril.

(**h**) During mineralization of osteoid the hole zones and the spaces between the collagen microfibrils and fibrils become filled with calcium hydroxyapatite crystals.

bones are made up of woven bone and are found, for example, in young subjects and at fracture sites. They also occur on the endosteal surfaces of medullary long bones and in some disorders of bone, e.g. hyperparathyroidism. Usually large numbers of osteocytes are present, which is indicative of high rates of bone turnover.

### Osteoclasts

The other main cell type in bone is the osteoclast. These are large multinucleated cells, $100\,\mu m$ in diameter. Osteoclasts are formed by fusion of mononuclear phagocytes from bone marrow. This has been shown in a number of ways. For example, in parabiotic animals (i.e. two animals whose blood circulation has been linked), where one has been irradiated to destroy bone marrow and the marrow cells of the other have been labelled with tritiated thymidine, then the osteoclasts in the irradiated animal are found to be derived from the marrow of its parabiont. Similarly, in chimeric transplants from quails to chick or mouse, the characteristic nuclei of the quail cells appear in the recipient's osteoclasts when haematogeneous transplants are made from the quail. Moreover, in osteopetrotic animals (i.e. those with dense bone and inadequate osteoclast activity) absorption of bone can be promoted in the osteopetrotic animal by transplantation of marrow or spleen cells, which act as precursors of osteoclasts.

Osteoclasts appear on the surfaces of bone, which is sub-sequently resorbed, especially under the stimulation of para-thyroid hormone. Barnicott, in a classical experiment, showed that parathyroid tissue cultured on calvaria induced bone re-sorption with the appearance of increased numbers of osteoclasts. The role of the osteoclast in the resorption and remodelling of bone is well established: they appear to break down bone components through the action of lysosomal enzymes which they release extracellularly.

Parathyroid hormone controls calcium levels of the body fluid principally by regulating the removal of calcium from bone. In mammals elevations of plasma calcium levels occur several hours after parathyroid hormone administration. Parathyroid hormone also increases osteoclast numbers and activity both *in vivo* and *in vitro*. However, these effects are usually noted long after the changes in plasma calcium levels have occurred, leading to the belief that, in mammals at least, osteoclasts are not rapidly responsive to parathyroid hormone and perhaps are not involved in the acute regulation of calcium metabolism. The situation appears to be different in birds where, during egg-laying, ad-ministration of parathyroid hormone induces functionally active osteoclasts within 20 minutes and at the same time causes a marked increase in the plasma concentration of calcium.

Calcitonin (see p. 208) reduces osteoclast activity. For example, if Barnicott's experiment of placing parathyroid tissue on calvaria in organ culture is repeated in the presence of calcitonin, bone resorption does not occur.

It will be appreciated that interference with any of the above processes (the synthesis and secretion of osteoid constituents, its eventual mineralization or of its resorption and remodelling) can lead to profound changes in bone structure and growth.

### Bone growth and remodelling

In the young, bone is growing, i.e. it increases in size, particularly in length. Apart from formation of new bone, there is remodelling of existing bone so that its formation and reabsorption are coupled. In the adult, bone turnover continues, albeit at a slower rate: in females, particularly after the menopause, reabsorption can exceed formation so that bone mass then becomes reduced.

A number of factors interact to regulate the balance of bone turnover. These include local factors (both chemical and mechanical) and hormonal factors (Fig. 6.3). The activity of bone-forming cells and bone-reabsorbing cells is coupled and, for example, osteoblasts produce an osteoclast activating factor, which acts locally. Production of this osteoclast activating factor is dependent upon a number of things, including parathyroid hormone and the active form of vitamin D, namely 1,25-dihydroxycholecalciferol.

So the action of parathyroid hormone in stimulating bone resorption is indirect, through its action on osteoblasts (Fig. 6.3). There are probably several osteoclast activating factors, including interleukin I, the production of which is stimulated by parathyroid hormone. The turnover of bone and its regulation is important to calcium homeostasis at all ages. Thus, if the parathyroid gland is removed in adult humans, serum calcium falls within 48 hours. This is because the return of calcium to the circulation is reduced since there is a reduction in bone resorption.

## The parathyroid glands

DEVELOPMENT AND MORPHOLOGY

The embryology of the parathyroid glands has already been dealt with in the chapter on the thyroid (Fig. 5.1a). Parathyroid glands are found in all classes of vertebrates from the Amphibia to the Mammalia, and there is a remarkable uniformity in their microscopic structure. Their number varies from two to eight and they may be either quite separate from the thyroid, attached to its surface, or embedded in it. In the human there are usually four glands but there may be additional accessory glands. They are small, approximately $6 \times 4 \times 2$ mm; each weighs about 40–60 mg; they are usually larger in women than in men. They lie on the posterior surface of the thyroid, between its

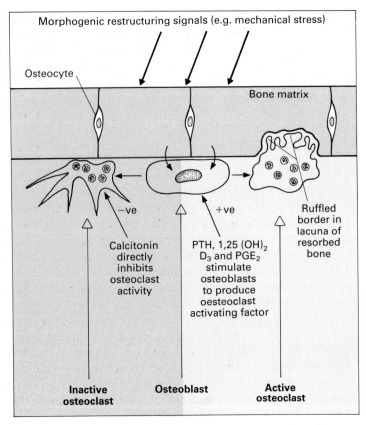

**Fig. 6.3** Factors that affect the remodelling of bone. Morphogenic restructuring signals such as mechanical stress can influence bone remodelling, while hormonal factors control osteoblast activity. Calcitonin has an inhibitory action, with formation of an inactive osteoclast. Parathyroid hormone (PTH), 1,25-dihydroxycholecalciferol $(1,25(OH)_2D_3)$ and prostaglandin $E_2$ $(PGE_2)$ act on the osteoblast to produce an osteoclast activating factor that stimulates bone matrix resorption by osteoclasts.

capsule and the surrounding cervical sheath. An important point to be noted is that variations in number, size and location of the parathyroids are common. Both the regularly occurring and accessory glands may be situated at some distance from the gland's normal location. It has been estimated that in man about one in ten glands is aberrant; they may be found down in the mediastinum or high up in the neck, but can also be found in the thyroid itself or, sometimes, posterior to the oesophagus.

There is a rich blood supply to the glands derived mainly from the inferior thyroid arteries, but also occasionally from the superior thyroid vessels. The venous drainage is via the superior, middle and inferior thyroid veins. Numerous lymphatics are present in the gland and although the sympathetic innervation derives from the superior and middle cervical ganglia, there is no secretomotor supply to the glandular tissue.

In man each gland is surrounded by a thin connective tissue capsule from which septa pass into its substance. There are two types of cell. The principal cell type is the 'chief' cell but just before puberty a second kind of cell appears, called the oxyphil cell. The cells are arranged in irregular, anastomosing cords and sheets or occasional acini, separated by vascular channels. After puberty fat cells appear among the parenchyma and in older people they may make up 60–70% of the volume of the gland.

## CHIEF CELLS

The chief cell occurs in the fetal, infantile, prepubertal as well as in the adult parathyroid and is responsible for the synthesis and secretion of parathyroid hormone. Ultrastructural studies on the developing gland indicate that most of the cells are inactive and they only become active as parturition approaches. Under the light microscope the cells are small, $4–8\,\mu m$ in diameter, and are usually polarized with respect to the adjacent blood supply. Two forms of the cell have been described which appear to be either dark or light. Dark (active) chief cells are characterized ultrastructurally by the cytological features of actively protein-synthesizing cells with vesicles and small membrane-bounded granules, $0.1–0.4\,\mu m$ in diameter, which may represent secretory granules. Large secretory granules are rare and cytoplasmic glycogen is sparse. Light (inactive) cells possess abundant glycogen and lipofuscin granules which are lysosomal residual bodies. These cells have little rough endoplasmic reticulum, a small Golgi complex and few associated vacuoles and secretory granules. These cells are inactive or resting cells which outnumber the active ones in the normal gland by a ratio of about 4:1. The active cells can be followed experimentally through a secretory cycle, from synthesizing, through packaging, secretion and then involution stages (light cells). Secretion appears to be by exocytosis and it seems likely that the microtubules and microfilaments found in chief cells play a role in the secretory process.

## OXYPHIL CELLS

The oxyphil cells begin to appear in the human parathyroid gland about the time of puberty and increase in number with age. They are characterized at the level of the light microscope by a smaller nucleus than that in the chief cell, an acidophilic cytoplasm and their larger size of about $10\,\mu m$ in diameter.

## Parathyroid hormone

This is made up of a single chain of 84 amino acids. The whole sequence of the molecule is not necessary for expression of full biological activity. The amino-terminal portion is the important part of the molecule. A synthetic peptide has been made which comprises the first 34 residues of the intact molecule. This one-third fragment of parathyroid hormone has full biological activity, and can not only raise serum calcium concentrations but also increase urinary excretion of phosphate (that is produce phosphaturia).

Parathyroid hormone is synthesized as a larger molecule and two precursor forms have been identified (Fig. 6.4). The smaller of these is called proparathyroid hormone and has been identified in extracts of parathyroid glands, though it is probably not secreted. It has an extra six amino acids at the amino-terminal end and thus has in total 90 amino acids. The larger precursor has only been identified in cell-free protein synthesizing systems which can make protein when an appropriate messenger RNA (e.g. extracted from parathyroid glands) is added. Under these circumstances a molecule known as pre-proparathyroid hormone is identifiable, having an extra 25 amino acids at the amino-terminus of proparathyroid hormone. Its existence illustrates the general phenomenon (see Chapter 1) that secreted proteins (including hormones) are synthesized in larger precursor forms. The 'pre' amino-terminal extension is more hydrophobic or

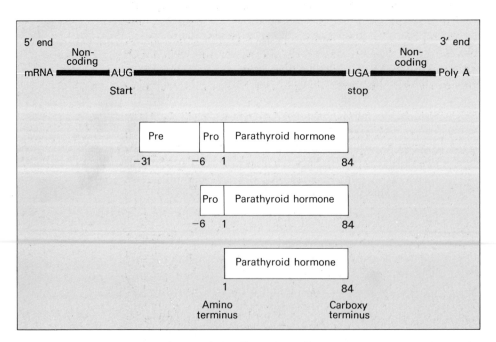

Fig. 6.4 Messenger RNA codes for the synthesis of parathyroid hormone which begins with creation of a signal peptide with 25 amino acids, −31 to −7, of pre-proparathyroid hormone. The signal peptide is normally removed before synthesis of the hormone is completed. Proparathyroid hormone has 90 amino acids, the first six of which are removed before the 1−84 hormone is secreted.

lipophilic (i.e. less water-soluble or more fat-soluble) and this is thought to facilitate translocation of the molecule from the ribosomes through the intervening membrane and into the lumen of the endoplasmic reticulum. The lipophilic extension is not required in the secreted molecule since it provides a signal to the membrane of the endoplasmic reticulum to permit passage of the newly synthesized molecule. According to this 'signal' hypothesis, the signal peptide leads the way through the endoplasmic reticulum membrane and it is then removed enzymatically, with release of the prohormone itself. The prohormone is packaged into secretory granules which are then passed into the cell cytoplasm: cleavage of the profragment usually occurs just before the hormone is secreted.

Messenger RNA has been isolated from normal parathyroid glands of cows and from human parathyroid tumours, allowing cloning of complementary DNA for bovine and human parathyroid hormones. With the complementary DNA it has been possible to establish the structure of the gene and investigate post-transcriptional modification of RNA (Fig. 6.5) and verify the structure of the hormone. The complementary DNA has also been used to study the regulation of messenger RNA. This has a long half-life of at least 24 hours in the parathyroid cell. Changes in secretion of hormone can occur much more quickly so that they do not depend on changes in synthesis but rely on the release of stored hormone, or possibly changes in the metabolism of the hormone within the parathyroid cell, which can break down the peptide hormone that it has synthesized. Accelerated or slowed break-down of parathyroid hormone would

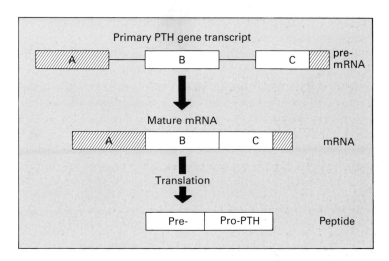

**Fig. 6.5** The transcription- and translation-products of parathyroid hormone. The gene comprises three exons and two introns on the short arm of chromosome number eleven. Segments B and C of the messenger RNA are translated to yield pre-proparathyroid hormone (PTH).

alter the amount available for secretion. Alterations in the processing of messenger RNA within the cell could alter the rate of synthesis of hormone and may be important to long-term adaption.

ACTIONS OF PARATHYROID HORMONE

There has for long been a debate as to whether the most important action of parathyroid hormone is on phosphate or on calcium, and whether the most important effects are those exerted on the kidney or those on bone. It was at one stage thought that the parathyroid glands might even produce two hormones, one controlling calcium and the other regulating phosphate. Since the synthetic 1−34 amino-terminal peptide affects both calcium and phosphate, that postulate is not necessary. It seems that these regulatory effects and the responses of bone and kidney are integrated. Both the phosphaturic and the hypercalcaemic effects have been used as the basis of bioassays for parathyroid hormone; those which depend upon changes in serum calcium have proved to be more reliable because a number of factors can affect phosphate excretion non-specifically. Of the many bioassay systems available, the most commonly used is that which depends on the known ability of parathyroid hormone to prevent the fall in serum calcium concentration in rats after parathyroidectomy. To increase the sensitivity of the bioassay, the rats are maintained on a diet which is low in calcium for 5 days; then the parathyroid glands are removed (either by surgery or by cautery). Parathyroid hormone is injected, and 5 hours later the serum calcium is measured. The potency of highly purified preparations of bovine, human or porcine parathyroid hormone which have been produced is about 2000 IU/mg.

The rise in serum calcium concentration after administration of parathyroid hormone is in part due to the direct effect of parathyroid hormone on bone, where it increases resorption. Parathyroid hormone also has a direct effect on the renal excretion of calcium: the net effect on the kidneys is a composite one. On one hand there may be a rise in renal excretion because of a greater filtered load induced by hypercalcaemia itself. In addition, parathyroid hormone stimulates the reabsorption of calcium in the tubules and this will reduce excretion. The overall effect of parathyroid hormone on urinary excretion of calcium is thus variable, depending upon the relative magnitude of the two effects.

In both bone and kidney the effects of parathyroid hormone are the results of hormone binding to a cell-surface receptor with activation of adenylate cyclase. In bone, specific competitive binding of parathyroid hormone to osteoblasts occurs, but not to osteoclasts. It is also worth noting that in contrast calcitonin only binds to osteoclasts (Fig. 6.3). In the kidney, binding of parathyroid hormone occurs to multiple cell types; but specific competitive binding occurs to the cell membrane of the primary foot processes of glomerular podocytes and to the antiluminal surface of all three segments of the proximal tubule. Both parathyroid hormone and calcitonin bind strongly to the peritubular surface of segment I of the proximal tubules where they are probably degraded in the kidney vacuolar lysosomal system. The increased intracellular concentrations of cyclic AMP specifically activate the target-cell, probably by modulation of protein kinase activity. In this respect, therefore, the action of parathyroid hormone in generating cyclic AMP is typical of most other peptide hormones (see Chapter 1). Specificity in the system is conferred at two sites—firstly at the receptor sites on the target-cell, which only respond to a particular hormone, and secondly within the cell since it is the specific properties of the target-cell produced by differentiation of the various tissues that are activated. Thus, the renal tubular system is activated by parathyroid hormone in such a way that the secretion of phosphate is increased, and the osteoclast can be stimulated to perform its specific function, which is resorption of bone. The effects of parathyroid hormone on adenylate cyclase in renal tubules can be used as the basis of *in vitro* bioassay; for this, isolated cell membranes from the renal cortex are used.

When cyclic AMP production is stimulated by parathyroid hormone *in vivo* some of the cyclic AMP escapes from the cell and there is a rise in the amount of cyclic AMP in blood and urine. This rise in cyclic AMP in blood arises largely from an action of the hormone on the kidney; this can be shown by following the appearance of cyclic AMP in the renal vein where its concentration rises more rapidly and to a higher value than elsewhere. The increase in renal excretion of cycle AMP is due to a direct excretion into the renal tubules, though a small part may also be due to the increased filtered load attributable to the rise in circulating cyclic AMP concentration. It should be noted that there is no known biological role for the cyclic AMP that appears in blood and in urine and that its principal role is within the cell. The extracellular changes in cyclic AMP serve, however, as a marker of the intracellular events; the changes in cyclic AMP precede all other responses which follow the administration of parathyroid hormone. In man the changes in cyclic AMP in plasma and urine (Fig. 6.6) occur within minutes, while phosphate excretion does not change for a few hours, and repeated injections of parathyroid hormone may be needed over 2−3 days before there are significant changes in serum calcium concentration.

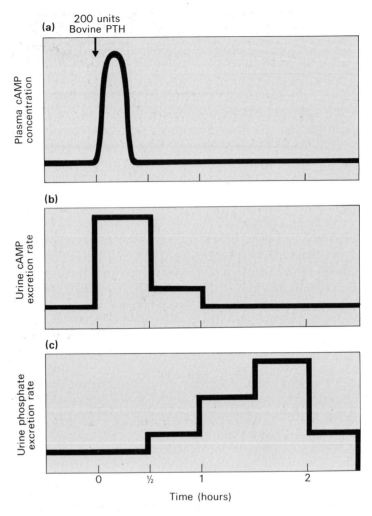

200 units
Bovine PTH

Plasma cAMP concentration

(b)

Urine cAMP excretion rate

(c)

Urine phosphate excretion rate

0      ½      1      2

Time (hours)

**Fig. 6.6** Injection of parathyroid hormone (PTH) intravenously in man increases the activity of renal adenylate cyclase and some of the cyclic AMP produced appears in blood (**a**) and urine (**b**). The phosphaturic response (**c**) then follows.

CONTROL OF THE SECRETION OF PARATHYROID HORMONE

Secretion of parathyroid hormone occurs continuously to maintain its concentration in the circulation, from which it is cleared rapidly with a half-life of about 5 minutes. Since parathyroid hormone is important in the regulation of calcium and phosphate metabolism, it might be expected that both of these would affect the activity of the parathyroid glands, possibly through feedback mechanisms. The most important regulator in the secretion of parathyroid hormone is the serum calcium concentration (Fig. 6.7); hypercalcaemia suppresses secretion, while hypocalcaemia (which can be produced by administration of an agent

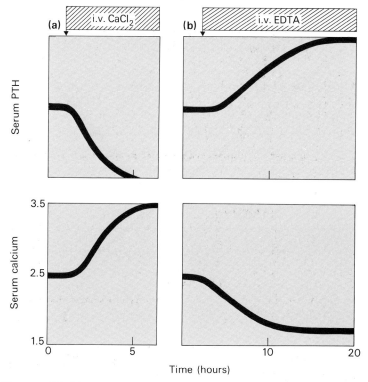

**Fig. 6.7** (a) Rise in serum calcium reduces the secretion of parathyroid hormone (PTH): this can be produced by infusion of calcium.

(b) Conversely, a fall in serum calcium (produced by infusing EDTA which complexes calcium) stimulates secretion.

such as EDTA which complexes calcium ions) stimulates secretion. The secretion of parathyroid hormone is proportional to the degree of hypocalcaemia (Fig. 6.8). Surprisingly, perhaps, it is not so clear that phosphate also has a regulatory action. When phosphate is infused there is stimulation of parathyroid glands but this is probably attributable to the hypocalcaemia that is induced as a result of the phosphate infusion, and if this is prevented then a high concentration of phosphate has no effect on parathyroid hormone secretion. Another divalent ion which does effect parathyorid gland secretion is magnesium; its effects are most easily studied with the parathyroid gland in tissue culture. The effects are similar to those of calcium, although on a molar basis, magnesium is less potent.

A number of other factors can be shown experimentally to modulate the activity of the gland. These include adrenaline, pressor amines and derivatives of vitamin D, but whether these are of physiological significance remains, however, to be established.

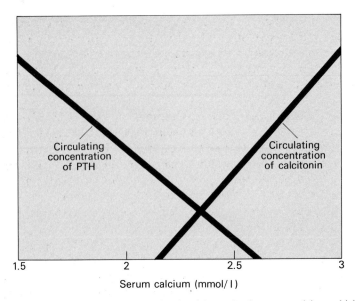

**Fig. 6.8** Calcitonin secretion is stimulated by a rise in serum calcium which suppresses secretion of parathyroid hormone (PTH). Conversely, hypocalcaemia stimulates parathyroid hormone release and reduces calcitonin release.

EFFECTS OF OVERSECRETION OF PARATHYROID HORMONE

Excessive parathyroid hormone causes hypercalcaemia and phosphaturia. This is most commonly due to a benign tumour of one of the four parathyroid glands, though sometimes it is due to hyperplasia of all four glands. This is called primary hyperparathyroidism, to distinguish it from the secondary overactivity of the glands that develops in an attempt to compensate for long-standing hypocalcaemia which can occur for example because of malabsorption of calcium. Secondary hyperparathyroidism can also be caused by chronic renal failure.

Primary hyperparathyroidism was first recognized by von Recklinghausen because of its effects on bone, causing resorption. The destruction of bone can sometimes be detected radiologically; for example, in the phalanges it causes subperiosteal resorption. Sometimes this is so extensive that it leads to cyst formation with development of a so-called 'brown tumour', for example in the skull or pelvis. Bone disease is the major feature in only about 15% of patients with primary hyperparathyroidism, causing bone pain and difficulty in walking. However, histologically the bone is abnormal in most cases of primary hyperparathyroidism. The basic changes found in longstanding cases of severe hyperparathyroidism are osteoclastic resorption of bone, progressive thinning of the cancellous and cortical bone structure, and fibrosis of the marrow. Bone is resorbed from the surfaces of the trabeculae with the formation of lacunae which produce severe distortion of the normally smooth outline of the bony seams. Increased numbers of osteoclasts are found in the lacunae. In some areas bone may be completely resorbed and replaced by soft tissue composed of a mass of mononuclear phagocytes, fibroblasts and multinucleate osteoclasts. Radiologically this area is detectable as a 'cyst'.

Renal calculi are much more common than bone disease, occurring in half of the patients with hyperparathyroidism. The renal stones are made of calcium and phosphate and hence are radio-opaque. The stone formation is presumably due to long-standing hypercalcaemia and hypercalcuria (increased urinary excretion of calcium) though the latter feature does not occur in all the patients. The stones develop in the calyces of the kidney and may move down the ureter, thereby causing renal colic; blood in the urine (haematuria) and recurrent infections of the renal tract (pyelonephritis) are consequences of the presence of stones. The kidneys may be damaged by presence of renal calculi, which may even lead to renal failure, if untreated. Hypercalcaemia *per se* can also impair renal function; thirst and polyuria can also occur.

Treatment of primary hyperparathyroidism is by surgery, with removal of the overactive parathyroid. Because of the embryological development of the parathyroid glands, it may be difficult to find the parathyroid tumour, which may be embedded within the thyroid, tucked away behind the oesophagus, or it may be down in the mediastinum, within the thymus. If possible, therefore, it is desirable to locate the overactive parathyroid gland preoperatively. The best means of doing this is by 'parathyroid venous sampling'; in this technique blood is taken from different points in the venous tree by cannulation of veins in the neck and the hormone content is measured (Fig. 6.9). The pattern of distribution of the hormone from different positions in the neck can indicate the probable location of the tumour, especially if samples have been taken from the superior, middle and inferior thyroid veins into which the parathyroid venous effluent drains.

CAUSES OF RISE IN SERUM CALCIUM

With the increased use and availability of biochemical screening tests, hypercalcaemia is often discovered 'accidentally' before it actually causes any symptoms. Apart from overactivity of the parathyroids, there are other mechanisms that can lead to hyper-calcaemia. For example, malignant cells (metastases) in bone cause destruction of the bone itself and release of calcium. Sometimes this is due to an 'osteoclast activating factor'. Tumours can also cause hypercalcaemia, without their having metastasized to bone, by secreting a 'parathyroid-hormone-related peptide'. This has been cloned and shown to have, in its amino-terminus, structural

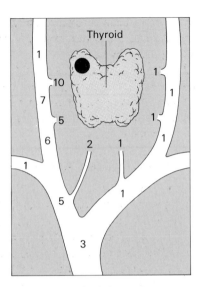

**Fig. 6.9** Parathyroid tumours can be localized by assaying parathyroid hormone in blood samples taken from cannulation of the great veins of the neck and the small thyroid veins. The numbers indicate the relative concentration of hormone in a patient with a tumour of the right upper parathyroid gland. The peak concentrations are in the right superior thyroid vein and the right internal jugular vein. The concentrations (shown in arbitrary numbers) are lower in the other veins such as the inferior thyroid veins and superior vena cava, thus pointing to the probable location of the tumour in the upper right parathyroid.

similarity to the amino-terminus of parathyroid hormone but the tumoral hypercalcaemic factor is larger. Excess thyroid hormone increases the turnover of bone, and occasionally thyrotoxicosis causes hypercalcaemia. Overdosage with vitamin D can also raise the serum calcium, partly by the physiological effect of vitamin D, which is to increase calcium absorption from the gut, and partly from a pharmacological effect in which stimulation of bone break-down occurs. Rarely, ingestion of large amounts of milk, or calcium-containing antacids taken for peptic ulceration, can cause hypercalcaemia, even though the body's homeostatic mechanisms can normally control wide variations in calcium intake.

EFFECTS OF UNDERSECRETION OF PARATHYROID HORMONE

Lack of parathyroid hormone causes hypocalcaemia and hyper-phosphataemia. The clinical effects are the consequence of a low serum calcium which results in an increased excitability of the tissue, causing paraesthesia (pins and needles) or attacks of tetany and even of epilepsy. Surgical removal of parathyroid glands causes hypocalcaemia and symptoms appear within 24–48 hours. The glands may be removed accidentally during an operation for thyroid disease because of the close physical relationship between the two glands. The parathyroids are only the size of a rice grain and may not be seen. Frequently, however, there is no known cause for failure of the parathyroids, so the condition is called 'idiopathic hypoparathyroidism'.

In assessing the significance of a low total serum calcium, account has to be taken, of course, of the concentration of albumin in the serum, since hypoproteinaemia can lead to a fall in total serum calcium. However, in this situation the ionized calcium will be unaffected.

### RESISTANCE TO THE ACTIONS OF PARATHYROID HORMONE

Failure of the tissues to respond to parathyroid hormone also leads to the development of hypocalcaemia. This occurs in a congenital condition which mimics the effect of idiopathic hypo-parathyroidism, and so is called 'pseudohypoparathyroidism'. In this condition the serum phosphate concentration is high and the serum calcium is low, and there is secondary hyperparathyroidism with high (rather than low) concentrations of circulating para-thyroid hormone. The patients may have mental deficiency and also other stigmata of the disease which may suggest the diagnosis: these include shortness of some of the metacarpals, particularly the 4th and 5th metacarpals and a characteristic roundness of the face. The patients are frequently mentally defective but whether this is due to the long-standing hypocalcaemia or to another associated genetic factor is not clear. Paradoxically, in patients with pseudohypoparathyroidism, there may be ectopic

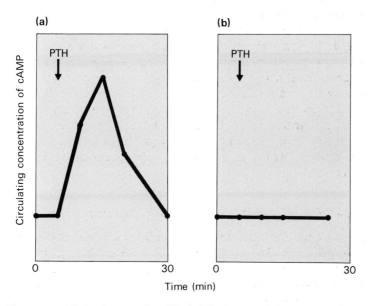

**Fig. 6.10** (a) In hypoparathyroidism following surgical removal of the parathyroid, the response to injected parathyroid hormone (PTH) is normal as shown by the rise in circulating cyclic AMP.

(b) In contrast, in a patient with pseudohypoparathyroidism there is no response because of resistance in the target-cells.

calcification, with deposition of calcium salts subcutaneously, in muscle and in brain, though the cause for this is not clear. The diagnosis can be established by showing that when parathyroid hormone is given, there is a lack of the normal response (Fig. 6.10). In pseudohypoparathyroidism administration of parathyroid hormone does not cause a rise in plasma or urinary cyclic AMP, although it will produce a normal response in patients with iodiopathic hypoparathyroidism or surgically induced hypoparathyroidism.

The resistance to the action of parathyroid hormone in pseudohypoparathyroidism is due to a defect in the target tissue, namely bone and kidney. The receptor in the target-cells (see Chapter 1) is on the external surface of the membrane while the catalytic unit (the adenylate cyclase) is on the inside. The receptors and the catalytic unit are normally linked by a third component of the system; this regulatory component is called the G-unit because it binds guanosine triphosphate—it is also called the N-protein because it binds nucleotides (see Chapter 1). In pseudohypoparathyroidism it seems likely that there is a defect in one part of the N-protein, at least in some patients, and this deficiency leads to the resistance to the action of parathyroid hormone.

EFFECTS OF CHANGES IN SERUM MAGNESIUM
CONCENTRATION

The effects of changes in serum magnesium in patients are complex. A fall in the concentration of magnesium can stimulate parathyroid hormone secretion, but if severe hypomagnesaemia develops then the stimulatory effect is lost. Moreover, there is loss of responsiveness to parathyroid hormone. Such patients develop hypocalcaemia which is difficult to correct. It is believed that this combination of abnormalities arises because magnesium is necessary not only for the action of adenylate cyclase but also for the regulation of the release of parathyroid hormone. Severe magnesium deficiency can arise in patients who receive no food by mouth and are being fed for long periods intravenously. Magnesium depletion can also occur as a result of malabsorption syndromes which cause diarrhoea. Correction of the magnesium depletion leads to a rapid rise in the concentration of parathyroid hormone in the circulation, within minutes, and the hypocalcaemia can be corrected simply by remedying the deficiency of magnesium.

## Calcitonin

The original demonstration of the existence of a hypocalcaemic factor, later called calcitonin, depended on the classical cross-perfusion studies of Copp. The thyroid and parathyroids of an animal were perfused *in situ*, and the venous effluent was pumped into a second animals. When the concentration of calcium in the original perfusate was raised, a fall in the serum calcium concentration was observed in the recipient animal. This was evidence for the production of a substance that was released into the circulation and which acted on distant tissues, thus fulfilling Starling's requirements for the use of the term 'hormone'.

Originally, the hormone was thought to be produced by the parathyroids but it was later shown that it came from the thyroid gland in mammals, and from the ultimobranchial body in birds and fish. The ultimobranchial bodies or glands were first described in elasmobranch fish by Van Bemmelen in 1886. Although there were earlier descriptions of the non-follicular cells of the mammalian thyroid gland, it was not until 1932 that Nonidez called them parafollicular cells and suggested that they could have an endocrine function: however, he had no idea as to the nature of their secretion. The embryology of the thyroid gland and ultimobranchial bodies has already been descibred (Fig. 5.1a). In amphibians, reptiles and birds the ultimobranchial bodies and the thyroid gland remain as quite distinct structures. However, in mammals the ultimobranchial bodies become fused with the thyroid and their cells become dispersed among the thyroid follicles as the parafollicular or C-cells. The ultimobranchial body and thyroid C-cells in all classes of vertebrates are ultimately derived from neural crest cells.

In the human, C-cells are largely restricted to the posterior part of the lateral lobes of the thyroid, usually in the region adjacent to the parathyroid glands, and it seems likely that during development some cells of the ultimobranchial body end up in these other sites rather than the 'normal' one, within the thyroid gland. Usually these ectopic C-cells go undetected, unless they become neoplastic and enlarge. The blood supply to C-cells is common with that of the thyroid follicular cells. C-cells in mammals are not innervated but in amphibia and birds the ultimobranchial calcitonin secreting cells do have a nerve supply.

MORPHOLOGY OF C-CELLS

C-cells can be found either closely adherent to thyroid follicles (parafollicular) or in an apparently interfollicular location, although this latter position may be due solely to the plane of section through the C-cells (i.e. tangential to the follicle wall). At the light microscope level they are difficult to identify in sections stained with haematoxylin and eosin but, as Nonidez showed, the intense argentophilia (i.e. silver staining) of their granules enables them to be easily demonstrated with silver impregnation methods. The origin of the C-cells of the ultimobranchial body from the neural crest was shown by Le Dourain who took cells from the neural crest of the quail and put them in place of the neural crest of chick embryos. The quail cells are readily recognizable because of their large nuclear chromatin mass. When the chick embryo developed the quail cells could be found in the ultimobranchial bodies.

The C-cells possess a number of cytochemical characteristics which are used as the paradigm for the class of cells known as the APUD system. This acronym APUD is derived from the words, *A*mine, *P*recursor-*U*ptake, *D*ecarboxylase. The significance of these is that the cells contain amines, they can take up amine precursors and they contain a decarboxylase. The amine is fluorogenic (such as catecholamine or 5-hydroxytryptamine) and the amine precursor can be 5-hydroxytryptophan (5HTP) or dihydroxyphenylalanine (DOPA). Thus, the characterization of the APUD cells is based on cytochemical characteristics. Also the cells generally possess sufficient concentrations of side-chain carboxyl groups to give marked metachromasia and they also contain esterases such as choline esterase and $\alpha$-glycerophosphatase.

Apart from the C-cells of the thyroid gland and ultimobranchial bodies which secrete calcitonin, the APUD system includes the adrenal medulla, and other peptide hormone secreting cells. The other endocrine cells that have the cytochemical characteristics of the APUD system include the anterior pituitary and the cells of the Islets of Langerhans in the pancreas and the cells that secrete hormones from the gastrointestinal tract (see Chapter 7). However, the origin of these does not seem to be from the neural crest. The various cell types that comprise the APUD system may give rise to a wide spectrum of neoplasias that maintain many of the phenotypic characteristics of their normal progenitor cells. In a patient more than one endocrine tumour may be produced and so they are called 'multiple endocrine neoplasias'. They have been grouped into two classes. Type I multiple endocrine neoplasias arise from those APUD cells that do not appear to be neural crest in origin (e.g. parathyroid, anterior pituitary, pancreatic Islet and gastrointestinal endocrine cells) while type II tumours arise from APUD cells of neural crest origin (e.g. thyroid C-cells and adrenal medullary cells). Tumours of the parathyroid glands can arise in patients with type I or type II multiple endocrine neoplasias.

Infusion of calcium into an experimental animal induces C-cell degranulation; for example, in rats infused with calcium the granule count per cell is halved 4 hours after the injection and many of the cells are completely degranulated. Long-term stimulation with high calcium concentration, either *in vivo* or in organ-cultured C-cells, leads to degranulation and an accompanying hyperplasia and hypertrophy of the cells. In particular, the rough endoplasmic reticulum and the Golgi complex become extensive and enlarged. On the other hand, low ambient calcium levels leave C-cells, either *in vivo* or in culture, largely unchanged.

Calcitonin is a peptide containing 32 amino acids, with a di-sulphide bridge yielding an amino-terminal circle of amino acids between residues 1 and 7; there is a proline amide group at the carboxy-terminus (Fig. 6.11).

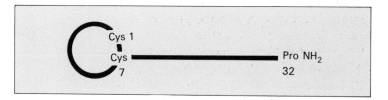

**Fig. 6.11**    The structure of calcitonin with its disulphide ring.

Apart from these features, there are considerable variations in the actual amino acid sequence of calcitonin in different species. The calcitonin gene lies on the short arm of chromosome 11 in humans. It has six exons and five introns (Fig. 6.12) and the gene encodes for a much larger peptide than calcitonin, i.e. 136 amino acid residues rather than the 32 amino acids of calcitionin. Demonstration that the gene encoded for a larger peptide led to the detection of previously unrecognized peptides, the so-called 'cryptic peptides', that included amino-terminal and carboxy-terminal peptides. The calcitonin gene is also transcribed in tissues other than the parafollicular cells of the thyroid and differential splicing of the exons can occur so that different peptides are made in diverse tissues (Fig. 6.12). One of these is a 'calcitonin gene-related peptide' (CGRP) that consists of 37 amino acids. Like calcitonin, it can be synthesized and secreted by the thyroid, but more is made in the nervous system, particularly in the hypothalamus and pituitary. Calcitonin gene-related peptide may be important as a neurotransmitter, and it also has very powerful vasodilator properties.

The hypocalcaemic effect of calcitonin depends primarily on its ability to inhibit the mobilization of calcium from bone, by suppressing the activity of the osteoclasts. It may also have some stimulatory effect on bone formation, and thus increase calcium uptake, although this is probably less significant. Secretion of calcitonin is stimulated by hypercalcaemia (Fig. 6.8) which at the same time suppresses secretion of parathyroid hormone.

Thus, calcitonin is capable of counteracting the effects of parathyroid hormone. It has been postulated that it is important in protecting the body from the effects of a sudden influx of calcium such as would be produced by drinking a pint of milk which contains 25 mmol (1 gm) of calcium and in patients who have been thyroidectomized where intravenous infusion of calcium causes a greater rise in serum than it does in normal subjects. Nevertheless the physiological role of calcitonin remains

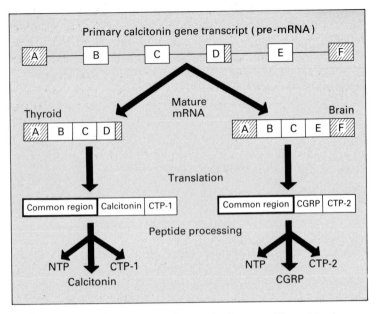

**Fig. 6.12** Peptides arising from the calcitonin gene. The calcitonin gene consists of six exons, shown here as A–F. These can be differentially spliced after transcription to give different forms of mature messenger RNA. The sequence of calcitonin is encoded in exon D; splicing of exons A, B, C and D gives a messenger RNA which, when it is translated, yields pre-procalcitonin. From this, an amino-terminal peptide (NTP), calcitonin and a carboxy-terminal peptide (CTP–1) are produced by post-translational processing. An alternative splicing process, using exons A, B, C, E and F, yields a different messenger RNA. The product of this has a common amino-terminal region, the 'calcitonin gene-related peptide' (CGRP) and a different carboxy-terminal peptide (CTP–2). The left hand pathway in the diagram predominates in parafollicular cells of the thyroid to yield calcitonin, while the CGRP pathway predominates in the brain.

uncertain, though increased concentrations of calcitonin are found in pregnant and in lactating women and so it may be more important under those conditions.

EFFECTS OF OVERPRODUCTION OF CALCITONIN

Overproduction of calcitonin occurs in patients who have tumours of the parafollicular cells of the thyroid: this is called medullary carcinoma of the thyroid. It was from such a tumour that human calcitonin was first isolated. The presence of this tumour can be a familial, inherited condition. However, it can also occur without there being any family history of such a tumour. Sometimes the presence of a medullary carcinoma of the thyroid is associated with the presence of another tumour, of the adrenal medulla, called a phaeochromocytoma (see Chapter 3), so that the patients have tumours of two groups of APUD cells. Patients with a medullary carcinoma of the thyroid usually present with a goitre in the neck, owing to enlargement of the thyroid gland. The concentration of calcitonin is very high in the circulation of these patients. Despite this, the serum calcium is entirely normal and there is no demonstrable abnormality of calcium homeostasis or in bone architecture. The reason for this observation is not clear, but because of it, there is doubt as to whether calcitonin has a significant role to play in calcium homeostasis, at least in man, though its role in animals may be greater: e.g. in egg-shell formation in birds. It may also be more important in growing children and in pregnant women, contributing to growth or preservation of the skeleton.

## Vitamin D

STRUCTURE AND METABOLISM OF VITAMIN D

Although known as a vitamin, and thus regarded as a compound that has to be provided in the diet, vitamin D can be formed in the skin. Exposure to ultraviolet light in sunshine converts 7-dehydrocholesterol to cholecalciferol (vitamin D3). Fig. 6.13 shows how irradiation with ultraviolet light opens the B-ring of the steroid nucleus to give previtamin D; then there is rotation of the A-ring to give vitamin D3. This can be absorbed into the circulation and is the natural form of vitamin D. Formation of cholecalciferol in the skin is important since the sources of vitamin D in the diet are limited, for example to fish and eggs. Ergocalciferol (vitamin D2) is a pharmaceutical product of plant origin—it is made by irradiation of ergosterol, which is found, for example, in extracts of wheat germ. Vitamin D2 is used in food fortification, for example, in margarine. In some countries, it is added to milk.

By 1965, because of the work of Kodicek in Cambridge and DeLuca in America, it was realized that vitamin D had to be further metabolized before it was capable of exerting its biological activity (Figs. 6.14 and 6.15). This involves the addition of hydroxyl groups. The first step occurs in the liver, in which an hydroxyl group is added to the side-chain, converting cholecalciferol to 25-hydroxycholecalciferol (i.e. 25-hydroxyvitamin D3) which is the major form of vitamin D in the circulation (unless the patient ingests ergocalciferol which is converted to 25-hydroxyergocalciferol, i.e. 25-hydroxyvitamin D2). Further metabolism of 25-hydroxycholecalciferol is necessary; this occurs in the kidney which adds an additional hydroxyl group in the A-ring to give 1,25-dihydroxycholecalciferol (also called calcitriol) (Fig. 6.14) which is the most potent form of vitamin D. Other circulating metabolites of vitamin D, formed from 25-hydroxycholecalciferol include 24,25-dihydroxycholecalciferol, made by 24-hydroxylation in the kidney. The concentration

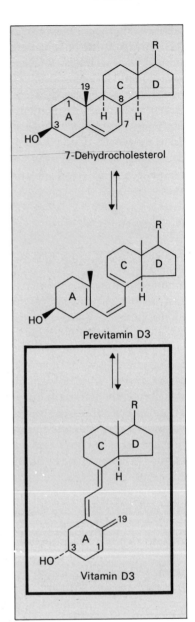

**Fig. 6.13** Ultraviolet irradiation, for example in skin, opens the B-ring of 7-dehydrocholesterol to give pre-vitamin D3: rotation of the A-ring then gives vitamin D3. In this illustration R is the side-chain of cholesterol, 7-dehydrocholesterol and vitamin D3 (see Fig. 6.14).

Projection of groups relative to the plane of the rings:

▶ forwards; ＿＿ backwards.

of 25-hydroxycholecalciferol in the circulation is quite high (3–30 ng/ml) but the concentration of 1,25-dihydroxychole-calciferol is very low (20–60 pg/ml). There is a circulating vitamin D-binding protein which has high affinity for 25-hydroxy and 24,25-dihydroxyvitamin D but low affinity for 1,25-dihydroxyvitamin D.

EFFECTS OF VITAMIN D

Under normal circumstances probably all the effects of vitamin D are due to 1,25-dihydroxycholecalciferol. It remains to be

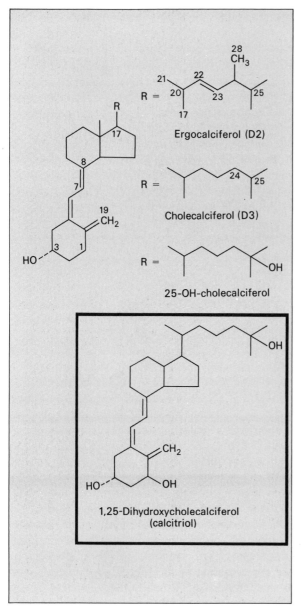

21
20
22
28 CH₃
17
23
25

R =

Ergocalciferol (D2)

24
25

R =

Cholecalciferol (D3)

R =

OH

25-OH-cholecalciferol

R
17
8
7
19 CH₂
3 1
HO

OH

CH₂

HO    OH

1,25-Dihydroxycholecalciferol
(calcitriol)

Fig. 6.14  The structures of vitamin D2, vitamin D3, 25-hydroxycholecalciferol and of 1,25-dihydroxycholecalciferol in the hormonal form (calcitriol). The hydroxy group is in the $\alpha$ orientation and so this compound is also called 1$\alpha$,25-hydroxycholecalciferol and the enzyme which produces it from 25-hyproxycholecalciferol is called 25-hydroxycholecalciferol, 1$\alpha$-hydroxylase.

established whether any of the other metabolites of vitamin D have a physiological role or whether they are break-down products. The main action of 1,25-dihydroxycholecalciferol is to stimulate calcium absorption. This occurs by a direct action on the intestinal mucosa where it acts, like a steroid hormone, on the nucleus. The effect of 1,25-dihydroxycholecalciferol on the nucleus leads to an increase in the synthesis of messenger RNA, which in turn leads to increased protein synthesis. Among the proteins formed in the intestinal cell is a calcium-binding protein which is believed to be important in transporting calcium across

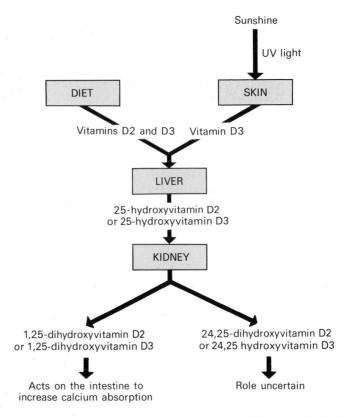

**Fig. 6.15** The sources and metabolism of vitamin D. The term vitamin D is used when it is not necessary to differentiate between vitamin D2 and D3.

the intestinal cell. The target-cells have a receptor protein for 1,25-dihydroxycholecalciferol with a molecular weight of about 60 000. The receptor site is in the carboxy-terminal part of the protein while the amino-terminal part of the molecule possesses a region that can bind specifically to DNA. Divalent cations such as zinc are important for binding to DNA, possibly by determining the conformation of the protein and giving rise to processes that can interdigitate between the helices of DNA. Binding of the receptor protein to DNA increases in the presence of 1,25-dihydroxycholecalciferol. As in the case of steroid hormones, the binding of the hormal form of vitamin D, i.e. 1,25-dihydroxycholecalciferol, occurs on the 5'side of the gene, upstream of the promoter region (Fig. 6.16). As a result, expression of the gene for calcium-binding protein is increased.

VITAMIN D AS A HORMONE—THE REGULATION OF
METABOLISM OF VITAMIN D

Since 1,25-dihydroxycholecalciferol is synthesized in the kidney and is secreted in the bloodstream to act on a distant tissue (the

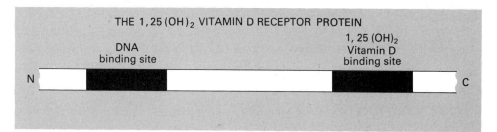

THE 1,25(OH)$_2$ VITAMIN D RECEPTOR PROTEIN

DNA
binding site

1,25(OH)$_2$
Vitamin D
binding site

N

C

**Fig. 6.16** A schematic representation of the nuclear receptor protein for 1,25-dihydroxyvitamin D, which is like the receptor for steroid hormones. There is a site which can bind 1,25-dihydroxyvitamin D: when that site is occupied, the receptor protein binds to DNA and ultimately stimulates the synthesis of calcium-binding protein for example.

intestine), it can be regarded as a hormone. In this sense the kidney is therefore an endocrine gland. This endocrine system is subject to feedback control. The activity of the 1-hydroxylase system is dependent on the serum calcium and phosphate concentrations (Fig. 6.17). Low calcium stimulates the 1-hydroxylase system, while high calcium activates the 24-hydroxylase that can convert 25-hydroxycholecalciferol to 24,25-dihydroxycholecalciferol. The latter is probably biologically inert and the formation of 24,25-dihydroxycholecalciferol is reciprocally related to the production of 1,25-dihydroxycholecalciferol. A low serum phosphate activates the 1-hydroxylase system. Parathyroid hormone stimulates and calcitonin suppresses the 1-hydroxylase. There may be other interactions between the

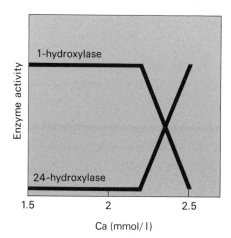
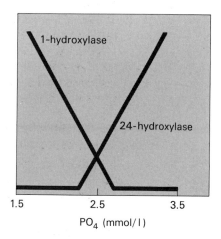

**Fig. 6.17** The effects of changing calcium and phosphate on the activity of renal hydroxylation of 25-hydroxycholecalciferol. Low calcium and low phosphate stimulate 1-hydroxylation which yields 1,25-dihydroxycholecalciferol, while high calcium and high phosphate increase 24-hydroxylation which yields 24,25-dihydroxycholecalciferol.

parathyroid glands and vitamin D endocrine systems, and it appears that derivatives of vitamin D can modulate the secretion of parathyroid hormone, so as to maintain calcium homeostasis.

EFFECTS OF DEFICIENCY OF VITAMIN D

Deficiency of vitamin D causes rickets in children; in adults the corresponding condition is osteomalacia. Both conditions are characterized by failure of calcification of osteoid, which is the matrix of bone and the manifestations depend on whether or not the bone is growing.

In children there is a failure of remodelling, so that the growing ends are swollen (Fig. 6.18). This can be seen at the wrists and at the costochondral junctions (the swelling of which leads to the development of what is called a rickety rosary). Endochondral ossification fails and this leads to excessively thick plates of epiphyseal disc cartilage, which is soft and poorly calcified. In addition, both the primary and secondary spongiosa are inadequately calcified so that the bone bends. This results in deformity, bow legs or knock knees. Radiologically it can be shown that the changes are greatest at the growing ends of bones. The x-ray appearance of rachitic bones is characterized by classical changes at the distal ends of long bones including cupping, fraying, widening, and generally decreased bone density.

In the adult the main feature is pain; the bone may partially fracture to give what is called a 'Looser's zone' or pseudofracture. In addition there may be profound muscle weakness, affecting particularly the hip and shoulder muscles, due to an associated proximal myopathy. Osteomalacic bones have generally decreased density, but since the epiphyses are closed in adulthood, rickets is not present. In the mature skeleton, osteomalacia leads to the production of wide layers of osteoid which eventually come to cover the vast majority of available bone surfaces. The simplest objective method of assessing the presence or absence of osteomalacia is to examine the calcified sections of biopsied bone under polarized light. More than four birefringent lamellae in the uncalcified osteoid on the surfaces of bone trabeculae or Haversian systems indicates the presence of osteomalacia.

In vitamin D deficiency the serum calcium may be low. This can cause tetany and increases parathyroid activity. Hypocalcaemia does not always occur, however, and so this cannot be the main cause for the failure of calcification of the osteoid in bone. It is likely, therefore, that vitamin D derivatives have a direct action on bone to induce mineralization, although it has been difficult to prove this *in vitro*.

Deficiency of vitamin D in the UK occurs in two groups of

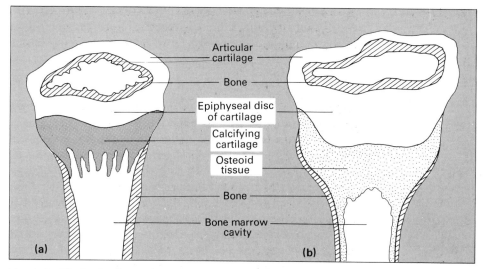

**Fig. 6.18** The heads of normal (**a**) and rachitic (**b**) growing tibia.

(**a**) A normal growing epiphyseal disc of cartilage is shown and the underlying zone of calcifying cartilage.

(**b**) The epiphyseal disc of cartilage is greatly enlarged and underneath it is a thick zone of osteoid tissue, i.e. uncalcified bone matrix. Note also the generally thickened epiphyseal region in the rachitic bone.

the population, the elderly and the Asian immigrants. In the former it is likely that the deficiency occurs because of a combination of dietary deficiency and lack of exposure to sunlight because of living indoors (the ultraviolet component of sunlight is filtered out by glass). The causes of vitamin D deficiency in Asians is less clear. It has been postulated that dietary factors cause rickets or osteomalacia by binding calcium, but this is not the case: nor is a low calcium diet the cause of failure of mineralization of bone.

The normal daily requirement in humans is 100–400 units of vitamin D daily and since the potency is 40 000 u/mg this corresponds to 2.5–10 μg/day. Vitamin D deficiency can be treated with small doses although the amount given is often rather greater than the normal requirement, say about 3000 u/day. Improvement occurs quite quickly, within weeks, but it takes a much longer time, perhaps a year, before the skeleton is entirely normal. The condition can be treated with smaller amounts of 1,25-dihydroxycholecalciferol, about 0.5 μg/day. When vitamin D3 is given orally to a vitamin D deficient patient, it is rapidly hydroxylated to 25-hydroxycholecalciferol, and then to 1,25-dihydroxycholecalciferol. The small doses that are used only give physiological concentrations of 25-hydroxycholecalciferol but quite quickly, within 48 hours, supranormal concentrations of 1,25-dihydroxycholecalciferol are produced. This is the result of increased 1-hydroxlase in the kidney. This overactivity persists for many months, presumably as a consequence of persistent secondary hyperparathyroidism.

OTHER CAUSES OF RICKETS AND OSTEOMALACIA

There are, of course, many other causes of rickets and osteo-malacia apart from a deficiency of vitamin D. Chronic renal failure is one cause; this is probably because there is a lack of the 1α-hydroxylase activity with the loss of functioning renal tissue. There is also a congenital disorder which is believed to be due to a lack of 1α-hydroxylase, and this is called pseudovitamin D deficiency rickets. This condition can be treated with small doses of 1,25-dihydroxycholecalciferol. Barbiturate and phenytonin therapy (for epilepsy) can cause rickets and osteomalacia; this may be related to the induction of enzyme systems by these drugs and interference with the normal metabolism of vitamin D.

Not all cases of rickets or osteomalacia are related to vitamin D. For example, phosphate depletion can be responsible, and this can arise in renal tubular disorders that result in excessive loss of phosphate and hypophosphataemia: this is sometimes called 'phosphate diabetes'. Even this type of rickets can, however, be treated with vitamin D, but the condition is resistant to vitamin D and so large doses are needed. One cause for this hypophos-phataemic rickets is a mutation on the X chromosome which causes an X-linked dominant disorder.

EFFECTS OF EXCESS VITAMIN D

Large doses of vitamin D can cause hypercalcaemia and this is referred to as 'vitamin D intoxication'. This can result from excessive ingestion of any of the forms of vitamin D that are available for therapeutic purposes (such as cholecalciferol, ergocalciferol, 25-hydroxycholecalciferol and 1,25-dihydroxy-cholecalciferol). They can be used, for example, to correct hypo-calcaemia due to hypoparathyroidism. Large amounts of vitamin $D_2$ or vitamin $D_3$ have to be given, e.g. 50 000−100 000 units (1.25−2.5 mg) daily. Much smaller amounts of 1,25-dihydroxycholecalciferol 0.5 μg/day) can be used: this increases calcium absorption and mobilizes calcium from bone. Intoxication of vitamin D causes nausea, vomiting and dehydration because of hypercalcaemia. If the hypercalcaemia is prolonged, calcification can develop within the kidney and renal function can be im-paired. Thus, careful monitoring of therapy is needed to avoid overdosage. If hypercalcaemia is produced by 1,25-dihydroxy-cholecalciferol therapy, it is less prolonged when the treatment is stopped than if vitamin D has been given. One important reason for this is that vitamin D and 25-hydroxyvitamin D are fat-soluble; they accumulate in the body while 1,25-dihydroxy-cholecalciferol does not accumulate in this way, nor is it protein-bound, so it can be cleared rapidly from the circulation with a half-life of about 6 hours.

## SUMMARY

Maintenance of calcium homeostasis is important for all cells, not merely for the skeleton. During growth, calcium balance is positive. In adult life there is an equilibrium between absorption from the gut and loss through urine. This is regulated by parathyroid hormone, vitamin D and possibly calcitonin. Parathyroid hormone acts primarily on bone and kidney. Vitamin D can also be considered as a hormone, the active form of which is 1,25-dihydroxycholecalciferol, which is produced in the kidney and acts largely on the gut to increase absorption of calcium.

## FURTHER READING

AURBACH G. D., MARX S. J. & SPIEGEL A. M. (1985) Parathyroid Hormone Calcitonin and the Calciferols. In *R. H. Williams' Textbook of Endocrinology*, 7th edn, Eds. J. D. Wilson & D. W. Foster. W. B. Saunders, Philadelphia & London.

DELUCA H. F. (1980) Vitamin D revisited. In *Clinics in Endocrinology and Metabolism*. W. B. Saunders, Philadelphia.

O'RIORDAN J. L. H. & PAPAPOULES S. E. (1984) Bone. In *Clinical Physiology* 5th edn, Eds. E. J. M. Campbell, C. J. Dickenson, J. D. H. Slater, C. R. W. Edwards & K. Sikora, pp. 310–42. Blackwell Scientific Publications, Oxford.

# 7   Pancreatic and gastrointestinal hormones

The disease now known as diabetes mellitus was probably described in the earliest known medical text, the *Papyrus Ebers*, which was written about 1500 BC, about a thousand years before the time of Hippocrates. Later Aretaeus described it vividly, in the 2nd century AD, and he wrote of the disease as 'being a melting down of flesh and limbs into urine' referring to the passage of large volumes of urine (polyuria) and also to the loss of weight that characterizes uncontrolled diabetes. He also referred to 'unquenchable thirst' and said that if patients do not drink 'their mouth becomes parched and their bodies dry'. He went on to say, 'hence the disease is described by the name diabetes', from the Greek word meaning a syphon. In the 16th century the Swiss physician Paracelsus thought that diabetes probably resulted from the presence of salt and noted that there was acid in the urine. However, Willis in London in 1684 stressed that in this condition (which he referred to as the 'pissing evil') the urine 'was wonderfully sweet as if imbued with honey or sugar'. In 1776 Dobson was the first to show that the urine of diabetics contained sugar, and thus the association of diabetes mellitus with a disturbance of carbohydrate metabolism became apparent. Then in 1788 Cawley related the disease to disorders of the pancreas.

A major portion of the pancreas (the 'exocrine pancreas') is responsible for secreting digestive enzymes in pancreatic juice into the upper intestine but there are also endocrine cells spread diffusely through the gland which are grouped in islets, named after their discoverer Langerhans who described them in 1869. Twenty years later von Mering and Minkowski showed that removal of the pancreas from dogs led to a condition resembling diabetes mellitus, with a rise in blood sugar and the appearance of sugar and ketones in the urine. At the beginning of this century it was shown that the Islet cells of diabetic patients were abnormal. At about the same time it was also found that destruction of the exocrine cells by ligation of the pancreatic duct did not cause diabetes, since ligation did not affect the endocrine cells. These observations later led to the postulate that diabetes was due to lack of a hypothetical internal secretion of the pancreas into the bloodstream. In 1921 Banting and Best destroyed the exocrine pancreas, by duct ligation, and extracted from the remaining tissue a substance that could lower blood sugar in dogs. This was the protein hormone insulin and soon, after sufficient had been purified for human use, insulin was being used to treat diabetes mellitus.

Subsequently, studies on insulin pioneered techniques which were later to advance other fields of endocrinology; for example, Sanger in 1955 determined the complete amino acid sequence of the polypeptide and in 1969 Hodgkin established the three-dimensional structure from crystallographic studies, and shortly after that Steiner showed that insulin was actually synthesized as a larger precursor molecule, pro-insulin.

With the discovery of insulin it was at first thought that this was the key to the origin of diabetes mellitus. However, the situation is not so simple, as was demonstrated by further experimental studies. For example, Houssay showed that the severe diabetes resulting from pancreatectomy in the dog could be greatly ameliorated by removal of the pituitary gland. Later, Long and Lukens demonstrated that improvement could also be produced by removal of the adrenal gland. Moreover, when the whole of the pancreas had been removed in man, the diabetes that developed was not so severe, at least as judged by the patient's insulin requirement. In addition, while most attention has been focused on effects on carbohydrate metabolism it should also be emphasized that insulin has important additional actions on protein and fat metabolism.

The pancreas also secretes a number of other hormones. Important among these is glucagon which is a smaller peptide than insulin. Its existence was first demonstrated when pancreatic extracts were fractionated and some were shown to raise blood sugar, unlike the insulin-containing fractions which lowered blood sugar. More recently other peptides have been isolated from the pancreas: these include somatostatin and another peptide which may be a hormone but which, at present, is known simply as pancreatic polypeptide.

## MORPHOLOGY OF THE PANCREAS

In man, the head of the pancreas rests in the loop of the duodenum (Fig. 7.1) and its body extends towards the spleen which is usually in contact with the tail of the pancreas. It is functionally and structurally segregated into two parts. The larger portion consists of exocrine cells arranged in acini; these produce digestive enzymes which are secreted into the pancreatic duct and thence channelled into the duodenum. Scattered through the exocrine pancreas are aggregates of endocrine cells forming the so-called Islets of Langerhans; these account for about 2% of the pancreatic mass. In the Islets there are three

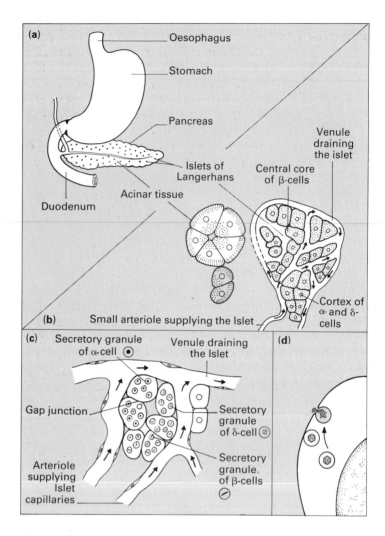

**Fig. 7.1** The endocrine pancreas.

(a) This consists of small groups of cells, the Islets of Langerhans, embedded in the exocrine pancreatic acinar tissue.

(b) Each Islet consists of a core mainly of $\beta$-cells surrounded by a rim or cortex of $\alpha$- and $\delta$-cells. The Islet is supplied with one or more small arterioles that penetrate the centre of the Islet and then break up into capillaries. These firstly supply the central $\beta$-cells and then flow to the periphery of the Islet to supply the rim of $\alpha$- and $\delta$-cells. The capillaries leave the Islet and form the draining venules. In this way the circulation ensures that the $\beta$-rich core of Islet cells are the first to be exposed to high glucose concentrations and the peripheral $\alpha$- and $\delta$-cells are exposed to high insulin concentrations from the inner $\beta$-cells.

(c) The three cell types of the Islet have distinctive secretory granules which enable them to be easily identified under the electron microscope. All three cell types have been shown to possess gap junctions, and thereby to be dye-coupled to one another. The cells therefore possess the means to interact intracellularly by direct transfer of substances from one cell to another.

(d) Part of a $\beta$-cell, showing a secretory granule discharging its contents in the process of exocytosis.

major cell types; these are known as the $\alpha$-, $\beta$- and $\delta$-cells, each containing distinctive secretory granules. The Islet cells can be distinguished from the acinar cells by a variety of histological techniques. They all have the cytological features that would be expected of cells which synthesize and secrete polypeptides, namely an extensive rough endoplasmic reticulum, a distinctive Golgi complex, and usually numerous secretory granules which are different in size, form and electron density for each of the three Islet cell types (Fig. 7.1c). Immunocytochemically, the $\alpha$-cells have been shown to contain glucagon, the $\beta$-cells insulin and the $\delta$-cells somatostatin in their respective granules. While the fine structure of the granules in $\alpha$- and $\delta$-cells does not differ greatly between species, the granules of the $\beta$-cells are usually characteristic of a particular species. The Islet cells release their hormones by exocytosis (Fig. 7.1d) and they then pass through two basement membranes into neighbouring blood capillaries and so into the circulation.

Developmentally, the pancreas arises from dorsal and ventral endodermal outgrowths from the foregut close to its junction with the midgut. These outgrowths form a branching duct system at whose termini the exocrine acini develop. From the ducts other cells bud off and form islets of cells, disconnected from their ductule origins. Eventually the three cell types characteristic of the Islets differentiate and become vascularized; sympathetic nerve terminals are found close to the Islet cells.

## SYNTHESIS AND SECRETION OF INSULIN AND GLUCAGON

Insulin is a polypeptide with a molecular weight of 6000 and consists of two chains, called A and B, which are linked by two disulphide bonds. A third disulphide bond links two cysteine residues within the A-chain. There is a larger precursor form of insulin which is called pro-insulin in which there is a connecting peptide (the C-peptide) between the A- and B-chains. Thus pro-insulin has the disulphide bonds of insulin, but instead of having two chains there is only a single chain of amino acids: pro-insulin has only minimal insulin-like activity. When the C-peptide is removed the single chain is broken and the amino-terminus of the A-chain and the carboxy-terminus of the B-chain become separated (Fig. 7.2).

In the $\beta$-cells of the Islets, the peptide which is actually synthesized on the ribosomes is a still larger peptide and is known as pre-pro-insulin. As the precursor molecule passes across the cisternal membrane of the rough endoplasmic reticulum, a chain of 24 amino acids is excised from the amino-

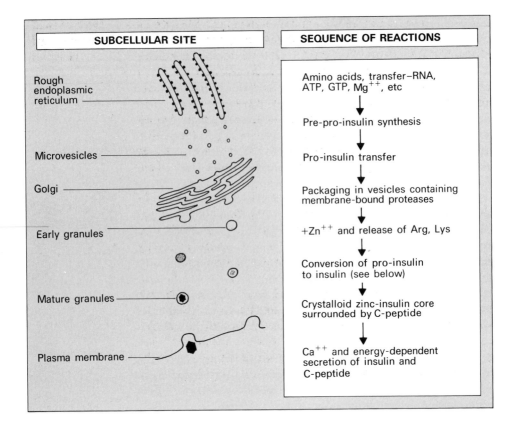

| SUBCELLULAR SITE | SEQUENCE OF REACTIONS |
|---|---|

**Rough endoplasmic reticulum**

**Microvesicles**

**Golgi**

**Early granules**

**Mature granules**

**Plasma membrane**

Amino acids, transfer–RNA, ATP, GTP, $Mg^{++}$, etc

↓

Pre-pro-insulin synthesis

↓

Pro-insulin transfer

↓

Packaging in vesicles containing membrane-bound proteases

↓

$+Zn^{++}$ and release of Arg, Lys

↓

Conversion of pro-insulin to insulin (see below)

↓

Crystalloid zinc-insulin core surrounded by C-peptide

↓

$Ca^{++}$ and energy-dependent secretion of insulin and C-peptide

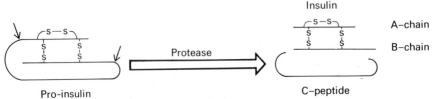

Pro-insulin → Protease → Insulin (A-chain, B-chain), C-peptide

**Fig. 7.2** Insulin synthesis and secretion from the $\beta$-cell of pancreatic Islets of Langerhans. Protein synthesis on the rough endoplasmic reticulum yields pre-pro-insulin which is transferred into the lumen of the endoplasmic reticulum. Hydrolysis yields pro-insulin which is then transferred to the Golgi apparatus, about 20 minutes after the initiation of protein synthesis. Pro-insulin is enclosed in vesicles which carry specific proteases bound to the membrane. Over a time period of about 30 minutes to 2 hours, the specific proteases act on pro-insulin to release the C-peptide and insulin within the granule. Progressive maturation and crystallization of zinc insulin takes place to yield a dense crystalloid region surrounded by a clear space containing C-peptide. When the cells are stimulated, an energy and calcium ion dependent fusion of the granules with the plasma membrane of the cell releases the contents into the bloodstream. Insulin and C-peptide are released in approximately equimolar amounts.

The lower portion of the illustration shows a schematic diagram of the structures of pro-insulin and insulin. Pro-insulin, on the left, is cleaved at two points (arrows) by specific proteases packaged into early $\beta$-cell granules. The C-peptide is cleaved from a single chain peptide to form insulin, which then has two chains, A and B, linked by two disulphide bridges and the A-chain also carries an intrachain disulphide bridge. Pro-insulin contains 86 amino acids while insulin has a molecular weight of 6000 with 21 amino acids in the A-chain and 30 in the B-chain.

terminus producing pro-insulin which is a single peptide with 81 or 86 amino acids, depending on the species, and with 3 disulphide bridges within the molecule. It is transported in microvesicles which arise from the endoplasmic reticulum to the Golgi complex of the cell where it is packaged, together with specific proteolytic enzymes which as yet are not activated, into so-called 'early' secretion granules. These have a light and uniform density in the electron microscope. Subsequently these granules mature into recognizable $\beta$-granules, during which time the proteases are activated and convert pro-insulin into insulin by specific cleavage of the C-peptide (Fig. 7.2).

Once the C-peptide is removed, the part of the insulin molecule which is important for biological activity becomes exposed. The newly formed insulin, as a hexamer, together with zinc atoms, constitutes the crystalline core of the $\beta$-granule; the C-peptide probably remains in the clear space surrounding the crystalline core (Fig. 7.2). Eventually, as a result of appropriate stimuli, the membranes of the mature $\beta$-granules fuse with the cell surface membrane and insulin is released into the bloodstream.

Rather less is known of the synthesis of glucagon, except that a larger precursor, proglucagon, is made in the $\alpha$-cells, and this is then split to yield the active hormone which has 29 amino acid residues arranged in a single chain.

## Human insulin

Human insulin differs in amino acid sequence from that in other species. It has been obtained in three ways. The first was by extraction from human pancreas; it was from this source that the structure of the molecule was determined. The second source is to modify porcine insulin from which it differs only at the carboxy-terminus of the B-chain, with threonine at B30 in the human insulin and alanine at B30 in porcine insulin. A transpeptidation reaction is used to substitute an amino acid: this is achieved with porcine trypsin in the presence of a large excess of an ester of threonine in an organic solvent-plus-water mixture along with porcine insulin. This combination was chosen to achieve efficient insertion of threonine (close to 100%) and it facilitates the subsequent purification of the product with removal of the ester group on threonine to yield human insulin.

The third approach is direct synthesis. This was first done chemically, making the A- and B-chains separately and then joining them together. While this chemical synthesis was a major achievement, it is not suitable for large scale production. Instead, therefore, genetic engineering techniques are now used. DNA sequences encoding the A- and B-chains of human insulin were synthesized chemically with an extra DNA triplet encoding methonine at the 5' end of the nucleotides. These synthetic nucleotides were then inserted into separate plasmids, adjacent to a tyrosine synthetase operon. This operon carries a promoter that is highly efficient and the recombinant DNA yields a 'chimeric' protein with a tyrosine synthetase sequence followed by either an A- or B-chain sequence. The proteins produced are so large that they precipitate in the cytoplasm of *E. coli* in which the cloning was performed, and the precipitated proteins are thereby protected from peptidases in the bacteria. The proteins were then isolated and treated with cyanogen bromide to cleave the chains at the methionyl residue and release the A- and B-chains of insulin. Cyanogen bromide converts the methionyl residue to homoserine which remains attached to the tyrosine synthetase while the insulin chains (which do not contain methionine) are freed. The separate A- and B-chains have then to be purified and joined together with the correct intra-chain and two inter-chain disulphide bonds. There are 12 possible combinations, and the best yield of the one form of insulin required was achieved at high pH and low temperature. These conditions are obviously very different from those in the pancreatic Islet, where the conformation of insulin is determined initially by the structure of pro-insulin with its C-peptide, which ensures that the correct disulphide bonds can be made. The genetically engineered product, however, after separation from bacterial proteins, is identical with insulin extracted from humans.

### Regulation of insulin and glucagon release

One of the main regulators of insulin and glucagon release is the amount of glucose in the blood. A rise in blood glucose stimulates the release of insulin while a fall in blood glucose suppresses its secretion. Conversely, the secretion of glucagon is stimulated by a fall of blood glucose and is suppressed by a rise in the concentration of glucose in the blood. Amino acids stimulate the release of *both* insulin and glucagon; stimulation of insulin secretion by amino acids ensures that they are taken up by the cells of the body while the simultaneous release of glucagon ensures that this is not accompanied by hypoglycaemia. There is also a neural component controlling the secretion of pancreatic hormones (Table 7.1). Stimulation of the vagus or pancreatic nerve which causes release of insulin can be blocked by atropine: thus, there is a parasympathetic, cholinergic innervation to the Islets. In the presence of atropine, stimulation of the pancreatic nerve also induces glucagon release through a sympathetic, adrenergic innervation mediated by $\alpha$-receptors which can be blocked with phentolamine. There is a sympathetic supply to the $\beta$-cells which appear to possess both $\alpha$- and $\beta$-adrenergic receptors (see Chapter 3). Noradrenaline ($\alpha$-receptor) at low doses within the physiological range increases insulin output. However, insulin release is inhibited by adrenaline from the

**Table 7.1** Some factors regulating insulin release from the β-cells of the pancreatic Islets.

| Increased by | Decreased by |
|---|---|
| Raised blood glucose | Low blood glucose |
| Amino acids | |
| Glucagon | Somatostatin |
| Gastrin, secretin | |
| Cholecystokinin | |
| Glucose-dependent insulinotrophic peptide (GIP) | |
| Sympathetic innervation (α-receptors) | Sympathetic innervation (β-receptors) |
| Parasympathetic (cholinergic) innervation | Stress (e.g. exercise, hypoxia, hypothermia, surgery, severe burns) |

adrenal medulla which acts at β-receptors, as do high doses of noradrenaline. *In vivo* the overall effect of sympathetic stimulation is to depress insulin release. It seems likely that the main role of the sympathetic supply is to modulate cell activity with respect to other stimulation. Adrenaline, which inhibits the secretion of insulin, also stimulates the secretion of glucagon and so increases blood glucose indirectly, quite apart from the direct effect that it has in stimulating the mobilization of glucose from glycogen in the liver.

Several of the gastrointestinal hormones, secretin, gastrin, cholecystokinin and glucose-dependent insulinotrophic peptide (GIP, also known as gastric inhibitory peptide) stimulate insulin secretion. Their release is stimulated by ingested food and an oral glucose load thus increases insulin secretion much more than glucose given intravenously.

## The regulation of blood glucose and its significance

The amount of glucose in the circulation depends on its absorption from the intestine, uptake by and release from the liver, and uptake by peripheral tissues (Fig. 7.3). Normally no glucose is lost in urine since all that is filtered in the glomeruli is reabsorbed in the renal tubules. In the fasting state, the concentration of glucose in blood normally lies between 3 and 5 mmol/l; it may rise to 7 mmol/l after a meal but has to exceed 10 mmol/l to produce glycosuria. In some healthy subjects the renal threshold is reduced and as a result glycosuria can occur when the blood sugar is normal.

Serum glucose concentrations rise following absorption of carbohydrate from the intestine. After a meal or an oral glucose load (Fig. 7.4) absorption occurs rapidly and blood sugar reaches a peak within an hour of ingestion of glucose. Absorption is more rapid in patients who have had part of the stomach removed

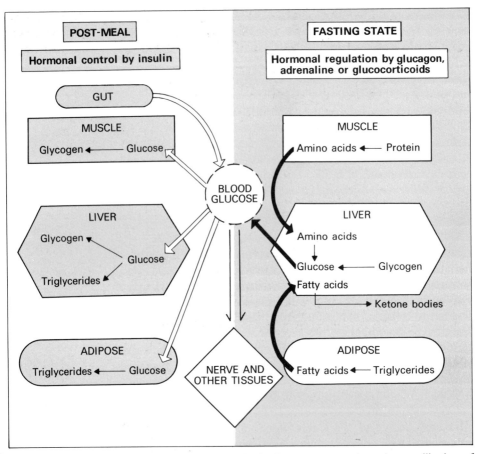

**Fig. 7.3** Regulation of blood glucose concentration: tissue utilization of metabolites after a meal and in a fasting state are contrasted. Food is absorbed from the gut and increases the blood glucose concentration. Insulin facilitates absorption and the control of the synthesis of glycogen and triglyceride storage depots in liver and adipose tissues. In the fasting state, amino acids are mobilized from muscle proteins to yield pyruvate in the liver, where gluconeogenesis and glycogenolysis are capable of maintaining the blood glucose concentration required for utilization by brain, nerve and other tissues. Various hormones, including adrenaline, glucagon and glucocorticoids, exert a regulatory action at different sites in these tissues. Fatty acids, mobilized from adipose tissues under the control of a number of hormones (adrenaline, adrenocorticotrophin, glucagon, growth hormone), provide a substrate for liver and muscle metabolism. Ketone bodies produced in the liver are normally also used as a substrate for muscle metabolism.

surgically (a partial gastrectomy) and so the blood sugar can rise to a peak within half an hour of administration of a glucose load and exceed the renal threshold and glycosuria can occur. Uptake of glucose by peripheral tissues is also regulated by the concentration of circulating insulin. The concentration of glucagon is important in the regulation of the amount of glucose in the circulation by decreasing its storage in the liver and is depressed

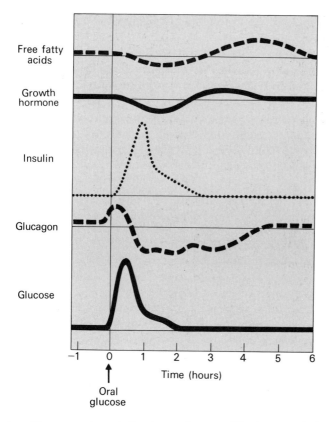

Free fatty
acids

Growth
hormone

Insulin

Glucagon

Glucose

Time (hours)

Oral
glucose

**Fig. 7.4** Hormone and metabolite changes in serum following an oral glucose load. In an oral glucose tolerance test a 50 g glucose load is administered to a normal adult at time zero, and the subsequent changes in serum concentrations of glucose, free fatty acids and three hormones are illustrated. Horizontal feint lines show the basal, fasting levels of the hormones or metabolites. Rapid absorption of glucose yields a peak in the serum concentration within the first hour, with a return to basal levels within 2 hours. Neural, anticipatory stimulation initially increases the glucagon concentration which is then suppressed by the increase in insulin that lags only slightly behind the glucose curve. High glucose concentrations suppress basal growth hormone release initially, but a small surge of growth hormone can be observed after 2−3 hours. Elevated insulin concentrations stimulate lipogenesis and hence cause a decrease in circulating free fatty acids. Growth hormone, probably via its action on the liver to stimulate somatomedin production (see Chapter 2), later causes a release of free fatty acid from adipose tissue for use by muscle and liver cells.

following the absorption of glucose as is shown in Fig. 7.4. However, the hormonal responses which occur after a protein-rich meal (or following administration of an amino acid-rich mixture) will induce different changes from those of orally administered glucose shown in Fig. 7.4. In particular, amino acids cause increased release of insulin and glucagon and also of growth hormone to stimulate uptake of amino acids into muscle cells, while maintaining the serum glucose concentrations which are required for utilization of the amino acids by peripheral tissues.

After a meal, glucose is converted to glycogen (in the liver and muscle) and to fat (in the liver and adipose tissue) as shown in Figs. 7.3 and 7.5 However, in the periods between meals or during a fast, the most tightly regulated process is the release of glucose from the liver. This is particularly important in maintaining the concentration of glucose in the circulation to supply tissues such as muscle and brain (which has limited ability for using other fuels). During fasting, amino acids are released from muscle and are used to form pyruvate in liver, from which glucose is formed by the enzymes of the gluconeogenic pathway (Fig. 7.5). At the same time glucose is produced from glycogen by activation of the enzyme phosphorylase, by a mechanism which is described below (Fig. 7.6), in order to maintain serum glucose concentrations. In addition, fatty acids are released from adipose tissue and they are metabolized in the liver where they are converted to ketone bodies. Fatty acids as well as ketone bodies are then used as an energy source in lieu of glucose by various tissues, especially muscle, thus reducing the amount of glucose which needs to be synthesized by metabolism of the amino acids from muscle cells. It should be noted that the synthesis of ketone bodies in normal individuals does not usually exceed the rate at which tissues can utilize them. Glucose normally provides a principal energy source of tissues of the body,

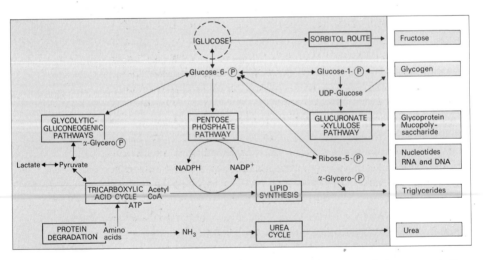

**Fig. 7.5** Interrelationships among alternative routes of glucose metabolism. The central role of glucose in carbohydrate, fat and protein metabolism is summarized. The principal metabolic pathways are shown enclosed in boxes in order to simplify the diagram; some key intermediates and products of metabolic interconversions are shown. The reversibility of certain reaction sequences implied by double-headed arrows is not necessarily intended to suggest that the same enzymes are involved in both the forward and reverse reactions.

and uptake by many peripheral tissues requires a minimal, though continuous, secretion of insulin. Thus, because of the dual and opposite actions of glucagon and insulin, hypoglycaemia does not normally develop even in the fasting state, or during exercise which can require the mobilization and utilization of grams of glucose.

Insulin and glucagon together control the metabolites required by peripheral tissues and both are involved in maintaining glucose homeostasis. Insulin is considered to be an anabolic hormone in that it promotes the synthesis of protein, lipid and glycogen, and it inhibits the degradation of these compounds. The key target tissues of insulin are liver, muscle and adipose tissue. Insulin promotes cell growth in many different cell types and is an absolute requirement for normal growth in all immature animals. In contrast, glucagon acts largely to increase catabolic processes, particularly in the liver. There is now strong evidence during transition from the fed to fasted state that liver glycogen and fat synthesis may be fuelled not directly by glucose but predominantly by lactate.

## Hormonal regulation of carbohydrate, fat and protein metabolism

The flux of glucose to and from the liver is closely regulated by several endocrine factors acting in concert to alter the activity of important intracellular enzymes. Insulin and glucagon being peptide hormones must act primarily on the cell surface. The precise way in which insulin modulates intracellular processes is not entirely known although activation of tyrosine kinase is essential as described in Chapter 1. Glucagon is known to activate adenylate cyclase in the membranes of its target-cells and so increase intracellular cyclic AMP. A number of the enzymes important in carbohydrate and fat metabolism can exist *in vivo* in an active or inactive form; these two forms are interconvertible by phosphorylation and dephosphorylation mechanisms. This is the so-called covalent modification of the enzymes; that is the chemical addition or removal of phosphate by protein kinases or phosphoprotein phosphatases respectively. This mechanism provides a basis for the regulatory process of carbohydrate and fat metabolism, although not all the effects of insulin and glucagon can at present be explained in this way.

Many of the enzymes involved in catabolic processes are activated by phosphorylation, while others (which are generally involved in biosynthetic reactions) are more active in the dephosphorylated form. Phosphorylation itself is catalysed by a group of enzymes known as protein kinases of which at least three classes exist. The first class of these enzymes is dependent upon the presence of cyclic adenosine monophosphate (cyclic

AMP) for activity while the second is active in the absence of this nucleotide; a third class of calcium ion-dependent protein kinases has been found which are regulated by alterations in the intracellular concentration of calcium (see Chapter 1). These kinases are reasonably specific, and phosphorylate either a single protein or a small group of structurally related proteins. The removal of phosphate is catalysed by phosphoprotein phosphatases which are much less specific than the kinases.

### Glycogen metabolism

The control of glycogen metabolism is dependent upon phosphorylation–dephosphorylation of the relevant enzymes. The rate-limiting enzymes of glycogen metabolism are the catabolic enzyme, phosphorylase (which is active in the phospho-form), and the anabolic enzyme, glycogen synthetase (which is active in the dephospho-form), as shown in Figs. 7.6 and 7.7 respectively. These reciprocal effects clearly can be interlinked: glucagon thus stimulates glycogenolysis with mobilization of glucose from glycogen, and adrenaline has a similar action which is also mediated by cyclic AMP.

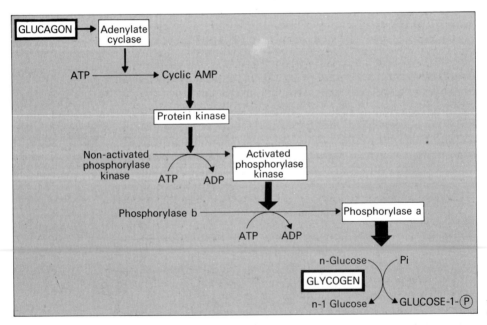

**Fig. 7.6** The cascade sequence for the glycogenolytic response stimulated by glucagon. Glycogen mobilization from the liver is largely regulated by glucagon, which activates adenylate cyclase to produce cyclic AMP from ATP. The cyclic AMP activates a protein kinase which converts inactive phosphorylase b to the active phosphorylated enzyme, phosphorylase a. By a cascade effect with three successive enzymes, the activity is amplified so that the production of glucose-6-phosphate from glycogen can be accelerated 1000-fold by glucagon.

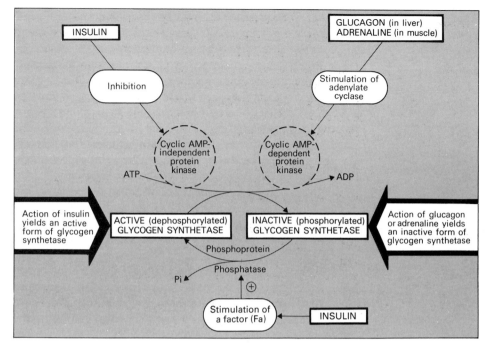

**Fig. 7.7** Regulation of glycogen synthetase activity by phosphorylation–dephosphorylation mechanisms. Glycogen synthetase is inactive in the phosphorylated form. Two protein kinases are capable of phosphorylating glycogen synthetase, one of which is cyclic AMP-dependent and the other is cyclic AMP-independent. Glucagon action on the liver or adrenaline action on muscle (*top right of illustration*) stimulates adenylate cyclase. The increased concentrations of cyclic AMP stimulate the cyclic AMP-dependent protein kinase which in turn inactivates glycogen synthetase: this reaction is required as part of the glycogenolytic action of these two hormones. The second protein kinase, which is cyclic AMP-independent, is inhibited by insulin action (*left of illustration*). The mechanism of inhibition is uncertain, but it may involve calcium ions or some other intracellular component which is produced by insulin action on the cell. Formation of inactive, phosphorylated glycogen synthetase is thus inhibited by insulin action, and glycogenesis is promoted. Insulin also activates a factor (Fa) which reacts with an inactive form of phosphoprotein phosphatase to produce the active form of the phosphatase. Insulin therefore acts on glycogen synthetase (a) by suppression of protein kinase activity and (b) by stimulation of phosphoprotein phosphatase activity, both of which favour the presence of the dephospho-form of the enzyme, and hence glycogenesis.

The converse process, that is the switch from glycogenolysis to glycogen synthesis, may be triggered either by a fall in the tissue content of cyclic AMP or by a rise in blood glucose concentration. The fall in tissue concentrations of cyclic AMP may result from a switch from a glucagon-dominated to an insulin-dominated state (Fig. 7.7). Alternatively, the rise in blood glucose itself after a meal may be critical, since it is possible that the attachment of a glucose molecule to the active form of phosphorylase a may modify its conformation so that it becomes a better substrate for phosphoprotein phosphatase which then dephosphorylates and inactivates it. With the removal of phosphorylase a (which is a potent inhibitor of glycogen synthetase phosphatase), there is not only a cessation of glycogen break-down but an activation of the synthetase phosphatase which converts glycogen synthetase to the active (dephosphorylated) form, thus leading to synthesis of glycogen (Fig. 7.7). Thus, both synthesis and breakdown of glycogen in the liver are controlled by the plasma concentrations of glucagon and insulin (Fig. 7.8).

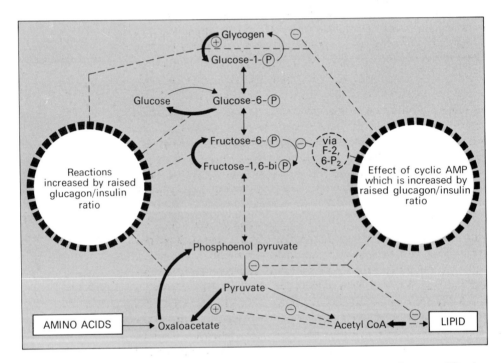

**Fig. 7.8** Influence of raised glucagon/insulin ratios on glucose mobilization from liver. Intracellular cyclic AMP concentrations are increased by glucagon. Glucose release from the liver is then increased as a result of increased glycogenolysis and gluconeogenesis; the latter results from increased amino acid metabolism. Those steps which show increased activity are indicated by heavy arrows. The rise in the concentration of cyclic AMP decreases the activity of those glycolytic steps shown by $\ominus$. The glycogenolytic step, mediated by phosphorylase, is specifically stimulated $\oplus$ by cyclic AMP (see Fig. 7.6). Acetyl CoA modulates the fate of pyruvate, hence it can stimulate pyruvate carboxylase $\oplus$ and inhibit pyruvate dehydrogenase $\ominus$ in an allosteric mechanism (Fig. 7.10). Conversely, insulin action on the liver decreases the intracellular cyclic AMP concentration and therefore favours glycogen synthesis (Fig. 7.7) and increases triglyceride synthesis from glucose (Fig. 7.3) Regulation of the interconversion of fructose-6-phosphate and fructose-1,6-biphosphate is mediated via fructose-2,6-biphosphate (F-2, 6-$P_2$), which is itself regulated by cyclic AMP.

Insulin affects the rate of lipogenesis in a number of ways and thus regulates triglyceride metabolism. A critical step in lipogenesis is the activation of an insulin-sensitive lipoprotein lipase in the capillaries with subsequent uptake of released fatty acids into adipose tissue. Lipogenesis is facilitated by uptake of glucose, because its metabolism via the pentose phosphate pathway provides reducing equivalents (i.e. NADPH) for fatty acid synthesis. The availability of glycerophosphate for esterification is also important for triglyceride synthesis. Many of the actions of insulin in stimulating lipogenesis (triglyceride synthesis) are opposed by glucagon.

In adipose tissue, triglycerides are stored as metabolic fuel depots and the maintenance and mobilization of these depots is under hormonal control. Mobilization of triglyceride from adipose tissue is dependent on an intracellular hormone-sensitive lipase which can be activated by a number of hormones including catecholamines, adrenocorticotrophin and glucagon. These hormones almost certainly act by stimulating formation of intracellular cyclic AMP which controls the conversion of the inactive form of the lipase to an active phosphorylated form via a cyclic AMP-dependent protein kinase. The enhanced release of free fatty acids from adipose tissue by this lipase can be reversed rapidly by insulin, although the mechanism of this antagonism is not yet clear.

Lipogenesis is also regulated by covalent modification, i.e. phosphorylation or dephosphorylation of the relevant enzymes, acetyl CoA carboxylase and fatty acid synthetase. These two enzymes, which together constitute the lipogenic pathway, are also subject to allosteric modification; their activity is also dependent on the supply of precursors from the glycolytic pathway or in the pathway of lipogenesis itself. The first enzyme in the pathway, acetyl CoA carboxylase, is subject to phosphorylation–dephosphorylation interconversion, at least in adipose tissue and in the mammary gland (Fig. 7.9). The phosphorylation (inactivation) is catalysed by a cyclic AMP-dependent protein kinase, while the converse reaction is catalysed by phosphoprotein phosphatase. Presumably, similar control mechanisms operate in the liver: phosphorylation of the carboxylase under the influence of a cyclic AMP-dependent protein kinase could explain the very rapid inhibition of fatty acid synthesis which occurs in liver following treatment with glucagon. A cyclic AMP-dependent protein kinase which can phosphorylate acetyl CoA carboxylase is also present, and this protein kinase may be the locus of control by insulin in stimulating fatty acid synthesis. A second locus could be on the phosphoprotein phosphatase, with dephosphorylation of acetyl CoA carboxylase in a manner analagous to that described for insulin action on glycogen synthetase (see Fig. 7.7).

The presence of both cyclic AMP-dependent and cyclic AMP-independent protein kinases controlling a single reaction provides an additional dimension to hormonal regulation of enzyme activity. When the concentration of glucagon is low and that of insulin is high (as can occur following a high carbohydrate load), both kinases could be inactive and acetyl CoA carboxylase would be converted to the active form with stimulation of lipogenesis. Regulation of the phosphatase by insulin can further accelerate this process, as could removal of long-chain acyl CoA derivatives (Fig. 7.9).

*Protein synthesis*
Insulin stimulates the uptake of amino acids into cells and in this way could stimulate protein synthesis by providing the precursor

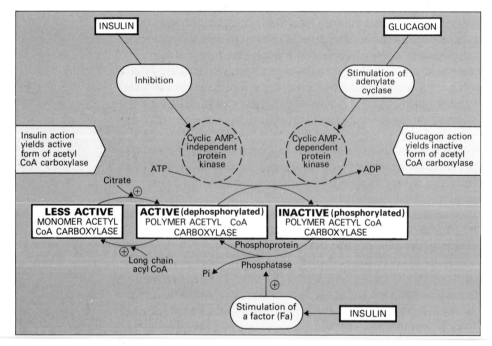

**Fig. 7.9** Regulation of acetyl CoA carboxylase by allosteric regulators and by phosphorylation–dephosphorylation mechanisms. Acetyl CoA carboxylase which is involved in fatty acid synthesis exists as a monomer and in two polymeric forms which are interconvertible by dephosphorylation. Citrate and long-chain acyl CoA control the relative proportions of the less active monomer and the active polymeric-form of acetyl CoA carboxylase by allosteric mechanisms. As in the case of glycogen synthetase (Fig. 7.7), two protein kinase enzymes are capable of regulating the conversion of active polymer acetyl CoA carboxylase to the inactive phosphorylated form of the enzyme. The cyclic AMP-dependent protein kinase may be activated by glucagon (*top right of illustration*), while the cyclic AMP-independent protein kinase is inhibited by insulin action on the target-cell (*top left of illustration*). Glucagon action on the cell hence decreases lipogenesis, while insulin action stimulates fatty acid synthesis.

amino acids required. It may also, however, have an additional effect on protein synthesis by regulating translation. The phosphorylation of ribosomal S6 protein is believed to be increased by insulin. As is described below (p. 244) insulin can increase polyamine synthesis which appears to be involved in synthesis of ribosomal RNA, and hence the effect on protein synthesis may be indirect.

## Ion transport

Insulin also modifies anion and cation transport into tissues. It counteracts the effects of glucagon and the cyclic AMP-induced release of potassium ion from perfused liver. Insulin may also alter $Ca^{2+}$ flux and ion binding in a number of tissues. Increase in the concentration of calcium ion within the mitochondria could play an important part in regulating the activity of pyruvate dehydrogenase and altering the conversion of pyruvate to acetyl CoA required for lipid synthesis, ketone body formation and for the tricarboxylic acid cycle (Fig. 7.10). Calcium ions have a dual action which provides for a rapid and effective switch-over mechanism; they accelerate the conversion of inactive pyruvate dehydrogenase to an active form (by activating a phosphoprotein phosphatase) and calcium ions simultaneously inhibit phosphorylation of the dehydrogenase. Pyruvate carboxylase, a key enzyme in gluconeogenesis, is activated by acetyl CoA; the latter metabolite at the same time inhibits pyruvate dehydrogenase via its action on the protein kinase, and thus the balance between the activity of these two key enzyme steps is regulated simultaneously (Fig. 7.10).

## Experimental diabetes mellitus

Originally von Mering and Minkowski produced diabetes mellitus by removal of the pancreas. Later it was found that the Islet cells could be selectively destroyed by the administration of alloxan or streptozotocin. In this way it has been possible to study uncontrolled diabetes and the sequence of events following administration of insulin in an otherwise intact animal. This has helped in understanding the interplay between adipose tissue and liver metabolism and has emphasized the importance of a number of metabolic intermediates in regulating tissue metabolism.

METABOLIC PATHWAYS INFLUENCED BY INSULIN

Within minutes of administration of insulin to a severely diabetic rat, there is a decrease in the cyclic AMP content of the liver, and metabolism in this tissue is converted from glucose production to glucose utilization. It is possible to outline the probable sequence of events which leads to this change-over from production to utilization of glucose following insulin administration. A

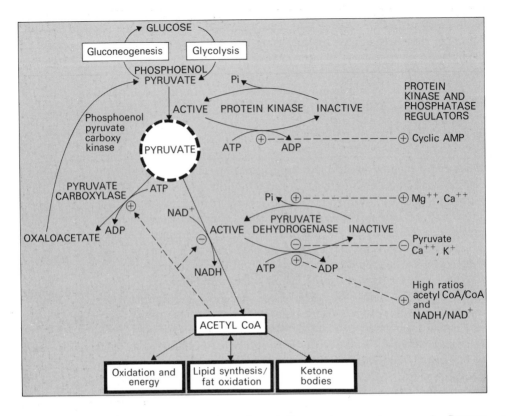

**Fig. 7.10** Regulation of metabolism at the pyruvate crossroads. Pyruvate occupies a central point in the metabolism of glucose which can result in gluconeogenesis, lipid synthesis, production of energy or ketone bodies. Acetyl CoA (*lower*) is derived from fatty acid oxidation or from carbohydrate catabolism; it acts as an allosteric regulator of the two enzymes pyruvate carboxylase and dehydrogenase which use pyruvate as the substrate. The production of acetyl CoA by pyruvate dehydrogenase is inhibited when excess acetyl CoA accumulates. However, acetyl CoA is an allosteric stimulator $\oplus$ of the second enzyme, pyruvate carboxylase, which yields oxaloacetate that may be converted to phosphoenol pyruvate and thence to α-glycerophosphate which is required for triglyceride synthesis. Pyruvate dehydrogenase itself is controlled by phosphorylation–dephosphorylation mechanisms (*centre right*). The protein kinase which inactivates pyruvate dehydrogenase is *not* regulated by a cyclic AMP-dependent protein kinase; however, it is stimulated $\oplus$ by high ratios of acetyl CoA:CoA and by high NADH:NAD$^+$ ratios, and it is inhibited $\ominus$ by pyruvate and calcium ions. Activation of phosphorylated pyruvate dehydrogenase by a phosphoprotein phosphatase is stimulated $\oplus$ by divalent metal ions. Production of pyruvate from phosphoenol pyruvate may be decreased by increasing the activity of a cyclic AMP-dependent protein kinase when a hormone (such as glucagon) increases the intracellular cyclic AMP concentration, yielding an inactive, phosphorylated phosphoenol pyruvate kinase. Thus, a fairly complex series of control mechanisms, some of which are interdependent, act at different sites around pyruvate to control the metabolic products in response to the prevailing metabolite, co-factor and hormone concentrations.

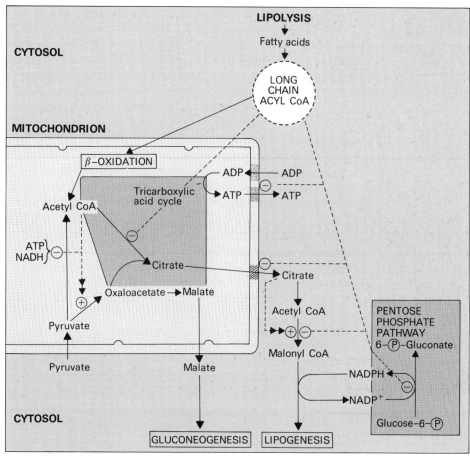

Fig. 7.11 Some sites of action of long-chain acyl CoA derivatives on the regulation of liver metabolism. Lipolysis yields fatty acids which are metabolized in the liver and they yield long-chain acyl CoA which is the substrate for $\beta$-oxidation in mitochondria. The illustration shows those metabolic steps which are under inhibitory regulation $\ominus$ from high levels of long-chain acyl CoA. The adenine nucleotide and citrate translocases (shown by hatched areas on the mitochondrial membrane), citrate condensing enzyme, acetyl CoA carboxylases (Fig. 7.9) and glucose-6-phosphate dehydrogenase are all inhibited by long-chain acyl CoA derivatives: this ensures that fatty acid metabolism does not also result in lipogenesis. Further regulation is achieved at the pyruvate crossroads (see Fig. 7.10), where acetyl CoA regulates the fate of pyruvate and causes a switch of metabolism to gluconeogenesis. When citrate accumulates in the cytosol it stimulates $\oplus$ acetyl CoA carboxylase, which controls lipogenesis by regulating the rate-limiting reaction which controls the formation of malonyl CoA.

decrease in the cyclic AMP of tissues reduces the rate of lipolysis in adipose tissue, which in turn reduces the amount of free fatty acids in the blood with a consequent reduction in the amount of long-chain acyl CoA derivatives available in liver (Fig. 7.11). The rate of liver break-down of glycogen falls while the synthesis of glycogen increases (Fig. 7.8). In addition pyruvate kinase activity increases when cyclic AMP concentrations fall and there is increased capacity in liver for lipid synthesis (from acetyl CoA and precursors in Figs. 7.10 and 7.11). A decrease in long-chain acyl CoA facilitates the transfer of ATP from mitochondria to the cytosol (Fig. 7.11) by relieving the inhibition of mitochondrial adenine nucleotide translocase.

In the cytosol, the increased ATP concentration and an increase in the cytosol $NAD^+/NADH$ ratio increases the glycolytic flux and decreases lactate formation; by these means energy-requiring processes such as lipogenesis, glycogen synthesis and protein synthesis are increased. At the same time, in liver mitochondria, there is increased flux through the tricarboxylic acid cycle and a decrease in mitochondrial acetyl CoA. With increased activity of pyruvate dehydrogenase and a decrease in pyruvate carboxylase activity, there is decreased gluconeogenesis and also ketone body formation. The release of inhibition of the lipogenic route and of citrate transport lead to increased lipid synthesis, which in turn requires a source of NADPH that is generated by an increased flux through the pentose phosphate pathway (Fig. 7.11).

*Effects of insulin on hexokinase and glucokinase*
The initial step of glucose utilization involves the transport and phosphorylation of glucose by ATP; this is catalysed by hexokinase (Fig. 7.5). The transport of glucose across certain cell membranes is regulated by insulin and there is evidence that this process may involve phosphorylation within the membrane. Those tissues in which insulin regulates glucose uptake (such as muscle, adipose tissue, heart and some peripheral nerves) are generally classified as insulin-sensitive i.e. insulin-dependent tissues.

Inside the cell there are four isoenzymic forms of hexokinase, and of these, three (types I–III) have a low $K$m for glucose and are markedly inhibited by glucose-6-phosphate. This direct feedback inhibition by the reaction product ensures that there is coupling between the rate of glucose phosphorylation and the rate of glucose utilization by the many pathways which rely upon this metabolite. A characteristic of insulin-dependent tissues is their high proportion of hexokinase type II, the content of which decreases markedly in diabetic animals: these changes are particularly significant in adipose tissue, heart and lactating mammary gland. Much of the hexokinase is bound to mitochondrial membranes, which is an advantageous site for the utilization of mitochondrial ATP. The enzyme can be displaced from mitochondria by glucose-6-phosphate and this displacement facilitates the inhibitory action of glucose-6-phosphate. Experimental diabetes reduces the binding of hexokinase to mitochondria, especially in adipose tissue and mammary gland.

Hexokinase type IV is also called glucokinase; this is found almost exclusively in the liver cytosol where it is particularly important in the regulation of blood sugar. This isoenzyme may account for 80% of the normal capacity of liver for phosphorylation of glucose. The kinetic properties of glucokinase are important in glucose homeostasis; it has a high $K$m for glucose of approximately 10mM, i.e. twice the normal glucose concentration. The enzyme comes into action when the glucose load reaching the liver via the portal circulation is elevated, as would occur following a high dietary carbohydrate intake. The high $K$m ensures that the enzyme is fully active only at high blood glucose concentrations: the activity of the enzyme at normal blood glucose concentrations is only a fraction of its maximum possible activity. Another important feature of glucokinase is that, unlike the other hexokinase isoenzymes, this enzyme is *not* inhibited by its product, glucose-6-phosphate. This feature highlights the importance of glucokinase in liver storage of glycogen and in the homeostasis and regulation of blood glucose concentration. The activity of hexokinase decreases rapidly in experimental diabetes, if an animal is starved or if it is fed a diet rich in fat.

*Effects of insulin deficiency on lipogenesis*
In diabetes, the activities of a group of enzymes involved in lipogenesis are reduced but can be restored by administration of insulin. The enzymes involved include ATP-citrate lyase, acetyl CoA carboxylase, fatty acid synthetase, NADP-malate dehydrogenase and enzymes of the pentose phosphate pathway, glucose-6-phosphate dehydrogenase and 6-phosphogluconate dehydrogenase (Fig. 7.11). Not only is the activity of these enzymes reduced, but the amount of enzyme present also falls because of a reduced rate of enzyme synthesis. The decrease in lipogenesis and increased lipolysis yields free fatty acids which are metabolized to ketone bodies in the liver.

*Actions of insulin on amino acid metabolism and urea synthesis*
Insulin has an important role in regulating amino acid uptake and protein synthesis. In diabetic animals, amino acids are mobilized from muscle and transported to the liver where they are deaminated; this leads to increased urea production (Fig. 7.5). The carbon skeleton arising from amino acids will contribute not only to gluconeogenesis but also to ketogenesis. Removal of the pituitary gland (hypophysectomy) in large measure restores the blood glucose of a diabetic animal towards normal, because of removal of growth hormone and adrenocorticotrophin which are involved along with insulin in regulating glucose homeostasis: while hypophysectomy can reduce the disturbance of carbohydrate metabolism in diabetic animals, protein synthesis remains disordered because of the absence of insulin.

The five enzymes of the urea cycle in the liver have increased activity in diabetic animals and there is additionally an increase in the activity of liver glutamate–pyruvate transaminase, an enzyme involved in the alanine cycle. Conversely, the activity of ornithine decarboxylase is reduced in a number of tissues. The activity of ornithine decarboxylase is rate-limiting for polyamine synthesis, which in turn can be correlated with the synthesis of ribosomal RNA. The latter may be important for the role which insulin plays in the regulation of protein synthesis, since ornithine decarboxylase can be induced by addition of insulin plus amino acids to tissue cultures.

GLUCOSE OVERUTILIZATION IN DIABETES

The characteristic changes occurring in uncontrolled diabetes are a rise in blood glucose and increases in glycogen breakdown, gluconeogenesis, fatty acid oxidation, ketone body production and urea formation. There is depression in the synthesis of glycogen, lipid and protein in the cells of those tissues which are normally dependent upon insulin.

Diabetes has classically been considered to be a disease with 'glucose overproduction' by liver and 'underutilization' by insulin-requiring tissues such as muscle and adipose tissue. The cells of those tissues which have an insulin-dependent glucose transport system are relatively unaffected by the high blood glucose concentrations in a diabetic, since the specific transport system for glucose into the cell is not active in the absence of insulin. This is not so, however, for the insulin-independent cells in which glucose entry is largely governed by the concentration gradient between the exterior and interior of the cell. In consequence, overutilization of glucose can occur in these tissues. Thus, in diabetes there appears to be diversion of glucose from insulin-dependent pathways to those not requiring the hormone. The facilitation of many processes in such insulin-independent tissues by the raised levels of intracellular glucose may result in some of the pathological phenomena associated with long-term diabetes (Fig. 7.12).

In uncontrolled or poorly controlled diabetes there is increased glycosylation of a number of proteins, including haemoglobin and the $\alpha$-crystallin of lens. In long-term diabetes, the glycosylated form of haemoglobin, $A_{1c}$, has altered affinity for oxygen and this may be a factor in tissue anoxia, while the glycosylation of $\alpha$-crystallin lens protein may lead to cataract formation; a glucosamine—protein complex is also formed in long-standing diabetes resulting in biochemical and morphological alterations to the capillary system, and there is some evidence that increased glycosylation of collagen is related to basement membrane thickening in the kidney.

A number of factors tend to promote the diversion of glucose into the sorbitol pathway leading to fructose. In diabetes, the most important factors are, first, the high level of intracellular

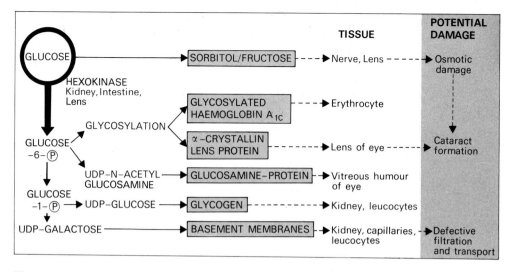

**Fig. 7.12** Glucose overutilization and induced pathological changes in tissues resulting from non-insulin requiring pathways. Glucose movement into many cells including those of the kidney, certain nerve tissues, the eye, seminal vesicle, erythrocytes and leucocytes is not dependent upon insulin: in diabetes, the concentration gradient between the extracellular and intracellular compartments is sufficient to drive glucose into these cells. The mass effect of a high intra-cellular glucose concentration drives the reactions summarized above through some of the key intermediates shown. The increased activity of the sorbitol and glycogenic pathways yields osmotic damage, while glycosylation reactions lead to alterations in the eye and basement membranes of cells which in turn affect permeability and transport mechanisms. These reactions may account for many of the pathological changes observed in severe diabetes.

glucose in tissues where the glucose transport system is insulin-independent, such as lens, liver and kidney, and second, the high $NADPH:NADP^+$ ratio which results from the decrease in the rate of other reductive synthetic reactions such as fatty acid synthesis. The accumulation of sorbitol could cause osmotic damage which may be important, for example, in the aetiology of cataract formation. The peripheral neuropathy and altered motor nerve conduction velocity that occurs in some diabetic patients may be linked to sorbitol accumulation and associated changes in myoinositol.

In some tissues, such as the kidney, which do not require insulin for glucose uptake but which rely on maintenance of the higher serum to tissue concentration gradient of glucose, changes in the activity of a variety of enzymes occur which facilitate rates of glucose utilization along specific metabolic routes. In diabetes, the increased activity of hexokinase in renal cortex, intestinal mucosa and lens may lead to glucose overutilization: the concentration of glucose-6-phosphate rises and this can in turn lead to an increase of glycogen and of components of basement membranes in these tissues (Fig. 7.12). An increase has also

245

been observed in the activity of enzymes of the pathway that lead to uridine diphosphate (UDP) glucose (used in glycosylation reactions), and of the glucuronate−xylulose pathway and the pentose phosphate pathway in kidney. The activity of the kidney glucosyl transferase is increased; this enzyme transfers glucose residues from UDP-glucose on to the galactosyl hydroxylysine residues which can thus be linked to thickening of the filtration basement membrane that occurs in diabetes, but which is reduced following insulin treatment. Hence, the increase in hexokinase which provides the precursor glucose-6-phosphate for these multiple pathways could be an important determinant in the subsequent metabolic response to diabetes; its increased activity may lead to structural changes in the tissues, and excessive glucose utilization in certain tissues may in the longer term be more damaging than glucose underutilization in the body as a whole.

### The effects of diabetes mellitus

Among the classical symptoms of diabetes mellitus are the passage of an increased volume of urine (polyuria) and thirst (polydypsia). Polyuria is a consequence of the elevation of the blood glucose, which induces an osmotic diuresis. This occurs because the renal threshold for reabsorption of glucose from the glomerular filtrate is exceeded and so glucose is excreted in the urine. The volume of water excreted has to rise, and the loss of water causes thirst which in turn stimulates the patient to drink more. Weight loss is another common feature and this can be attributed to the combination of loss of glucose in the urine and to the increased break-down of fat and protein. Urine containing large amounts of glucose can induce infection with irritation of the vulva in women and of the foreskin in men, and the presence of glucosuria predisposes to infections of the urinary tract. Testing for the presence of glucose in the urine is used as a screening procedure to identify potential diabetes; the diagnosis can then be confirmed by showing that the blood sugar is elevated.

Under some circumstances severe uncontrolled diabetes leads to diabetic ketosis, or ketoacidosis. Rapid mobilization of triglycerides releases fatty acids into the circulation where they are taken to the liver and metabolized. $\beta$-hydroxybutyric acid and acetoacetic acid (often called 'ketone bodies') are produced far in excess of the ability of the tissues to use them, and their concentration in the circulation rises rapidly. They can cause nausea, vomiting and in addition cause a serious disturbance of acid−base metabolism which leads to metabolic acidosis. The respiratory centre is stimulated and this produces a characteristic, deep sighing respiration (Kussmaul breathing).

Uncontrolled insulin-deficient diabetes leads to a very high blood glucose concentration and a profuse osmotic diuresis with loss of large amounts of water, sodium and other electrolytes in urine. This in turn depletes the extracellular fluid and the plasma volume falls, leading to a reduction of blood pressure and of glomerular filtration. Break-down of intracellular protein leads to a loss of cell water and electrolytes, and if the glomerular filtration rate is reduced because of the decreased extracellular fluid volume then the plasma potassium may rise. At the same time, increased deamination of the amino acids released from the cells may contribute to a rise in blood urea and a serious negative nitrogen balance results. Dehydration is caused by the passage of large volumes of urine and contributes to the rise in blood urea. Total body water may fall by as much as 6 litres, half of this coming from the extracellular and half from the intracellular compartments. Before the discovery of insulin this condition was usually fatal: even now, one in 20 patients with severe diabetic keto-acidosis dies.

The main principles of treatment of diabetic ketoacidosis are based on an understanding of the pathophysiology of this condition. Fluid has to be given intravenously, as saline, to restore extracellular fluid volume and maintain the circulation and blood pressure and so restore the glomerular filtration rate. Secondly, it is necessary to give sufficient insulin to control the unrestrained gluconeogenesis by the liver and to restore glucose metabolism to insulin-dependent tissues; this will arrest lipolysis and ketone body production. At an early stage, administration of potassium is required to restore the intracellular losses of this ion; this can be done safely when glucose is entering cells under the influence of insulin and when renal function is satisfactory.

There are two other less common forms of diabetic coma. The first is called 'hyperosmolar non-ketotic diabetic coma' and the second is due to 'lactic acidosis'. The former usually follows a period of uncontrolled diabetes in which the patient has attempted to alleviate thirst by drinking fluids containing glucose. The blood sugar rises to a very high level, between 80 and 100 mmol/l; the patient becomes very dehydrated and drowsy and may then become comatose. Plasma osmolality is high (up to 450 mosmol/kg) and this is believed to be the cause of the coma and cerebral dysfunction. A logical treatment of this disorder is to give hypotonic fluid as well as insulin. Lactic acidosis caused coma in diabetics who were treated with Phenformin (a biguanide that is no longer used) which lowered blood sugar in part by reducing aerobic glycolysis. It also occurs in association with severe illness in which poor cardiac output and hypoxia usually play a part. Lactate accumulates in the circulation with acidosis and the patient develops acidotic breathing without having ketone bodies in plasma or urine, and the blood glucose concentration is not necessarily raised. The treatment of this condition requires administration of large amounts of alkali intravenously, as sodium bicarbonate solution.

Overproduction of some hormones can give rise to diabetes mellitus because their actions are opposite to those of insulin. Thus, acromegaly with excessive growth hormone concentrations may lead to the development of diabetes mellitus. Also, excessive production of adrenaline, for example by a phaeochromocytoma which is a tumour of the adrenal medulla (see Chapter 3), can give rise to diabetes mellitus, as can overproduction of cortisol from the adrenal cortex or the administration of large amounts of glucocorticoids. In the latter circumstances, whether the excess glucocorticoid comes from endogenous production or from administration of pharmacological amounts of glucocorticoid, the picture of Cushing's syndrome is identical. Overproduction of glucagon only rarely causes diabetes, but severe damage to the pancreas by disease or surgery can produce diabetes from a deficiency of insulin. A disturbance of liver function may disturb carbohydrate metabolism to produce diabetes.

There are two principal types of diabetes. The first is juvenile or type I diabetes in which there is usually total, or nearly total, failure to secrete insulin. It is in this group of diabetics that ketoacidosis can develop. The cause of the disorder is auto-immune destruction of the insulin-secreting cells in the Islets of Langerhans. The second major group of patients with diabetes mellitus develop a condition in which an inadequate amount of insulin is secreted even though the insulin-secreting cells are structurally intact. The condition, type II diabetes, is often familial. This is the most common form of the disease and it usually develops in later life; late onset (or maturity onset) diabetes, which develops between the ages of 40 and 70, is most common in obese subjects; obesity has been found to lead to resistance to the action of insulin.

Genetic factors are important in the genesis of diabetes. It has long been known that there is a tendency for diabetes to run in families, and analysis of the contribution of genetic factors has been helped by studying identical twins. These twins have the same genetic make-up so if one identical twin develops diabetes and the condition really is inherited, then the other twin should develop it within a few years. In the older group of non-insulin-deficient diabetics the condition is found to be concordant, i.e. both twins are affected, but in the insulin-deficient, usually younger diabetics, only half the twins are concordant and the other half are discordant. This led to the supicion that there were other factors that cause insulin-deficient diabetes apart from heredity.

There is a possibility that virus infections may be important and some of these may affect the Islets of Langerhans in the pancreas. Autoimmune disease, which may or may not be virus initiated, contributes since antibodies against pancreatic Islet cells have been found in patients with insulin-deficient diabetes. In most of these patients the antibodies are only found in the circulation at the time that symptoms of diabetes appear and diagnosis is made, and then they disappear.

Studies of human leucocyte antigen (HLA) markers have indicated that there is a relationship between these antigenic determinants and type I diabetes. The class II antigens DR3 and DR4 are associated with an increased risk of developing insulin-deficient diabetes. As with autoimmune thyroid disease, the expression of the DR antigen by 'injured' $\beta$-cells may be the mechanism by which the autoimmunogen is presented to the T-lymphocytes and the autoimmune process is thus initiated.

DIAGNOSIS AND TREATMENT OF DIABETES MELLITUS

Diabetes can be diagnosed if the blood glucose is very high, i.e. greater than 11 mmol/l. If a young person is given 75 g of glucose orally, within two hours the blood sugar should have returned to less than 5.5 mmol/l (Fig. 7.4). Glucose tolerance declines with age and in an older person the blood sugar at two hours after oral glucose often lies between 5.5 and 10 mmol/l; therefore, one can only say in this group that there is impairment of carbohydrate tolerance rather than overt diabetes. However, if the blood glucose remains above 10 mmol/l two hours after a glucose dose then diabetes can be diagnosed.

If a patient is completely deficient in insulin, there is no alternative but to treat the individual with injections of insulin, since the polypeptide would be degraded if given by mouth. However, if the patient is resistant to insulin, particularly if this is associated with marked obesity, then reduction of body weight is the best treatment and seems to lead to restoration of insulin sensitivity; diabetes many even disappear as long as the patient remains thinner. Between these two extremes there are patients who are partially insulin-deficient and there are drugs available which stimulate the pancreatic Islet cells to secrete more insulin. These drugs are helpful in avoiding the need for injections of insulin, particularly in a number of middle-aged diabetics who are not overweight. Sulphonyl ureas such as tolbutamide, chlorpropamide and glibenclamide stimulate secretion of insulin and may even cause hypoglycaemia. Biguanides, in contrast, act by increasing glucose uptake in tissues and reducing appetite.

When insulin was first isolated it was hoped that diabetics would no longer die from infections and diabetic ketosis and that they would be able to lead a normal life. It is now possible to relieve the symptoms of diabetes, and to reduce the incidence of ketosis by treating the disease. Nevertheless, long-standing diabetes may lead to a number of complications. Some of these are due to deposition of cholesterol in the arteries causing atheroma of the coronary arteries or the large blood vessels of the legs. In addition, there may be damage to the nervous system, including the autonomic nervous system. The eyes and kidneys may also be affected, owing to changes in the lens and basement membrane of small blood vessels (Fig. 7.12): the development of some of these complications may be attributable to overutilization of glucose by some tissues as discussed above. The risk of development of these complications is greater if the diabetes is poorly controlled, and measurement of the glycosylated form of haemoglobin, $A_{1c}$, may be useful in assessing the degree of control being maintained over a fairly long period of time.

As has already been described, the normal pattern of insulin release after a meal results in a very rapid rise, with a peak between 30 and 60 minutes and then a rapid fall until the next meal is taken (see Fig. 7.4). Insulin is released into the portal vein so that it can act directly on the liver, and blood glucose is controlled between very narrow limits, usually between about 3 and 5 mmol/l in a normal subject. Subcutaneous injections of insulin cannot mimic this pattern, since serum insulin rises and remains elevated longer than in the normal subject and all tissues of the body are exposed to the same concentration; it is not possible to reproduce selectively the higher concentration in the portal vein. Insulin replacement therapy therefore is very different from the physiological release of insulin from the pancreas of the healthy subject, and this may contribute to the failure to achieve glucose homeostasis. Initially, insulin used for therapy was mainly of bovine origin, but porcine insulin has advantages since it is closer in structural identity to human insulin. Even so, it can be antigenic in humans and can therefore cause antibody production and local reactions, and synthetic human insulin that has been made by genetic engineering techniques is now available for therapeutic purposes.

**Effects of excess insulin**

Excess insulin causes a fall in the concentration of blood sugar. The brain is extremely sensitive to the lack of glucose and this goes some way to explain the symptoms of hypoglycaemia, which include blurring of vision, slurring of speech and unsteadiness of gait: cerebral tissue may be irritated and epilepsy can result. If the blood glucose concentration remains very low, the patient becomes unconscious. This combination of symptoms is sometimes referred to as 'neuroglycopenia' or a 'hypoglycaemic attack'. Sympathetic activity is increased and this, with increased adrenaline concentrations, will produce glycogenolysis and release glucose from the liver. At the same time the patient sweats profusely and there is tachycardia and often tremor. While the sympathetic nervous system can respond rapidly, other regulatory mechanisms such as glucagon from the pancreas, cortisol from the adrenal cortex and growth hormone from the pituitary all contribute more slowly to glucose homeostasis.

Hypoglycaemic attacks can occur in diabetic patients who are being treated with insulin. Most commonly this occurs if they do not have enough food after an injection of insulin or if they exercise excessively; if it is known that exercise is to be more vigorous than usual, the patient should either reduce the dose of insulin or take extra carbohydrate. In addition, hypoglycaemic attacks can be caused by a tumour of the Islet cells of the pancreas which secretes insulin; such a tumour is called an insulinoma. The symptoms may be precipitated by a prolonged fast or by exercise, and the blood glucose can fall to below 2 mmol/l. Investigation of a patient with an insulinoma will show that at a time when the blood sugar is low there is still insulin detectable in the circulation. If the blood sugar falls in a normal person, the secretion of insulin is suppressed, but in a patient with an Islet cell tumour producing an excess of insulin, normal regulation fails. The blood sugar of a patient with an insulinoma is not continuously low and it is important, if possible, to measure the blood sugar and the concentration of insulin present during a period when the patient has hypoglycaemic symptoms. If this is not possible it may be necessary to provoke hypoglycaemia and at the same time see whether the production of insulin by the pancreas is suppressed. This is best achieved by administration of insulin to provoke hypoglycaemia and then measure the amount of C-peptide in the circulation. If endogenous secretion of insulin from an insulinoma continues, then at the same time there will be release of C-peptide into the circulation in approximately the same proportion to the insulin released: this can be measured to distinguish endogenously produced insulin from that administered exogenously.

Since the insulin-producing Islet cells are more commonly located in the tail of the pancreas, an insulinoma is more likely to be found there. However, the Islet cells are scattered through the pancreas and there may be more than one tumour present. It is possible to locate the tumours before surgery by arteriography, computer assisted tomographic scanning or by ultrasound. The tumours may be very small and difficult to find and it may not be possible to remove them; occasionally they are malignant and there may be metastases which secrete insulin. In either case there is an alternative form of therapy which is to administer the drug diazoxide orally: this inhibits insulin secretion and prevents the production of hypoglycaemia.

# OTHER HORMONES SECRETED BY THE PANCREAS

SOMATOSTATIN

This peptide which consists of 14 amino acids arranged in a single chain, is secreted from the δ-cells of the Islets of Langerhans and is stored in the granules of the δ-cells (Fig. 7.1). Somatostatin can inhibit the release of insulin and glucagon from the pancreas and so, perhaps, is part of a 'local hormone system' (the paracrine system). Somatostatin probably acts only on the cells in its immediate environment in the pancreas. It has also been localized in gut cells and in peripheral nerves; with such a distribution it could act as an endocrine, paracrine or neurotransmitter substance (see Chapter 1).

Somatostatin was first isolated from the hypothalamus, where it proved to be an inhibitor of the release of growth hormone from the anterior pituitary. Pharmacological doses of somatostatin inhibit virtually all gastrointestinal functions. Exocrine and endocrine secretions from the gastrointestinal tract, and also intestinal absorbtion, are reduced even when stimulated by maximal doses of the appropriate hormones (e.g. gastrin and cholecystokinin). Synthetic somatostatin is now available, and infusions that yield plasma concentrations similar to those found after the ingestion of a meal induce several of the inhibitory effects noted above. In addition, somatostatin may physiologically inhibit the secretion of gastric acid, gastric emptying and the release of gastrin. The secretion of pancreatic bicarbonate and enzymes is reduced, as is gall bladder emptying. The release of pancreatic polypeptide, motilin, and glucose-dependent insulinotropic peptide (GIP) is inhibited, as is the absorption of glucose, xylose and triglycerides.

Somatostatin has also been shown to exert effects on Brünner's glands in the rat. These glands produce a mucous alkaline secretion that forms a protective layer for the duodenal mucosa. The secretion also contains an epidermal growth factor which is capable of stimulating cell growth and differentiation and thus provides further protection for the duodenum. Brünner's gland secretions are stimulated by secretin and vasoactive intestinal peptide (VIP). If the latter hormone is infused (see Table 7.2) the volume and output of bicarbonate and epidermal growth factor increase (although the bicarbonate concentration does not change). When somatostain and vasoactive intestinal peptide are infused together the secretions from the Brünner's glands are greatly reduced. Infusion of an antiserum to somatostatin induces a pronounced increase in secretion, which suggests that endogenous somatostatin may have a role in the normal regulatory mechanisms that control secretions from Brünner's glands.

A mixed meal elicits an increase in plasma somatostatin concentrations. The peptide is released from both the stomach and pancreas following the administration, either intragastrically or intraduodenally, of proteins, fats or carbohydrates. Acid in the duodenum is also a very potent stimulus, making somatostatin a strong candidate for a role in the 'bulbogastrone mechanism' in which there is a reduction in gastric acid secretion during the acidification of the duodenal bulb. It would appear that the biological role for somatostatin is to prevent exaggerated responses following a meal.

As somatostatin has so many inhibitory effects, it is hardly surprising that its potential use as a therapeutic agent has been considered. However, a limitation is that somatostatin is cleared from the circulation in a matter of minutes. This has restricted the peptide's therapeutic use. A synthetic octapeptide with two D-amino acid substitutions has been developed and called minisomatostatin. Although not a long-acting substance, it does provide therapeutic efficacy with only two daily subcutaneous injections (a situation comparable to the administration of insulin to a diabetic patient). Patients with life-threatening diarrhoea associated with gut or pancreatic tumours (e.g. gastrinoma or 'VIP-oma') can be treated with this analogue. The results so far have been dramatic: the peptide is well tolerated, the stool volumes are greatly reduced and liquid excretions are replaced by semi-formed and normal stools.

## PANCREATIC POLYPEPTIDE (PP)

This peptide is produced by endocrine cells which are found in small clusters between cells of the Islets of Langerhans and also between the acinar cells of the pancreas. Pancreatic polypeptide is a powerful inhibitor of the secretion of enzymes by the pancreas and it also blocks the contraction of the gall bladder and hence the secretion of bile. These effects might at first appear strange. However, pancreatic polypeptide concentrations remain high for several hours after a meal, long after other hormone concentrations have reverted to their basal levels observed during the inter-digestive period. By this means, pancreatic polypeptide may help to conserve digestive enzymes and store bile for a subsequent meal. As in the case of insulin, the secretion of pancreatic polypeptide increases after a meal, particularly of meat or fish. Unlike insulin, however, this stimulation is not dependent upon the concentration of glucose in the circulation and the regulation is partly under neural control and partly under hormonal control. Stimulation of the vagus nerve produces secretion of pancreatic polypeptide, and there is an endocrine regulatory system as well in which hormones (such as cholecystokinin which is itself released by food) stimulate the release of pancreatic polypeptide. The role of pancreatic polypeptide remains uncertain; it is often produced in large amounts by pancreatic endocrine tumours but there are no symptoms or metabolic disturbances that can be attributed yet to this overproduction.

## HORMONES FROM THE GASTROINTESTINAL TRACT

It was possible at one time to argue that hormonal control of the gastrointestinal tract could be accounted for by three hormones: secretin, gastrin and cholecystokinin (also called pancreozymin) (Table 7.2). Since 1970, however, a large number of hormones has been detected in the gastrointestinal tract, in which they have also been shown to exert effects. In many instances, though, it still remains to be determined whether those effects are physiological or pharmacological.

Hormones of the gastrointestinal tract are difficult to study because they are not produced by discrete groups of cells organized into glands. Instead, they are released from single cells scattered along the digestive tract. Furthermore, as several of these peptides are found both in specific endocrine cells and in neurones and their nerve terminals, it is difficult to establish which effects are dependent on peptide release from nerve terminals and which of them represent endocrine activity. Because of this, many would prefer to group the biologically active peptides together as 'regulatory peptides', rather than describe, with uncertainty, an agent as having endocrine or neurotransmitter activity. Certainly in this chapter, several peptides are considered which might appear to be out of place in a text book of endocrinology. However, the relationship between the nervous and the endocrine systems is clearly so intimate that substances previously regarded as hormones have also been found to have roles as neurotransmitters or neuromodulators, so their inclusion is thus justified.

**Table 7.2**  Principal hormones of the gastrointestinal tract.

| Hormone | Origin | Released by | Produces |
|---|---|---|---|
| Secretin | Proximal small intestine | Acid in duodenum | A bicarbonate-rich pancreatic secretion |
| Gastrin | Gastric antrum | Distension of stomach and peptides | Stomach contractions and gastric secretion |
| Cholecystokinin Pancreozymin | Proximal small intestine | Products of fat and protein digestion | Gall bladder contractions An enzyme-rich pancreatic secretion |

SECRETIN

In 1902 Bayliss and Starling demonstrated that the pancreas could respond to stimuli applied within the duodenum even when the pancreas was denervated, and in this way they showed that Pavlov's theories had to be modified. Pavlov had established that the physiological responses of the body appeared purposive: for example, meat placed in the duodenum evoked enzyme secretions, and acid produced an alkaline secretion. He therefore thought that nervous regulation was the most likely mechanism of control. However, since the denervated pancreas still responded and extracts of the duodenum could also stimulate the pancreas, it was clear that nervous control could not account for all the findings. Bayliss and Starling deduced that the duodenal mucosa must normally release some active principle into the blood to control pancreatic function. Eventually secretin was isolated and shown to be a peptide with 27 amino acids arranged in a single chain. It is produced by endocrine cells in the duodenal and jejunal mucosa (Fig. 7.13), which appear to be replaced every 120 hours.

Secretin stimulates the pancreas to elaborate a fluid rich in bicarbonate. Such a fluid contributes to the neutralization of acid chyme released from the stomach and it provides a medium of suitable pH for digestion of food by pancreatic enzymes. The threshold for secretin release is pH 4.5 and it is maximally secreted in the range of pH 1 to 3, but only limited areas of the proximal small intestine are transiently exposed to such a low pH. Plasma concentrations of secretin are reduced when meal-induced acid secretion is prevented or inhibited from reaching the duodenum by aspiration, the use of antacids, or the action of an $H_2$-histamine receptor antagonist (which inhibits gastric acid secretion). Postprandial changes of secretin concentrations in man are small, but there is a positive correlation between the load of acid entering the duodenum and the circulating concentration of secretin. The most rapid rate of acid disappearance and the maximal secretin concentration occur 1.5 to 2 hours after a liquid meal, suggesting that the peptide is important in the postprandial period. Antiserum against secretin reduces postprandial bicarbonate secretions by more than 80%.

Potentiation between different agents can occur. Thus, the response to secretin and Caerulin (a cholecystokinin analogue) is greater than the sum of the individual responses to either agent given alone. In addition, secretin can increase hepatic bile production, so that when acid gastric juices enter the duodenum the release of secretin also stimulates the release of bile which helps to return the pH to neutrality.

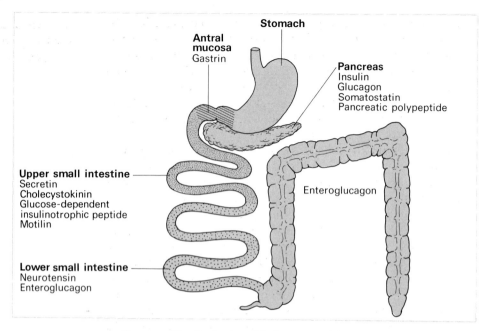

**Fig. 7.13** The distribution of the hormones of the pancreas and gastrointestinal tract. The approximate location of hormones are shown by shaded areas. Insulin, glucagon and somatostatin are synthesized in cells of the pancreatic Islets of Langerhans, and pancreatic polypeptide is found in endocrine cells scattered throughout the pancreas. Gastrin is located in the antral mucosa of the stomach, while the other peptide hormones are found in endocrine cells in the upper or lower small intestine, as shown in the diagram. Enteroglucagon is quite widely distributed throughout the small intestine as well as in the mucosa of the colon and rectum.

CHOLECYSTOKININ (CCK, ALSO CALLED PANCREOZYMIN)

The name cholecystokinin refers to the action of this hormone in causing contraction of the gall bladder, as was first described in 1928. It is synthesized in the endocrine cells of the mucosa of the upper small intestine and the peptide can also be detected in neurones of the small and large intestine. In 1943 an active principle that was capable of stimulating the pancreas to produce enzymes was also found in the upper small intestine and this was called pancreozymin. However, when cholecystokinin was finally purified in 1964, cholecystokinin and pancreozymin were found to be the same substance. Cholecystokinin, which is the name most commonly used, exists in a number of forms. The largest has 39 amino acids arranged in a single chain; there is another peptide consisting of 33 amino acids and this was the first to be isolated. However, only the last eight amino acids, in the carboxy-terminus of the peptide, are necessary for full activity and this octapeptide also occurs naturally. All these peptides have the same spectrum of biological activity although the smaller forms are more rapidly destroyed. A synthetic octapeptide can be used to test the ability of the pancreas to secrete enzymes. Cholecystokinin is unstable in the circulation. Its release is stimulated by fat and protein present in a meal. Cholecystokinin stimulates the release of pancreatic juice rich in enzymes, e.g. amylase, or inactive enzyme precursors, e.g. trypsinogen. These enzymes are the most versatile of those encountered along the digestive tract in that they are capable of hydrolysing the two major classes of nutrients, carbohydrates and proteins. It induces the contraction and evacuation of the gall bladder, with the release of bile into the duodenum. Cholecystokinin may control the motility of the sphincter so as to prevent the emptying of bile into the duodenum being too rapid.

Cholecystokinin has other important properties. It appears to be the most powerful stimulator of pancreatic growth, causing increases in pancreatic weight, DNA and enzyme content. It may also produce a sensation indicating that enough food has been eaten and so determine 'satiety' and appetite. Finally, the peptide may have a role in intestinal transport; both sodium and water absorption have been found to increase in response to cholecystokinin.

## Other hormones secreted by the stomach and gastrointestinal tract

### GASTRIN

Gastrin is secreted by the specialized endocrine cells that are located in the antral part of the gastric mucosa (Fig. 7.13 and Table 7.3). These are called the G-cells. In the fetus, but not in the adult, gastrin cells are also found in the pancreas. The main action of gastrin is to stimulate the gastric parietal cells to secrete acid. Secretion of gastrin is stimulated by distension of the stomach and by the presence of small peptides and amino acids in the stomach. Gastrin increases the blood flow to the gastric mucosa and has a direct effect on the gastric glands themselves. Presence of food in the stomach will release gastrin, as will also the thought, sight, smell and taste of food, as well as chewing and swallowing (the cephalic phase) through activation of the vagus. When the pH of the gastric contents falls below 2.5 the release of gastrin is inhibited. It is thought that acid acts directly on the G-cells and terminates the gastrin-stimulated phase of gastric digestion.

Gastrin also influences gastric peristalsis. The frequency of this event depends on rhythmic waves of depolarization and repolarization that originate in smooth muscle on the superior curvature and pass towards the lesser curvature and pyloric region. The term 'basal electrical rhythm' (BER) has been used

257

**Table 7.3** Actions of gut hormones on the gastrointestinal tract.

| Hormone | Site of action | Effect |
|---|---|---|
| Secretin | Pancreatic acini | ↑ $HCO_3$ rich secretion |
| Secretin | Liver | ↑ Bile secretion |
| Cholecystokinin (pancreozymin) | Gall bladder<br>Pancreatic acini | ↑ Contraction<br>↑ Enzyme secretion |
| Gastrin | Stomach (parietal cells) | ↑ Gastric acid secretion |
| Glucose-dependent insulinotrophic peptide | Pancreas (Islets of Langerhans) | ↑ Insulin secretion |
| Motilin | Stomach, duodenum, jejunum, oesophagus | ↑ Smooth muscle contractions |
| Enteroglucagon | Stomach and rest of GI tract | ↑ Mucosal growth |
| Neurotensin | Stomach | { ↓ Gastric acid secretion<br>{ ↓ Smooth muscle motility |
| Vasoactive intestinal peptide | Stomach<br>Liver<br>Pancreas | ↓ Gastric acid secretion<br>↑ Glucose release<br>{ ↑ Insulin release<br>{ ↑ $HCO_3$ rich secretion |

to describe these waves: they are not muscular contractions. These electrical changes do not necessarily lead to contractions but they do set the frequency of gastric peristalsis (about two per minute) and they hence coordinate it. If the stomach is stimulated when the smooth muscle is in a state of maximal depolarization a contraction is more likely to occur. Gastrin produces a greater force of contraction and can also increase the frequency of the basal electrical rhythm.

As in the case of cholecystokinin, gastrin can exist in a number of forms. The largest has 34 amino acids but peptides with 17 and 14 amino acids are secreted as well. In fact, it is only the 4 amino acids at the carboxy-terminus that are required for full biological activity and a synthetic tetrapeptide is fully active. The only difference between these forms is that the larger ones are less rapidly degraded and so their action persists for longer. The same four amino acids that constitute the active form of gastrin are also present in cholecystokinin; therefore, large amounts of cholecystokinin can stimulate acid production, and the enzyme-secreting cells of the pancreas can respond to large amounts of gastrin.

The concentration of gastrin is normal in patients who have

duodenal ulcers, but if attempts are made to neutralize gastric acid by administration of antacids then the secretion of gastrin increases. The gastrin-secreting cells may be removed by surgical excision of the gastric antrum which thereby diminishes not only the production of acid but also the secretion of gastrin. Over-production of gastrin is found in patients with tumours of the G-cells. This syndrome was first described by Zollinger and Ellison and is associated with severe ulceration of the stomach and duodenum. This condition may be treated by removal of the tumour, but if this is not possible, then removal of all acid producing cells by total gastrectomy may be required. However, it is often possible to treat the condition satisfactorily by giving large oral doses of a histamine-blocking agent such as Cimetidine or Ranitidine which are $H_2$-antagonists.

GLUCOSE-DEPENDENT INSULINOTROPHIC PEPTIDE
(GIP OR GASTRIC INHBITORY PEPTIDE)

This hormone is found in the endocrine cells of the upper small intestine, and it can stimulate the release of insulin but only if blood glucose is raised: the latter feature obviously provides a safety mechanism since stimulation of insulin secretion when blood glucose is low would be undesirable. Glucose and fat in the lumen of the intestine can stimulate release of glucose-dependent insulinotrophic peptide. It has been known for some time that glucose given by mouth produces a far greater rise in the secretion of insulin than the same quantity of glucose infused intravenously. Glucose-dependent insulinotrophic peptide is not an insulin secretagogue but it augments glucose-stimulated insulin release when the plasma glucose concentration is about 20% above the fasting level. The correlation between glucose-dependent insulinotrophic peptide and insulin release has been convincingly demonstrated in man using a 'glucose clamp' technique, in which constant hyperglycaemia is created by continuous intravenous glucose infusion. This produces a typical biphasic insulin response. Glucose at a dose of $40 \, g/m^2$ of body surface area is then ingested. Although plasma concentrations of immunoreactive glucose-dependent insulinotrophic peptide change little before glucose ingestion, there is a pronounced increase following an oral glucose load. Insulin concentrations also rise strikingly above the elevated levels induced by hyperglycaemia alone. The time-courses for the rises in concentrations of glucose-dependent insulinotrophic peptide and insulin are nearly identical. Glucose-dependent insulinotrophic peptide therefore has an important role in signalling to the pancreas that a significant carbohydrate or fat load is present in the gut which will require metabolic disposal. The release of insulin is reduced when there is disease of the upper intestinal mucosa; this may contribute, for example, to the development of diabetes mellitus in subjects with coeliac disease. Glucose-dependent insulinotrophic peptide also inhibits the secretion of gastric acid, and so when first discovered it was referred to as gastric inhibitory peptide. However, in man, any effect of the inhibitory peptide on gastric secretion is thought to be weak and it is perhaps compensated by an intact vagus.

MOTILIN

This is a peptide which can stimulate the smooth muscle of the stomach and upper small intestine. It is secreted by specific endocrine cells found in the mucosa of the duodenum and jejunum (Fig. 7.13) and the hormone is present in the circulation, even in the fasting state. Administration of motilin increases the contractions of the stomach and small intestine, even in the fasting state, when it is thought that it acts to keep the lumen of the bowel free of secretions and debris. Motilin also increases the rate of gastric emptying after a meal. It may stimulate the lower oesophageal sphincter to prevent reflux of acid into the oesophagus. The concentration of motilin increases only slightly after a meal, however. In old people there may be inadequate secretion of motilin and this may contribute to stasis and the development of bacterial overgrowth in the lumen of the bowel; this may damage the mucosa and cause malabsorption. Intravenous infusion of glucose or amino acids suppresses the release of motilin, and it may therefore have a role in regulating contractions of the gut and adjust them to the rate of absorption of food.

ENTEROGLUCAGON

Extracts of the small intestine contain enteroglucagon which has not been fully characterized, but it appears to be a peptide that is similar, although not identical, to pancreatic glucagon. The similarities are sufficient for immunological assays for glucagon to be used in measurement of enteroglucagon. The properties of enteroglucagon are different from those of pancreatic glucagon and it does not, for example, stimulate the release of glucose from the liver. Moreover, enteroglucagon is released by ingestion of fat and glucose, two substances which depress the release of glucagon from the pancreas. Enteroglucagon is secreted from the endocrine mucosal cells which are found throughout the small intestine and also in the mucosa of the colon and rectum (Fig. 7.13): it is therefore the most distal of the gastrointestinal hormones. The secretion of enteroglucagon rises quite rapidly after a meal and is continued for many hours: fasting for several days is necessary to obtain a truly basal state. The concentration of enteroglucagon in the circulation is raised in those diseases that cause damage to the intestinal mucosa; this may be associated with increased turnover of the mucosal cells and enteroglucagon may, therefore, be a growth factor for the small intestinal mucosa. Support for this theory is obtained in animal studies in which enteroglucagon secretion rises with high food intake, a situation which is known to cause an increase in growth of the intestine; conversely, starvation which is associated with atrophy of the intestinal mucosa, results in lower concentrations of entero-glucagon.

*Pancreatic and gastrointestinal hormones*

## HORMONES THAT OCCUR IN BOTH THE GASTROINTESTINAL AND NERVOUS SYSTEMS

A number of hormones have been found in both the gastrointestinal system and in the nervous system. Cholecystokinin, for example, has been found in the neurones and fine nerves of the brain and in the peripheral nervous system. In the nervous system the major form of cholecystokinin appears to be the octapeptide; it is rapidly destroyed and this form is, therefore, appropriate to a role as a neurotransmitter. It may well be that the function of neural cholecystokinin is quite different from that of the larger peptide released from the intestinal endocrine cells. Injection of cholecystokinin into the brain indicates that it may be important in the control of appetite and this may link its function in the nervous system with its role in the intestine.

Somatostatin was first isolated from the hypothalamus as described above in studies of the regulation of the secretion of growth hormone, and only subsequently was it shown that it could inhibit the release of almost all the gastrointestinal hormones in addition to blocking the effects on their targets organs, such as enzyme secretions. In the brain somatostatin is localized in neurones of the central nervous system, but in the periphery it is mostly found in endocrine cells.

### NEUROTENSIN

This peptide was first discovered in extracts of brain which were found to affect blood pressure. However, when the head of rats and the rest of the body were extracted separately and assayed for their content of neurotensin, it was found that most of the neurotensin occurred in the body and it was then identified in the intestinal mucosa. Intravenous infusions of neurotensin inhibit the secretion of gastric acid and inhibit the emptying of the stomach: vasodilation also occurs in the mucosa. Thus, absorbtion of food may be enhanced by delaying internal transport so that more time is available for mucosal transport to occur: a steep lumen-to-blood concentration gradient is maintained for the digested nutrients. The peptide consists of 14 amino acids and is produced by specialized neurotensin endocrine cells in the ileum (Fig. 7.13). It is released into the bloodstream after a meal and the amount secreted depends on the size of the meal: the larger the meal the greater the release of the peptide. Neurotensin may be important in regulating the release of food from the stomach and hence the passage of food along the small intestine, thus avoiding an overload to the system. The release of neurotensin is disturbed after gastric surgery for duodenal ulcer: in this situation the remnants of the stomach may empty rapidly and the food may be 'dumped' too quickly into the intestine.

### 'SUBSTANCE P'

This was the first peptide to be located both in the brain and in the gut. In the brain it is synthesized in neurones, stored in axonal synapses and acts as a neuromodulator or a neurotransmitter. Its function in the brain and spinal cord appear to be closely related with the sensation of pain. In the periphery, particularly in the gut, substance P is found in neurones and occasionally in endocrine-type cells. It is not clear yet whether it is released only locally or also into the circulation, i.e. whether it is part of the paracrine or endocrine sysem. Substance P also may be the excitatory transmitter for neurones in the gut.

### VASOACTIVE INTESTINAL PEPTIDE (VIP)

This peptide was originally found in the gut but was later also isolated in considerable quantities in the central nervous system. In both gut and brain, this peptide is found mainly in neurones and their synapses. In the gut these neurones are found between the muscle layers, in the myenteric or Auerbach's plexus and in the submucosa, the Meissner's plexus. Pharmacologically, vasoactive intestinal peptide can cause release of glucose from the liver and inhibit gastric acid production while stimulating pancreatic bicarbonate production and insulin secretion. These actions are normally expressed by the hormones glucagon, secretin and glucose-dependent insulinotrophic peptide (GIP). As the amino acid sequence of these peptides is very similar, it has been suggested that they have evolved from a single precursor hormonal peptide and thus there may be an evolutionary relationship between these hormones and the neurotransmitters. Vasoactive intestinal peptide is present in many other tissues apart from the gut, and like acetylcholine its role at each anatomical location is quite different. The general capacities of vasoactive intestinal peptide for stimulating hormone secretion and relaxing blood vessels and smooth muscle gives some indication of the possible diversity of its roles.

For example, it seems likely that vasoactive intestinal peptide released from postganglionic neurones produces salivary vaso-dilation. It also has a role in relaxing the so-called 'cardio-oesophageal' sphincter and the stomach during gastric filling. Vasoactive intestinal peptide also affects intestinal blood flow during digestion. Mechanical stimulation of the mucosa results in the release of 5-hydroxytryptamine from enterochromaffin cells that activates a VIP-dependent process whereby vasodilation occurs. Overproduction of vasoactive intestinal peptide occurs in the presence of a neural tumour, a ganglioneuroma. This causes severe watery diarrhoea with low blood pressure and flushing attacks. The diarrhoea can be so severe that the patient can die of hypokalaemic paralysis (due to potassium deficiency) or renal failure. This syndrome was first described by Verner and Morrison; resection of the tumour cures the symptoms.

BOMBESIN AND RELATED PEPTIDES

In 1971 bombesin was isolated from frog skin. Surprisingly, it was found to be a powerful stimulant of gastric acid secretion. In addition, it elicited a flow of pancreatic juice rich in protein and it caused the gall bladder to contract. Interest increased when bombesin-like immunoreactivity was discovered in nerves throughout the human gastrointestinal tract. The agent responsible appears to be a neuropeptide and it is regarded as a strong candidate for a role in the release of gastrin by the vagus.

ENKEPHALIN

Enkephalins are present in the nerve fibres of the myoenteric and submucous plexuses of the gastrointestinal tract. Presumably endorphins can exert local effects and this may explain why morphine derivatives are so effective in the treatment of diarrhoea since there must be receptors there.

# SUMMARY

Endocrine control of metabolism involves the integrated action of several hormones including secretin, cholecystokinin, insulin, glucagon, adrenaline, cortisol, growth hormone and the thyroid hormones. The steroid and thyroid hormones act at nuclear receptor sites, while insulin and growth hormone influence cellular permeability as well as intracellular events. The insulin receptor has tyrosine kinase on its cytoplasmic end, and this phos-phorylates proteins (see Chapter 1). The other hormones act by binding at target-cell receptors to stimulate production of the 'second messenger', cyclic AMP. Intracellular control of metabolism of carbohydrates and fats by insulin, glucagon and adrenaline involves groups of protein kinase enzymes within the cell; these kinases may be classified as being cAMP dependent or independent; the latter can be activated by calcium ions. Protein kinases and phosphatases regulate the activities of other key metabolic enzymes by a phosphorylation–dephosphorylation mechanism (called 'covalent modification'): some of the more important steps controlled by these mechanisms have been described in this chapter.

The hormones of the gastrointestinal tract regulate the activity of the stomach and the intestine. For example, gastrin controls acid production and secretin controls pancreatic exocrine secretion. Pancreatic endocrine function is also modulated by events in the stomach, via the hormone glucose-dependent insulinotrophic peptide. Many of the hormones of the gastrointestinal tract and pancreas are also found in the central or peripheral nervous system. These include: somatostatin, gastrin, cholecystokinin and vasoactive intestinal peptide; the brain also contains insulin and calcitonin. However, the role of these peptides in the nervous system is not clear. Some of the peptides may be important for the transmission of nerve impulses at synapses, but unlike classical neurotransmitters such as acetylcholine or nor-adrenaline, they are not synthesized in the nerve terminals: they are made in the cell bodies and are transported along the axons to the synapses. Even if the peptides are not essential for transmission at certain synapses, they may be important in modulating transmission at the synapse.

Shortly after Bayliss and Starling did their classical experiments, Sherrington published his classical book on the *Integrative Action of the Nervous System*. Now it can be seen that the secretion of hormones is also closely integrated. Moreover, the actions of the endocrine system are coordinated with those of the nervous system.

## FURTHER READING

BLOOM S. R. & POLAK J. M. (1981) *Gut Hormones*. Churchill Livingstone, Edinburgh.

BROWNLEE M., VLASSARA H., & CERAMI A. (1984) Nonenzmatic glycosylation and the pathogenesis of diabetic complications. *Annals of Internal Medicine* 101, 527–37.

COHEN P. (1985) The role of protein phosphorylation in the hormonal control of enzyme activity. *European Journal of Biochemistry* 151, 439–48.

DENTON R. M., BROWNSEY R. W. & BELSHAM C. J. (1981) A partial view of the mechanism of insulin action. *Diabetologia* 21, 347–62.

HARVEY B. F. (1983) Gut peptides and the control of food intake. *British Medical Journal* **287**, 1572–4.

HERS H-G. (1984) The discovery and the biological role of fructose-2,6-bisphosphate. *Biochemical Society Transactions* **12**, 729–35.

HOUSLAY M. D. (1984) The search for a molecular mechanism for the action of insulin. *Biochemical Education* **12**, 49–56.

HOUSLAY M. D. (1986) Insulin, glucagon and the receptor-mediated control of cyclic AMP concentrations in liver. *Biochemical Society Transactions* **14**, 183–192.

HUNTER T. (1985) Cell-surface proteins: at last the insulin receptor. *Nature* **313**, 740–41.

JEFFERSON L. S. (1980) Role of insulin in the regulation of protein synthesis. *Diabetes* **29**, 487–96.

KATZ J., KUWAJIMA M., FOSTER D. W. and MCGARRY J. D. (1986) The glucose paradox: new perspectives on hepatic carbohydrate metabolism. *Trends in Biochemical Sciences* **11**, 136–40.

NIMMO H. G. & COHEN P. T. W. (1987) Applications of recombinant DNA technology to studies of metabolic regulation. *Biochemical Journal* **247**, 1–13.

# Index